A TEXTBOOK OF
IMMUNOLOGY

For Undergraduate and Postgraduate Students of Life Sciences

Dr. P. MADHAVEE LATHA
M.Sc., M.Phil., Ph.D.
Associate Professor (*Zoology*)
Dr. S.R.K. Government Arts College
Yanam, Puducherry

S. CHAND
PUBLISHING

S Chand And Company Limited
(ISO 9001 Certified Company)

S Chand And Company Limited

(ISO 9001 Certified Company)

Head Office: D-92, Sector–2, Noida – 201301, U.P. (India), Ph. 91-120-4682700

Registered Office: A-27, 2nd Floor, Mohan Co-operative Industrial Estate, New Delhi – 110 044, Phone: 011-49731800

www.**schandpublishing.com;** e-mail: **info@schandpublishing.com**

Marketing Offices:

Chennai	:	Ph: 23632120; chennai@schandpublishing.com
Guwahati	:	Ph: 2738811, 2735640; guwahati@schandpublishing.com
Hyderabad	:	Ph: 40186018; hyderabad@schandpublishing.com
Jalandhar	:	Ph: 4645630; jalandhar@schandpublishing.com
Kolkata	:	Ph: 23357458, 23353914; kolkata@schandpublishing.com
Lucknow	:	Ph: 4003633; lucknow@schandpublishing.com
Mumbai	:	Ph: 25000297; mumbai@schandpublishing.com
Patna	:	Ph: 4011400; patna@schandpublishing.com

First Edition 2012
Reprints 2015, 2016, 2017 (Twice), 2018 (Twice), 2019, 2020 (Twice), 2021, 2022 (Twice), 2023, 2024

Reprint 2025

ISBN: 978-81-219-3918-8 **Product Code:** H6IMG68LFSC10ENAA12O

PRINTED IN INDIA

By Vikas Publishing House Private Limited, Plot 20/4, Site-IV, Industrial Area Sahibabad, Ghaziabad – 201 010 and Published by S Chand And Company Limited, A-27, 2nd Floor, Mohan Co-operative Industrial Estate, New Delhi – 110 044.

PREFACE

Medicine and biology are inseparable branches in life sciences. Coordination of biologists and medical professionals is indispensable in the advancement of medical research.

Immunology, a broad branch of biomedical science covers the study of all aspects of the immune system in all organisms. It reveals astonishing things about the immune system that defends from harmful foreign agents, much like a country's military which defends from invaders.

It has made numerous important advances over the past decades and is at the forefront in uncovering the mechanisms of human immunological disorders and in eradicating pandemic infectious diseases. Immunological advances have also revealed the mystery of life and death and provided insights into creating a better environment for contemporary human existence. An immunologist with general perspective is helpful in the diagnoses and treatment of the broad spectrum of immunologic diseases and makes its impact on medicine as a whole. Researchers in the field of immunology often aid in the solution of human health problems.

Hence most of the Universities have introduced immunology as one of the subjects in their under graduate and post graduate courses related to life sciences. Today immunology is on the cutting edge of research that is important in our lives.

The present book is intended to provide the reader with comprehensive information on immunology. A fresher to the subject finds it difficult to understand its new terminology usually coupled with medicine. While writing this book, every attempt has been made to explain each new term in boxes. To facilitate the level of understanding the subject and recollecting the same at the time of examination each topic is profusely illustrated with explanatory figures colour photos and flow diagrams. The book has been organized into 23 chapter's each one prepares the ground for understanding the following chapter.

Constructive suggestions from readers will be always welcomed for the improved use of the work.

Dr. P. Madhavee Latha

THANKS

I owe my deep sense of gratitude to my teacher Prof K.Jayantha Rao Dept of Zoology., S.V.University, Tirupathi., for his constant encouragement and moral support.

I wish to express my sincere thanks to Mr.R.V.Gopala Rao Head, Dept of Zoology Dr.S.R.K.Govt college Yanam U.T. of Puducherry., for his kind co-operation.

I express my wholehearted gratitude to my brother Dr. K. Sankaraiyah for his support and timely services.

Last but not least I am grateful to my Husband Mr.K.Suryanarayana Rtd Manager BHEL R & D, Hyderabad and my children Dr. Kavya and Sravya for their co-operation and support.

Dr. P. Madhavee Latha

CONTENTS

1

IMMUNOLOGY INTRODUCTION

IMMUNOLOGY INTRODUCTION

"In the struggle for survival, the fittest win out at the expense of their rivals because they succeed in adapting themselves best to their environment". -- Charles Darwin

All living beings follow survival of the fittest and struggle for existence laws of Charles Darwin at all levels of evolution. Microbes which existed long before humans on our planet are the best examples for the statements of Darwin. For their survival microbes obtained various adoptive modification, parasitism is one of their modifications. The parasitic modifications of microbes posed great threat to the life of the remaining organisms. As a part of their struggle for existence higher animals acquired a defense system known as "immune system". It is made up of a network of cells, tissues, and organs that work together to protect the body.

In biology a separate branch "immunology" has been developed to study and understand this natural defensive mechanism. The term immunology has been derived from the Latin term "immunus", which means "freedom from" or "exempt". Immunity provided by immune system is the state of protection from infections and diseases causing agents. Birth of the subject immunology took place in the 18th century through the efforts of an English physician Edward Jenner, when he tried to highlight the protective role of vaccine against smallpox disease. Louis Pasteur's accidental discovery of techniques that can minimize the virulence of pathogenic microbes strengthened the roots of immunology.

IMMUNITY

The extraordinary coordination of different cells, proteins, tissues, and organs of immune system provide immunity to the body against infectious organisms and other invaders. Blood and lymph systems play a vital role in coordinating the function of immune system. Since the pathogens that can cause disease arrive from different parts of the biological kingdom, immune systems response is not similar every time. This response depends upon various factors such as mode of entry of pathogen, type of pathogen, behavior of pathogen etc. In spite of the surveillance done by the immune system, certain pathogens manage to enter into the body and cause diseases. Skin and mucosa are general possible pathways for the entry of pathogens.

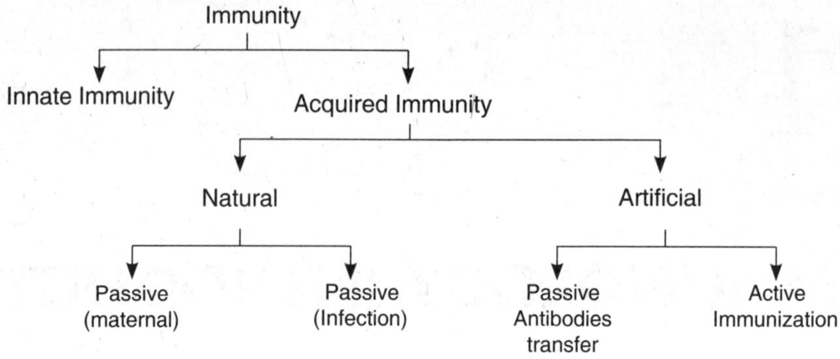

Fig. 1.1

POSSIBLE ROOTS OF PATHOGEN ENTRY:

1. SKIN: Even though the skin is tough and intact to prevent the entry of pathogens, some of the pathogens (eg. Hook worms, Schistosoma larvae) can penetrate through the skin or settle on the skin (warts causing virus, some of the fungal agents) and generate pathological conditions.

2. MUCOSA: Since respiratory tract, urinary tract, ureter, urethra, vagina etc. are open to the out side; pathogens can penetrate very easily through this path. Even though, mucosa layer lining the tract prevents adherence of pathogens and their entry, various pathogens manage to enter through different means and produce infection. For example Meningococus bacteria pass through epithelial cells and cause meningitis in humans. Some more examples are mentioned in Table 1.1.

Table 1.1

Pathogen	Disease	Mucosal site of entry
Rhinovirus	Common cold	Nasal epithelium
Influenza virus	Influenza	Upper respiratory tract
Bordatella pertussis	Whooping cough	Lower respiratory tract
Salmonella spp	Food poisoning	Small intestine
Rotavirus	Diarrhoea	Small intestine
E coli	Urinary tract infection	Bladder, Ureter
Neisseria gonorrhoeae	Gonorrhoeae	Vagina, Urethra

When the physical barriers skin and mucosal layers are damaged, different pathogens that generally cannot enter into the body in normal conditions can enter into the body through the damaged skin and mucosal layers and root pathogenesis. Hence infections simple to dreadful are common in burn and injury cases. The severity of the infection depends upon the intensity of the loss of natural barrier, general health condition and social conditions of the individual (surrounding environment also play a role in the maintaining health). Burn and cuts may lead to the *staphylococus, streptococcus, pseudomonas* and *clostridium* tetanus like infection.

Transmission of disease causing pathogens from animals to human is possible through their bites, scratches or through physical contact to human. Entry of some of the disease causing pathogens takes place through vectors.For example ***Malaria, Filariasis, Dengue*** etc. causing parasites enter in to their host man through mosquito bites.

Generally when pathogens enter into the body, they cause disease/ infection in the area where they managed to enter into the body. For e.g. cold virus develops uneasiness in mucosal layers of nose (entry point). Pain and itching develops due to pathogens entry in the injured area. Immune system attempts to eliminate the pathogens that managed to enter in to the body through different ways. The resistance provided by the immune system depends upon various factors such as physical condition, age, nutrition, genetic, social factors, nature of the pathogen etc. If immune system fails to wipe out the pathogens, the pathogens move deep into the body and multiply in different regions of the body ensuing simple to serious pathological changes. Septic, swelling of the whole part having the wound, severe pain, fever etc. are common if the wounds are neglected. Intensity of symptoms is high especially in old and diabetic people. Respiratory Bronchitis followed by common cough and cold is another well known example for failure or improper immunological response.

As the ultimate aim of immune response is to prevent the entry and multiplication, in initial stage response of immune system to different pathogens is common. In later stages immune response is very specific to each type of pathogen, to mount specific and suitable action against a particular pathogen population. Broadly speaking immunity varies for different pathogens in diverse conditions. With reference to the immune response, immunity can be broadly classified into Natural immunity and Acquired immunity.

1. Natural immunity:

Natural immunity is also known as innate immunity or non specific immunity. It is a pre-existing and natural defense mechanism inherited from parents to offspring. It is different in different species, races and even in different individuals of the same species. Generally it depends on various other factors such as age, physical fitness, nutrition, social condition etc. also. For example infants and old peoples are more susceptible to diseases than the remaining age groups. Since it is natural and pre-existing it is not specific for any particular pathogen. The non specific immunity provides protection through different types of natural barriers such as anatomical, mechanical, physiological, phagocytic, inflammatory etc.

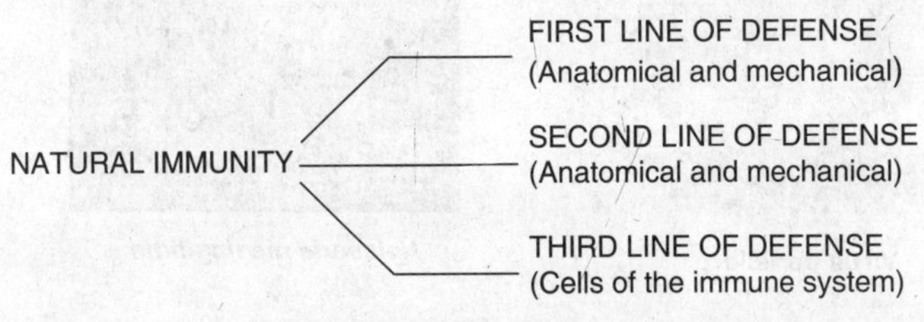

Fig. 1.2

Since anatomical and mechanical barriers are preventing the entry of pathogens, protection provided by these barriers is considered as the "first line of defense". Defense provided through enzymes and phagocytes following the entry of pathogen are referred as second line of defense and the protection in the later stages through inflammation involving natural killer cells, mast cells etc. is considered as third line of defense.

First Line of Defense: It is the protection provided by anatomical and mechanical barriers. Skin, surface mucosal linings of gastro intestinal track, urinogenital track, and respiratory track are considered as anatomical barriers. Mechanical actions such as coughing, sneezing, peristaltic movements etc. are the mechanical barriers that obstruct the pathogens entry in to the body.

Skin: Skin The impermeable nature of skin with epidermis and dermis and low PH (3 to 5) due to sebum secretions from the sebaceous glands prevents entry and growth of most micro organisms. If pathogens managed to enter into the body, they are removed by the circulating immune cells in the blood vessels of dermis.

Mucus membrane: - The mucosal lining of respiratory, urinogenital, gastrointestinal etc. tracts open to the external environment prevents adherence of microbes to the epithelial layers by trapping them in their sticky substance - mucus. The movements of cilia present on epithelial membrane of respiratory track helps in the removal of microbes trapped in mucus.

Mechanical actions: Mechanical actions like coughing, sneezing, peristaltic movements etc. help in driving out the foreign agents from respiratory and digestive tracks of animals.

Since all living beings follow the law of evolution "survival of the fittest" some microbes acquired adaptations to cross over the defensive barriers. They adhere to the mucosal layer either with their modified body structures or surface characters. For example in case of the bacterium *Neisseria gonorrhoeae* the pathogenic mechanism is involved in the attachment of the bacterium to nonciliated epithelial cells via pili (fimbriae) and the production of lipopolysaccharide endotoxin. The fimbriae, which play a major role in adherence, extend several micrometers from the cell surface (Fig 1.3). The lipopolysaccharide produced by *Neisseria*

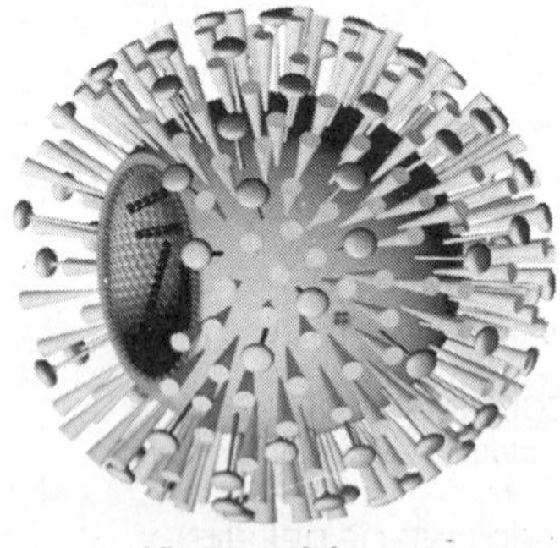

Virus particle

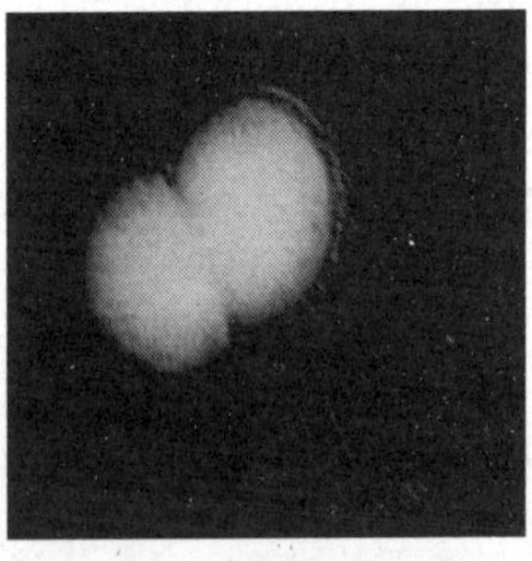

Neisseria meningitidis

Fig. 1.3

meningitidis is highly toxic, and it has an additional virulence factor in the form of its antiphagocytic capsule.

Virus particles attaches to their host cells through surface particles often called as viral attachment proteins. In enveloped viruses the surface glycoproteins oligomerizes to form spikes that protrude from the surface and help in their attachment to host cells.

SECOND LINE OF DEFENSE:

The action of certain physiological and biochemical barriers like temperature, pH etc., substance such as enzymes of complement system, natural antibodies e.g. blood group antibodies, interleukins and phagocytic cells present in body fluids (humus) provide second line of defense. An alteration in the body temperature affects the growth rate of microbes. For example high body temperature in birds prevents growth of the bacteria that can cause *anthrax*. Hence raise in temperature of the body during infection is an attempt to inhibit the growth of certain infection causing agents. PH of the surroundings also influences growth of microbes. For example presence of microbes is almost nil in the stomach region due to low PH in the presence of gastric acid – HCL. Occurrence of fungal infections in foot is due to absence of sebaceous glands that can create low PH environment. Hydrolytic enzymes found in saliva, tears, breast milk can kill microbes and work as anti microbial agents and prevent entry and multiplication of microbes into the body. Enzymes of complement system, and interleukins secreted by different immune cells further help in killing and removal of pathogens.

Phagocytosis is one of the defense weapons used by the immune system to remove the pathogens entered in to the body successfully. A group of immune cells such as Neutrophiles, basophils, eosinophils, macrophages, monocytes, natural killer cells etc. phagocytise the pathogens. The phagocytic cells reach the foreign agent with the help of chemotaxis.

THIRD LINE OF DEFENSE :

Third line of defense involves various cells of the immune system. Immune response to small wounds or injuries or mild infections involving various immune cells is routinely carried in all individuals in the same way. Different cells of immune system move to the region of infection or damage through chemotactic action to remove pathogens and damaged tissue. The whole procedure of immune response is known as "inflammation". Vasodilatation, marginalization, erythema, edema, and diapedesis are some of the common reactions that take place in the body during inflammation.

ACQUIRED IMMUNITY:

In addition to normal innate immunity, every individual develops resistance to certain infectious agents following exposure to them. Since the immunity is acquired by the individual following exposure to that particular pathogen, it is referred as acquired immunity. It is not natural, but adopted by the individual, and is very specific for the pathogen to which he has been exposed. Hence this kind of immunity is also referred as adoptive immunity or specific immunity.

TYPES OF ACQUIRED IMMUNITY :

Acquired immunity for specific pathogen can be developed through natural way by getting infection or artificially through vaccination. Based on the way of acquiring the immunity and the role of immune system, acquired immunity can be classified in to four types. They are Natural acquired active immunity, Natural acquired passive immunity, Artificial acquired active immunity and Artificial acquired passive immunity.

1. Natural Acquired Active Immunity:

Following pathogens/antigens entry in to the body by natural processes (as infection) immune system of the host body produces antibodies and cytotoxic cells to get rid of the pathogens. Subsequent to recovery some of the antibody producing plasma cells and cytotoxic cells are retained as memory cells. Memory cells provide immunity to the same pathogen in later period. The acquired immunity may be life-long as with smallpox, measles, chickenpox, yellow fever etc. or may be lost after few years e.g. diphtheria, tetanus or even for lesser period e.g. influenza, pneumonia etc.

2. Natural Acquired Passive Immunity

If antibodies produced by an individual (called donor) in response to a pathogen are naturally transferred to other individual (called recipient), the latter develops immunity. In this process recipients acquire immunity with out the involvement of their own immune system. Since the recipient's immune system is not involved in this process and transfer of antibodies taking place quite naturally it is referred as "natural acquired passive immunity". Immunity acquired by babies through natural transfer of antibodies from mother via placenta and breast milk is the best example for this type of immunity. These maternal antibodies remain with the child for about three to six months or sometimes twelve to fifteen months. The maternal antibodies generally provide resistance against whooping cough, diphtheria, German measles, disease of respiratory and gastrointestinal tract, etc.

Artificial Acquired Active Immunity: Vaccination also induces immunity. The pathogens or parts of the pathogens present in the vaccine induce immunity for that specific pathogen in vaccinated persons. Even though the exposure is not natural, immune system responds to the pathogen administered into the body and develops immunity. Since the vaccinated individual's immune system is involved in the development of immunity it is referred as "artificial acquired active immunity". Immunity acquired through vaccines for various infectious diseases such as cholera, tuberculosis, plague, pneumonia, smallpox, polio, tetanus, influenza, measles, rabies, yellow fever etc. belongs to this kind of immunity only.

Artificial Acquired Passive Immunity: Immunity acquired through direct injection of antibodies and sensitized cells collected from donors is known as "artificial acquired passive immunity". Since recipient's immune system is not involved in the production of antibodies and sensitized cells, it remains for a short period. In the absence memory cells, immunity developed by this method is purely temporary (only for two to three weeks). Earlier this kind of immunity was an important therapeutic device for disease treatment. Still it is under use for various viral diseases such as hepatitis B, chicken pox, arthropod-borne encephalitis, and bacterial disease such as diphtheria, tetanus, staphylococcal-poisoning etc. As the above mentioned diseases are very dangerous and fatal, injection of antibodies present in pooled serum into the blood of the susceptible individual saves the life. The immune fractions and cells can be collected from hyper immune serum of animals or human or from convalescent serum or from pooled sera of healthy individuals.

- Convalescent serum: The serum of the blood of one or more patients recovering from infection.
- Hyper immune serum: An antiserum possessing very large quantities of specific antibodies. It can be raised by repeated administration of a series of attenuated or live pathogens into the volunteers or animals. In earlier days antibodies for treatment of tetanus, diphtheria, gas gangrene, snake bite, etc. are produced in this way.

Since there is a possibility of rejection reaction for the serum raised in other animals, now a day's treatment with hyper immune serum is replaced by the antibodies raised through recombinant DNA technology.

Recombinent DNA technology: Joining together of DNA molecules from two different species that are inserted into a host organism to produce new genetic combinations that are of value to science, medicine, agriculture, and industry.

Adoptive immunity is not independent of innate immunity, in fact it is an extend reaction of immune system. Since the rate of multiplication of pathogens that entered into the body is very high, nonspecific innate immunity may not be effective. Host has to generate specific mechanism to get rid of the pathogens. As re attack by the same pathogen is possible, memory of that pathogen is necessary for a faster action. In addition to this, tremendous pressure imposed by the pathogens with their enormous ability to undergo mutations and molecular heterogenesity insisted evolution of acquired immunity in the higher vertebrates. The phagocytic cells and the chemicals substances released from pathogens and damaged cells are intimately involved in initiation of specific/ acquired immune reactions. Hence, both innate and acquired immunity work together to get rid of the foreign agents and the total work is regulated carefully.

2

IMMUNE SYSTEM

One of the biggest threats to survival is infection. To continue existence and to overcome the threat of infection, organisms have developed passive and aggressive defense mechanisms. Host defense mechanisms have been evolved since the first organisms encountered each other, hundreds of millions of years ago. Even simple unicellular organisms like bacteria also possess defense mechanisms to get protected against their pathogens (phage virus) that can cause infections. Complexity of defense mechanism increases with the increased complexity of body, ensuing development of a complex system known as "immune system" in multi cellular organisms. Evolution of the immune system is a direct consequence of microbes-exerted selection pressure on multi cellular organisms.

IMMUNE SYSTEM

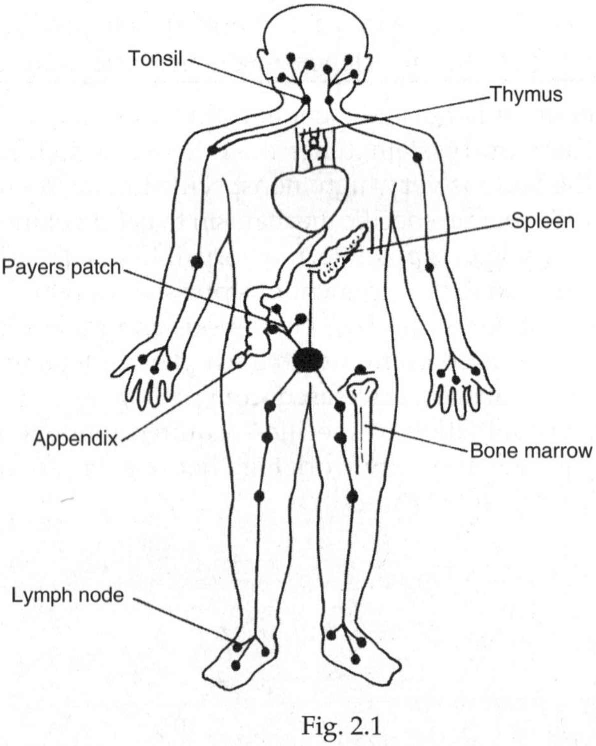

Fig. 2.1

By tracing the evolution of invertebrate immune system, it can be seen that it largely followed bi-directional "predator-prey" relationships. The vertebrate immune system was to some extent inherited from invertebrates, whereas a part of it has advanced considerably in the course of its own evolution. Although certain vertebrate-specific properties such as immune recognition and immune memory have also been identified in invertebrates in rudimentary forms, it is particularly those qualities like progressive development of humoral and cellular adoptive immunity, Major Histocompatibility Complex (MHC), variable class I and class II genes, precise mechanisms of immune recognition and long-term immune memory, reflect the fundamental evolutionary advancement of the vertebrate immune system.

The mammalian immune system is an incredibly complex and intricate system that can recognize non-self and provide protection from a wide variety of pathogens. In humans, the immune system begins to develop in the embryo. By the time a baby is born, the immune system becomes a sophisticated collection of tissues, organs and enzymes. Even the skin is considered as a part of the immune system.

ORGANS OF IMMUNE SYSTEM

Since lymphoid tissue and lymphoid organs form the core of immune system, immune system is also referred as lymphoid system. The organs of the immune system may be in compact form such as thymus, spleen, lymph node etc. or in diffuse form like gut associated lymphoid tissue, bursa equivalent region of bone marrow etc. Irrespective of their morphology, organs of immune system are classified functionally into primary and secondary lymphoid organs.

PRIMARY LYMPHOID ORGANS:

Primary lymphoid organs are also known as central lymphoid organs. These are the organs where differentiation, proliferation and maturation of pleuripotent stem cells into immuno competent cells take place. Thymus and avian bursa of Fabricus or bursa equivalent tissue in the bone marrow are categorized as primary lymphoid organs. Thymus helps in the differentiation and maturation of hemopoitic stem cells in to T cells. Bursa of fabricus or its equal region in bone marrow is responsible for the differentiation and maturation of B cells. Even though T and B cells in primary lymphoid organs are competent, they don't show any immune response. Since interaction with antigens is necessary for immune response, in the absence of antigens immune cells in primary lymphoid organs remain inactive.

THYMUS:

In mammals thymus is a flattened, grayish, bi lobed organ with lymphoepithelial tissue. It is located in the thorax immediately below to the sternum and above the heart with its upper narrower part extended into the neck. In the early stages of development, it is entirely an epithelial structure derived from the third and fourth pharyngeal pouches. This epithelial structure gradually grows and descends to thorax losing its connection with the pharyngeal pouches. Progenitor lymphocytes of hemopoitic stem cells migrate from bone marrow to the thymus through blood stream for differentiation and maturation into immuno competent lymphocytes. The fully developed thymus is encapsulated by connective tissue and becomes a bilobed structure. The number of lobes in thymus varies in different animals. For instance it is seven lobed in chick; ten lobed in pig and bilobed in man. The connective tissue of capsule penetrates deep into the lobes, dividing each lobe incompletely into many lobules. The strands of connective tissue in between the lobules are known as "trabeculae". Each lobule in thymus is organized into an outer cortex and inner medulla. The cortex or peripheral part of each lobule is densely populated with differentiated but immature "T cells or Thymocytes" and the medulla or central portion of the lobule is packed with loosely arranged mature lymphocytes. Since mature T cells are noticed in both cortex and medulla, the sequence of maturation of T cells within the thymus is not completely understood.

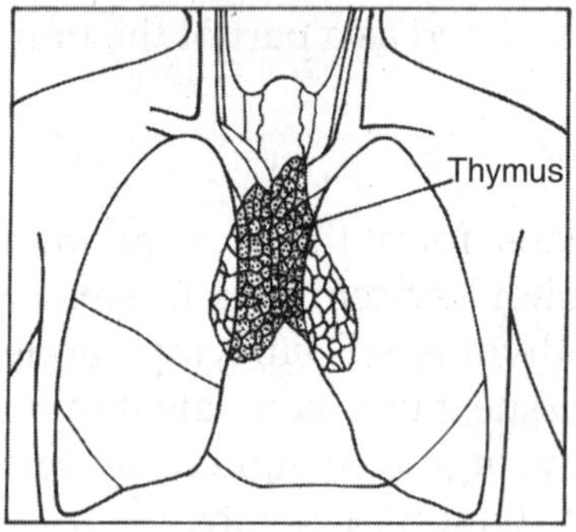

Fig. 2.2 Thymus Location

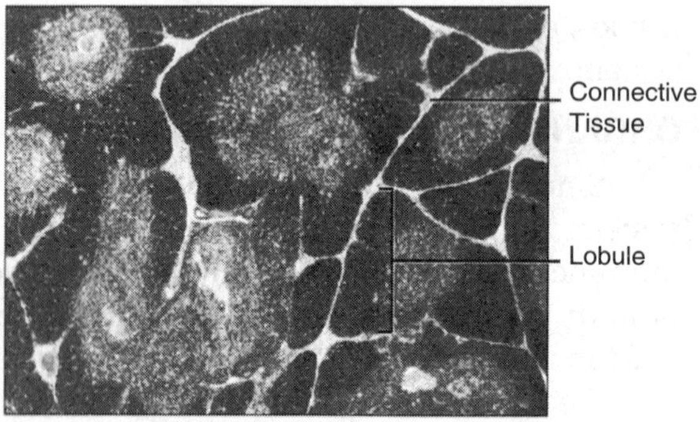

Fig. 2.3 T. S of Thymus

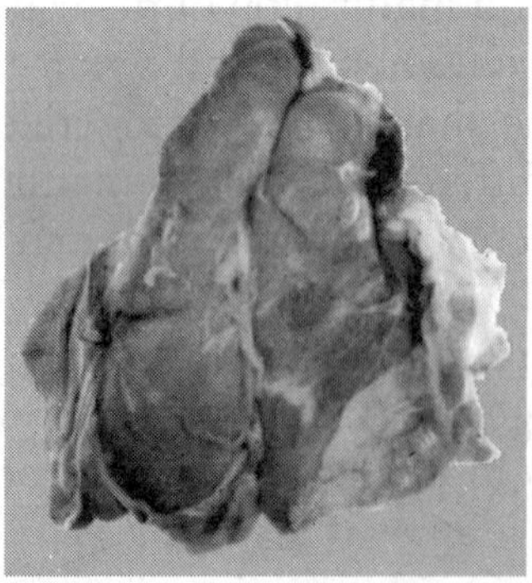

Fig. 2.4 Human Thymus

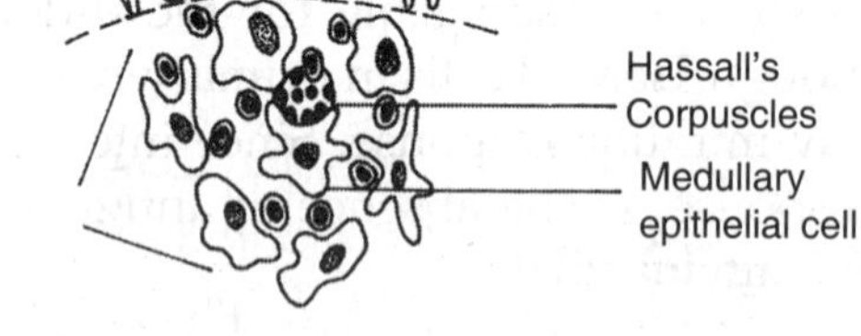

Fig. 2.5 Thymus diagram

The lymphocytes in thymus multiply rapidly, but majority of the cells (about 90-95%) die within 3 to 4 days leaving only a small fraction (about 5%) of cells for maturation. The hormone thymosin secreted by thymus epithelial cells might be helping in the differentiation and maturation of T lymphocytes. The matured T lymphocytes with longer life span leave the thymus to circulate in peripheral blood and lymph, and colonise in the thymus dependent areas of secondary / peripheral lymphoid organs. On interaction with antigens the T cells in secondary lymphoid organs become active and offer cell mediated immunity.

The reason for death of large number of developing T cells in thymus might be a selection process during the maturation of T cells. T cells that fail to react with antigens and the cells that can react with self antigens might be identified for elimination in the selection process to avoid any irregularity in the function of immune system.

A three dimensional network composed of inter digitating dendritic cells, stromal cells, epithelial cells and macrophages are present in thymus as a structural frame work of the organ. Some of the epithelial cells in the cortex show long membrane extensions that surround as many as 50 thymocytes. The membrane extensions of epithelial cells surround the blood vessels and lymph spaces of the cortex and medulla also. The possible function of this membrane is to prevent the macro molecules (including the antigens) of the blood to contact lymphocytes of the thymus. Hence they are referred as nurse cells. Their membrane may be responsible for nonexistence of immune reactions in thymus. Some concentric layers of degenerating epithelial cells referred as "Hassall's corpuscles" are found in the medulla of thymus. The function of Hassall's corpuscles is not clearly understood.

The thymus activity reaches peak in childhood but attains its largest size by puberty, later it shows **atrophy** (decrease in size) and becomes extremely small in old age. Hence aging is accompanied by a decline in thymus function and immunity. Significant decrease in cortical and medulla cells, increase in the total fat content of the organ, results in atrophy of the organ.

T cells are essential for cell mediated immunity, removal or defective formation or function of thymus affects immunity mediated by T cells. Experimental study of neonatal thymectomy (surgical removal of thymus) in mice has revealed deficiency of T cells and cell mediated immune response. **Aplasia** of thymus (Failure of development of thymus) also results in defects in cell mediated immune reactions. As T cells are involved in immunity to cancer, bacterial, viral, and fungal attacks, a person with T cells deficiency is vulnerable to many diseases and cancer. A baby born with Aplasia of thymus may die due to infections. Replacement of thymus or supplement of thymic hormone can correct the problems developed in the absence of thymus. Thymectomy in adolescence may not be fatal, but lead to gradual reduction in cell mediated immune response and affects resistance to infections. This is due to long life of lymphocytes and memory cells that are developed earlier than thymectamy. Since death of established lymphocytes is inevitable, cell mediated protection may not continue for longer time in the absence of T cells replacement, and there is a gradual reduction in cell mediated immune response.

BURSA OF FABRICUS AND ITS EQUIVALENT:

Bursa of Fabricus is primary lymphoid organ in birds. Differentiation, maturation and proliferation of B Lymphocytes take place in this organ. B Lymphocytes are responsible for the production of antibodies and humoral immunity. Bursa is seen only in birds and it is named after the person Fabricus, who invented the organ in birds. Like thymus, bursa of Fabricus is an epithelial structure developed as epithelial diverticulum from the dorsal region of cloaca. Development of this organ in birds takes place on about 15th day of development and by the time of hatching it develops into a fully functional organ. It attains maximum size (about 3 cm in diameter) in 4 months of age; later like thymus it also shows atrophy.

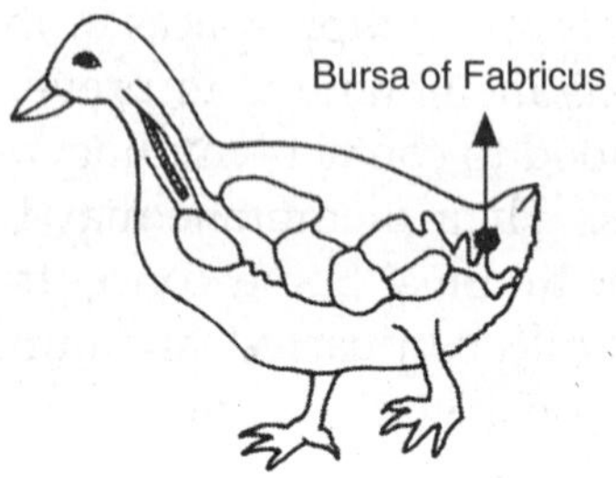

Fig. 2.6

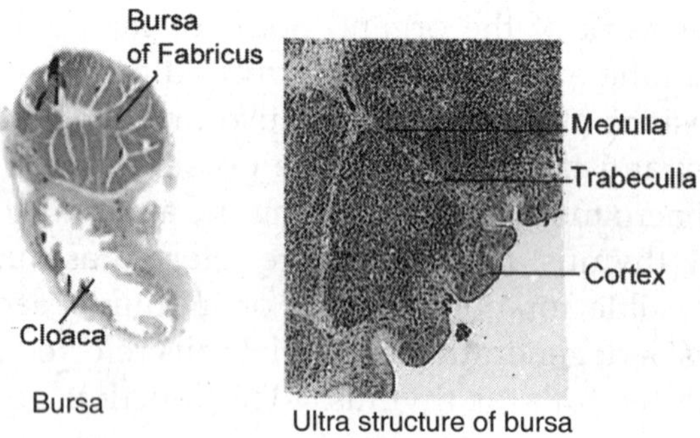

Fig. 2.7

Similar to the development of thymus, epithelial diverticulum from cloaca region is colonized by pleuripotent stem cells to undergo proliferation and differentiation to become immune competent lymphocytes known as "B cells" (B stands for bursa). Histological study of bursa shows similar characteristic features of thymus. Like thymus, bursa is divided into follicles by connective tissue and each follicle has cortex and medulla regions. The differentiated B cells show morphological similarity with T lymphocytes, but show significant difference in their surface markers and function.

The mature and immune competent B cells leave the primary lymphoid organ to reach secondary lymphoid organs through blood circulation. In secondary lymphoid organs the immune competent B lymphocytes produce antibodies in response to antigenic stimulus to provide humoral immunity.

In mammals and other vertebrates, bursa of Fabricus is absent, but certain regions of bone marrow serve as the bursa equivalents for differentiation and production of B lymphocytes. In early embryological stages spleen and ileal Peyer's patch act as primary lymphoid organ for differentiation, maturation and proliferation of B cells. In bone morrow, the stromal cells influence the differentiation and maturation process through their cytokines.

Bursectomy:

Neonatal bursectomy in birds has shown profound effect on antibodies production and humoral immune response, but the cell mediated immune response is unaffected. Germinal centres in secondary lymphoid organs failed to develop in bursectomized birds.

SECONDARY LYMPHOID ORGANS:

Secondary lymphoid organs: Secondary lymphoid organs are also known as peripheral lymphoid organs. These are the organs or regions where the mature and immuno competent lymphocytes colonize and function in response to antigenic stimuli. The mature lymphocytes from primary lymphoid organs migrate to secondary lymphoid regions through blood circulation to give protection from invading foreign agents. The secondary lymphoid organs are the regions, where the immune competent lymphocytes interact with foreign agents and execute immune response. Production of antibodies from activated B cells, activation of cytotoxic T cells in response to antigens takes place in the secondary lymphoid organs.

The secondary lymphoid organs may be encapsulated to have a specific shape or may be in the form of diffused tissues. Spleen, lymph nodes, adenoids, tonsils are the encapsulated secondary lymphoid organs. Mucosa associated lymphoid tissue distributed throughout the body such as alimentary canal, respiratory and urinogenital tracts etc. are the diffused secondary lymphoid regions. Efficiency of antigen trapping is same for both capsulated organs and diffused tissue. The secondary lymphoid organs are usually small and poorly developed at the time of birth but unlike primary lymphoid organs they show progressive growth with age. Out of all, lymph nodes and spleen are highly organized structures.

LYMPH NODE:

Lymph nodes are complex, bean shaped and encapsulated organs. The connective tissue capsule encloses the reticular net work packed with lymphocytes, macrophages and dendritic cells. They are clustered at the junctions of the lymphatic vessels and act as filters of lymph. If pathogens enters the body via respiratory or gastrointestinal tracts they must pass through the regional lymph nodes. During their passage through the lymph node, pathogens might be trapped by macrophages for phogocytization or initiate immunological response in T and B cells. The size of lymph nodes in humans varies from 1 to 25 mm. The indentation of the lymph node from which the blood vessels enter and leave the node is known as "hilus". Several afferent lymphatic ducts carry lymph into the organ, but a single lymph duct with filtered lymph leaves the node from hilus region.

The internal environment of lymph node shows three histologically different regions - cortex, para cortex and medulla. Like thymus, at certain regions the outer collagenous layer of capsule penetrates deep into the cortex and paracortex regions ensuing incomplete division of the organ. The connective tissue partitions are referred as "trabeculae". The cortex region of lymph node accommodates B cells, macrophages and follicular dendritic cells arranged as primary follicles. Antigenic challenge leads to enlargement of primary follicles into secondary follicles with a germinal center. Development of two germinal centres indicates

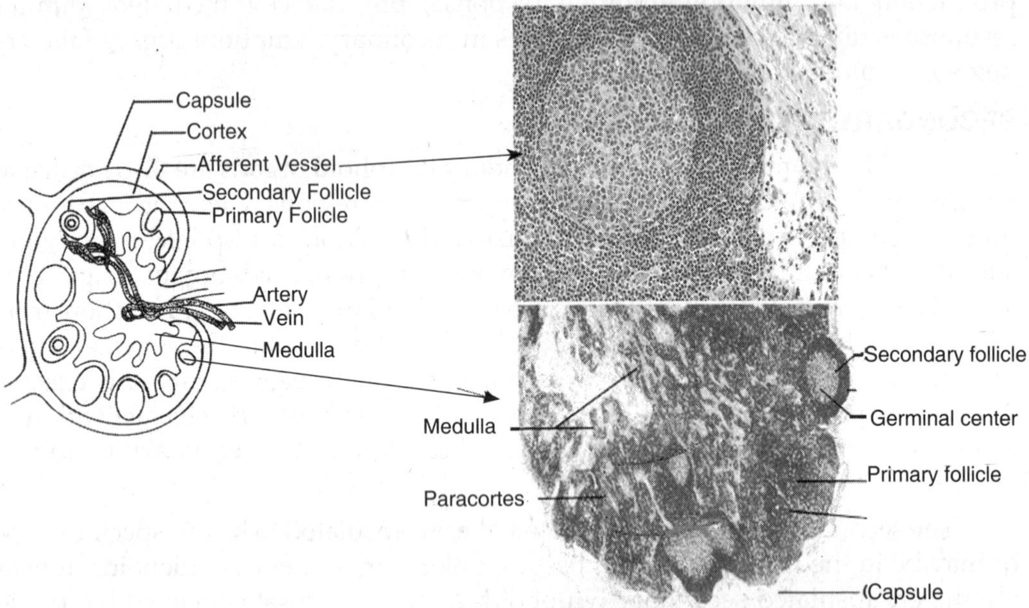

Fig. 2.8 Lymphnode

intense activation and differentiation of B cells followed by antigenic challenge. Secondary follicles with germinal centres appear more frequently in secondary immune response than in the primary response. Paracortex next to the cortex region is richly populated by T lymphocytes and inter digitating dendritic cells. The inter digitating cells with high levels of MHC class II molecules (Refer MHC Complex in chapter 11) process the antigens that enter the lymph node and present them to the T cells for further reactions. B cells confine to the edges of the paracortex, and both activated T and B cells confer proliferating foci. The foci reach maximum size within 3 to 4 days of antigen challenge and some of the B cells differentiate into plasma cells and start producing antibodies. (Refer B cell activation and differentiation in chapter 5). The antibodies bind to the antigens resulting in the formation of antigen antibody complexes. Follicular dendritic cells trap these antigen antibody complexes and retain for long periods to enhance B cells activation. The dendritic cells with antigen antibody complexes release growth factors that play an important role in B cell activation.

The medulla region of the lymph nodes shows medullary cords formed by connective tissue fibers and sinuses in between them. The medullary sinuses contain plasma cells derived from activated B cells. Phagocytic cells stretch out the margins of medullary sinuses.

When lymph enters into the sub capsular area of the lymphnode through various afferent lymphatic vessels, it slowly percolates in to the cortex, paracortex and medulla, exposing the pathogens moving within, to different immune cells present in the lymph node. Interaction of pathogens with immune cells initiates both humoral and cell mediated immune reactions. The lymph leaving the lymph node through single efferent lymphatic vessel carries not only lymph but also antibodies and activated lymphocytes produced against the foreign agents after antigenic challenge. The antigenic challenge sometimes initiates migration of lymphocytes from different regions of the body into the lymph nodes. The increase in the number of lymphocytes results in swelling up of the lymph node. Hence swollen lymph nodes generally indicate presence of pathogens and infection in the body.

Lymph: Lymph is a clear, colorless liquid with a composition similar to blood plasma. It is nothing but the clear, watery blood plasma leaked out through the capillary walls to flow around the cells. It contains oxygen, proteins, glucose and white blood cells. All the cells bathed in this fluid receive their nutrients and oxygen from it. Tubular vessels transport lymph back to the blood, ultimately replacing the volume lost during the formation of the interstitial fluid. Unlike the cardiovascular system, the lymphatic system is not closed and has no central pump. Lymph movement occurs despite low pressure due to peristalsis, valves, and compression during contraction of adjacent skeletal muscle and arterial pulsation.

SPLEEN:

Spleen is a large, red coloured, oval shaped, encapsulated secondary lymphatic organ, situated in the left side of abdominal cavity below the pancreas. It acts like a filter for the pathogens present in the blood. Spleen responds to systemic infections due to its communication with the main arterial circulation. Histological study of spleen reveals the penetration of connective tissue from capsule to the interior of spleen body in the form of trabeculae to divide spleen into centrally connected compartments. Each compartment shows two different regions "the red pulp and the white pulp". The red pulp is non lymphoid in function and consists of a net work of sinusoids enriched with RBCs and macrophages. Destruction of old and defective RBC's takes place in the red pulp. The red pulp is site, for haemopoiesis in early developmental stages (till 5th month of development). Later bone marrow seizes blood cells production. In adults during emergency spleen also produces RBC's, in addition to bone marrow to face the crisis.

The white pulp in spleen is lymphoidal in function. Major portion of lymphoid tissue arranges around a central arteriole forming a periarterial lymphatic sheath (PALS). Since the arrangement of lymphocytes is first described by Malphigi, it is also known as Malphigian body. In Malphigian body, the marginal zone located next to the PALS is made up of B cells, organized in the form of lymphoid follicles. T lymphocytes are distributed along with dendrite cells and the inter digitating cells are present around the arteriole. The blood born antigens enter Malphigian body of the spleen through an artery. The inter digitating dendritic cells trap the pathogens that are present in the blood and process them for submitting to T cells. Antigen presentation by antigen presenting cells (dendritic cells) activates the T cells and the activated T cells in turn stimulate B cells. Immunological response of both T and B cells helps in the removal of foreign agents from the blood. The

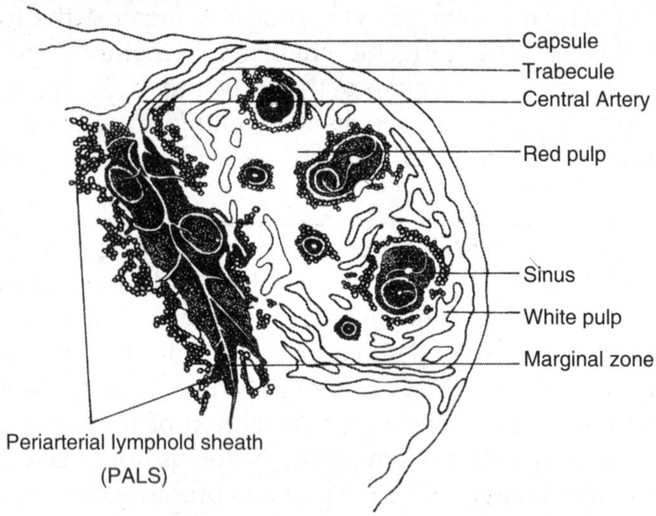

Fig. 2.9

primary follicle following antigenic stimulation may transform into secondary follicle with dense clusters of concentrically arranged lymphocytes.

Splenectomy in young children may lead to an increase in blood born diseases.

Tonsils:

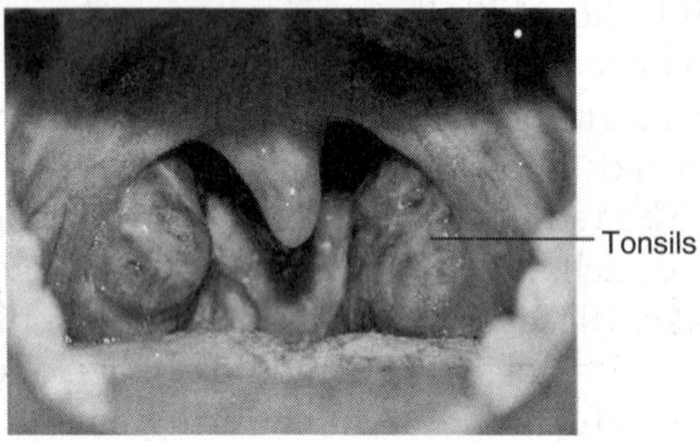

Fig. 2.10

Tonsils are the encapsulated secondary lymphoid organs found in three different regions, such as root of the tongue (lingual), at the back of the mouth (palatine) and in the roof of nasopharynx (adenoid). Unlike other lymphatic glands, tonsils do not show any separate cortex and medulla regions. Presence of crypts (pits) on the surface and stratified epithelial covering are identifying features of tonsils. The lymphoid cells in tonsils appear either in the form of dense islands, or scattered cells. The mucus glands of tonsils open either on to the surface or into the crypts of tonsils. The mucus secretion washes away the microorganisms. Accumulation of micro organisms in the lumen of crypts causes inflammatory reactions.

Mucosa associated lymphoid tissue (MALT):

The mucosa associated lymphoid tissue (MALT) appears as intra epithelial lymphoid region. Majority of cells in this MALT are T cells. The lamina propria that lies beneath the epithelial layer contains large number of B cells, activated T_H cells, and macrophages in the form of loose clusters. The sub mucosa layer beneath the lamina propria contains payer's patches, (nodules of 30-40 lymphoid follicles). A specialized cell group known as M cells (microfold cells) are present in mucous membrane to carry the antigenes from surface to the under lying mucosa associated lymphoid tissue. Analogous to the function, structure of M cells is also different; unlike epithelial cells of mucosal layer M cells are flat without any microvillie. The baso lateral membrane of the cells form pockets and accommodate clusters of B cells, T cells and macrophages in it. The phagocytes formed from the surface with antigen fuse with the membrane of pockets and release the phagocytized antigen in to it, for immunological reactions. The activated B cells differentiate in to plasma cells and secrete Ig A antibodies. These antibodies then transported out to the lumen through epithelial cells as secretory Ig A, to interact with the antigens in the surrounding areas of lumen.

Like mucosal layer the skin also is provided with lymphocytes for primary defense. The Keratinocytes (epithelial cells specialized for immunity) are capable of inducing inflammation with their secretions in the presence of a pathogen. The dendritic langerhan cells of epidermis can engulf pathogen and move to regional lymph nodes to present the antigen to T_H cells. The intra epidermal lymphocytes also check the pathogen entering through the skin. The vermiform appendix is also very rich in lymphoid tissue and is considered as "abdominal tonsil".

3

CELLS OF THE IMMUNE SYSTEM

Immune system conveys its work through different cells and soluble molecules secreted by them. Both morphologically and functionally different cells of the immune system develop from hemopoitic stem cells of bone marrow. The hemopoietic stem cells of bone marrow are pleuripotent in nature, under the influence of different environments they differentiate into different immune cells such as T lymphocytes, B lymphocytes, different granulocytes, mast cells, macrophages, megakaryocytes etc. The stem cells are self renewable; hence their number increases according to the need. The stromal cells of the bone marrow support the growth and differentiation of pleuripotent stem cells.

Generally differentiation of pleuripotent stem cells takes place in two different directions to produce lymphoid and myeloid groups of cells. When a stem cell differentiates into a progenitor cell it loses its pleuripotent character and is committed to produce a specific type of cell. Alterations in the micro environment of progenitor cell influence the process of differentiation. The lymphoid progenitor cells produce B lymphocytes, T lymphocytes and natural killer cells. Myeloid progenitor cells produce progenitors of red blood cells and different white blood cells (Eosinophils, basophils, neutrophils, mast cells, monocytes etc.)

HAEMATOPOIETIC STEM CELLS:

A haematopoietic stem cell is a cell isolated from the blood or bone marrow that can renew itself, can differentiate to a variety of specialized cells, can mobilize out of the bone marrow into circulating blood, and can undergo programmed cell death, called apoptosis. They are ultimately responsible for the constant renewal of blood cells. Out of of billions of new blood cells produced each day, 1 in every 10,000 to 15,000 bone marrow cells is thought to be a stem cell. In the blood stream the proportion falls to 1 in 100,000 blood cells. The classic source of haematopoietic stem cells (HSCs) is bone marrow. With regard to morphology, haematopoietic stem cells resemble lymphocytes. They are non-adherent, and round, with a rounded nucleus and low cytoplasm-to-nucleus ratio.

CELLS OF LYMPHOID LINEAGE:

Production of lymphocytes from pleuripotent hemopoietic stem cells is known as lymphopoiesis. Lymphocytes are the chief constituents of the immune system. The oligopotent (In biology, oligopotency is the ability of progenitor cells to differentiate into a few cell types) lymphoid progenitors derived from pleuripotent haemopoitic stem cells generate 3 types of cells through an orderly change; they are T Lymphocytes, B Lymphocytes and Null cells. Local hormones or cytokines influence the differentiation of lymphoid stem cells into different lymphocytes. Even though all the lymphocytes are derived from the same oligopotent lymphoid stem cells, their function and the surface receptors / markers differ. The micro environment of lymphoid stem cells influences the differentiation of stem cells. Hence the T and B Lymphocytes appearing morphologically similar differ in their functional characteristics and surface markers.

Since both T and B lymphocytes are morphologically similar, it is impossible to distinguish T cells and B cells in a peripheral blood smear. The surface receptors present on the lymphocytes confer specificity for antigen and immune response. The affinity of receptors for the different antigens varies. As the lymphocytes with the highest affinity for the most abundant antigens help in defense, their progeny are preferably generated. This kind of multiplication of specific lymphocytes is known as clonal expansion. Unlike T and B cells, null cells do not show any specific surface markers.

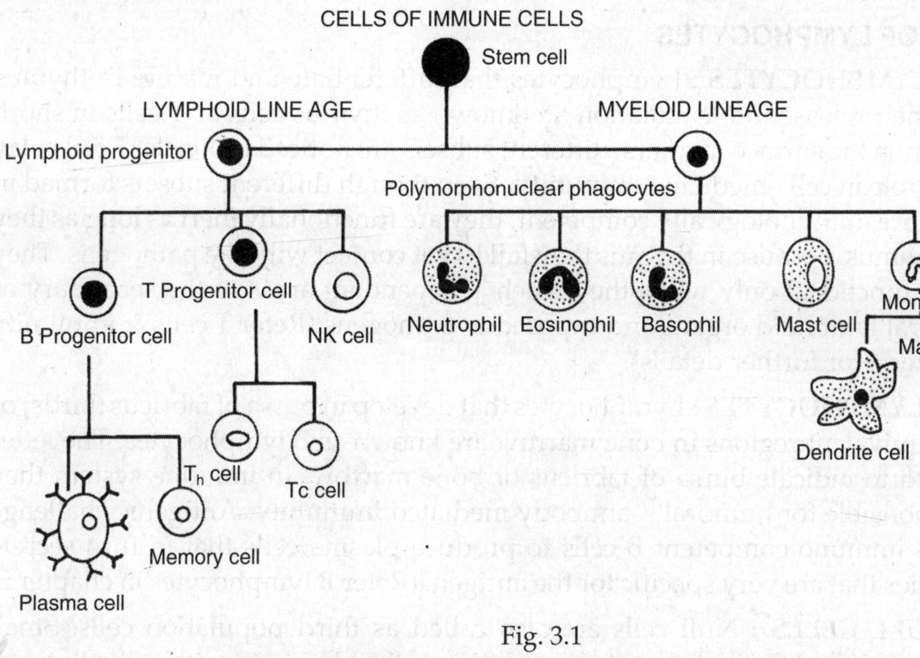

Fig. 3.1

A normal lymphocyte shows large, darkly stained nucleus with little to no basophilic cytoplasm. In normal situations, the coarse, dense nucleus of a lymphocyte is approximately about 7 micrometers in diameter. Some lymphocytes show a clear perinuclear zone (or halo) around the nucleus or could exhibit a small clear zone to one side of the nucleus. Presence of polyribosome is a prominent feature in the lymphocytes.

The lymphocytes following exposure to an antigen differentiate further to effector and memory lymphocytes. Function of effector lymphocytes is elimination of antigens, either by releasing antibodies (in the case of B cells), cytotoxic granules (in the case of cytotoxic T cells) or by signalling to other cells of the immune system (helper T cells). Memory cells remain in the peripheral tissues and circulation to respond readily to the same antigen upon future exposure.

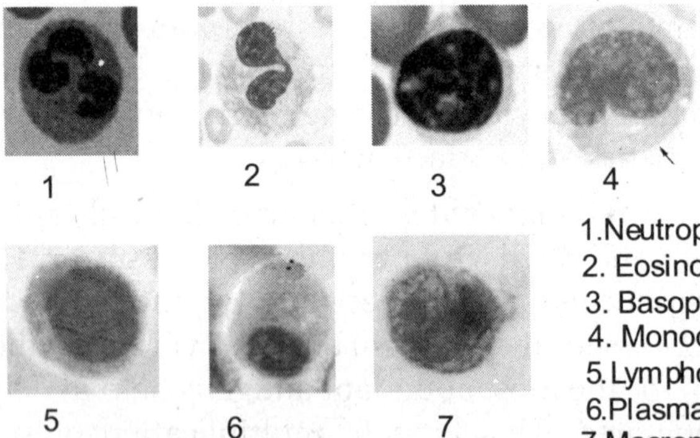

1.Neutrophil
2. Eosinophil
3. Basophil
4. Monocytes
5. Lymphocyte
6.Plasmacell
7.Macrophage

Fig. 3.2

TYPES OF LYMPHOCYTES

T LYMPHOCYTES : Lymphocytes that differentiate and mature in thymus before their release into circulation are known as thymus cells or T cells in short. Based upon the surface markers, different subsets are noticed in T cells. T cells play a major role in cell –mediated immunity. Even though different subsets formed in thymus are immunologically competent, they are functionally inert as long as they are in thymus. Because in thymus they fail to get contact with the pathogens. They become functional only when they reach T dependent areas of the secondary or peripheral lymphoid organs and exposed to pathogens (Refer T cells & immunity in chapter 4 for further details).

B LYMPHOCYTES : Lymphocytes that develop in bursa of fabricus (birds) or bursa equivalent regions in bone marrow are known as B lymphocytes. The letter B is used to indicate bursa of fabricus or bone marrow. In immune system they are responsible for humoral / antibody mediated immunity. Antigenic challenge initiates immuno competent B cells to produce plasma cells that in turn secrete antibodies that are very specific for the antigen. (Refer B lymphocytes in chapter 5)

NULL CELLS : Null cells are also called as third population cells. Small fractions (~2%) of the lymphocytes circulating in the blood are neither T cells nor B cells. Most of these are called natural killer (NK) cells because they are specialized to kill certain types of target cells, especially host cells that are infected with virus or modified to tumor cells. Unlike T and B cells, null cells lack immunologic memory and specificity. The specificity of the receptors with which NK cells recognize potential targets are not diversified like the T and B cells. Comparatively null cells are large in size with large granules of perforin and granzymes in their cytoplasm. They produce a number of immunologically important cytokines and play regulatory role in both cell mediated and humoral immune response. Stromal cell secretions in the surroundings of null cells play a vital role in their maturation. NK cells contain "activating receptors" and "Killer Inhibitory Receptors" (KIRs). When an NK cell binds to a target cell without class I MHC molecules, the activating receptors trigger the killing activity in NK cell. Killer inhibitory receptors (KIRs) convey an inhibitory signal to the NK cells if they encounter class I MHC molecules on target cell surface. Since viruses often suppress the expression of class I MHC in host cells, the virus-infected cells happen to be susceptible for NK cells killing activity. In the same way, cancer cells showing reduced or no class I MHC expression are vulnerable to killing by NK cells.

Lineage of NK cells is not clearly understood, however genes for NK receptors illustrate polymorphism. Hence the variety of NK receptors differs from person to person. Research information in this field has shown that IL-15 (interleukin –15) potentially promotes NK cells development from NK precursors (NKPs) and IL- 2 could maintain NK cell's survival and drive their development from committed precursors. Hence IL- 2 and IL - 15 are vital for NK cell generation. Absence of IL – 15 signalling cause severe reduction in the number of NK cells. Even though they possess certain T lymphocyte markers they are independent of MHC molecules to execute their lytic function on target cells. Because of this character NK cells provide first line of defense. When NK cells adhere to the target cell, they release perforin and granzymes at the junction of their interaction. The perforin causes pore formation on the target cell that results in its death through leakage of its contents and the granzymes induce apoptosis of the target cell.

Since NK cells are preprogrammed to recognize their targets, they are able to respond rapidly, thus providing an important tool in innate immunity. In addition to killing target cells, NK cells secrete cytokines such as anti-viral cytokine IFN-γ and inflammatory cytokine TNF-α. Since surface receptors of different null cells are different, their functions also vary. Based on functions null cells can be broadly divided in to two groups (a) Natural Killer cells, (b) Killer cells.

(a) Natural killer cells or NK cells: - They are about 15μm in diameter with a kidney shaped nucleus and azurophilic granules in their cytoplasm. NK cells are morphologically distinguishable from the other lymphocytes through the presence of 2 or 3 large granules in their cytoplasm. They exhibit spontaneous killer activity against any foreign cells, tumor cells, pathogen infested auto cells etc., even in the absence of prior stimulation. Therefore NK cells represent first line of defense to infections, tumor growth and other pathogenic alterations in tissue homoeostasis. NK cells are non phagocytic and non adherent to surfaces, but release perforin in close proximity to a cell selected for killing. Perforin forms pores in the cell membrane of the target cell through which the granzymes and associated molecules can enter inducing apoptosis.

Granzymes are serine proteases that are released by cytoplasmic granules within cytotoxic T cells and natural killer cells. Granzyme B (GrB) and perforin were found to coexist as multimeric complexes with the proteoglycan serglycin (SG) in cytotoxic granules, and cytotoxic cells were observed to secrete exclusively macromolecular GrB-SG. Their purpose is to induce apoptosis within virus-infected cells, thus destroying them.

Since they are capable of identifying alterations in surface markers of the auto cells, NK cells provide natural toxicity. Different surface receptors for activation and inhibitory signals are identified but the exact regulatory mechanism of NK cells is not yet clearly understood. Even though all NK cells are equally efficient in cytolytic activity, the mode of activation is different. Certain sub sets of NK populations show priority in killing tumor cells and others kill virus or bacteria infected cells. Irrespective of their killing priority they do not require any support from T cells or antigen presenting cells for their function or activation.

Azurophil is the term used to refer to objects that are readily staining with an azure dye. The term is used especially in reference to certain cytoplasmic granules in white blood cells, particularly hyperchromatin and reddish purple granules of certain blood cells.

(b) Killer Cells (or) K Cells: - K cells are antibody dependent for their activity. Due to this character K cells are also referred as antibody dependent cytotoxic cells (ADCCs). They possess receptors for Fc region of antibody; binding of antibody through Fc region to these receptors induces release of cytotoxic substances such as perforin, granzymes etc., in close proximity of antibody bound target cell. The released cytotoxic substances are responsible for lysis of target cell. Compliment fixation is not required for the lytic action of K cells. Like T cells, K cells can react with sheep erythrocytes and form rosettes.

MYELOID LINEAGE

Myeloid progenitor cells produce phagocytic cells and the remaining accessory cells. Different phagocytic cells of myeloid lineage can be classified into polymorphonuclear phagocytes and mononuclear phagocytes with reference to the nucleus structure. Monocytes and macrophages are included in mononuclear phagocyte cell group. Neutrophils, basophils, eosinophils are included into polymorphonuclear phagocytes group because of varying shapes of their nucleus. The accessory cells are the cells that help immune system in various ways such as processing and presenting the antigens to immunocompetent T cells, enhancing the immunologic response through secretion etc. Different cells of myeloid lineage are as follows.

Granulocytes: - About 60-70% of total leucocytes are granulocytes. They contain multilobed nucleus and many granules. Hence they are referred as polymorpho nuclear granulocytes (PMN or PML). They are short lived with a life span of about 2-3 days. They are not specific for antigens but play an important role in immunity. On the basis of morphology and staining characters the granulocytes are classified into three types namely neutrophils, eosinophils and basophils.

Neutrophils: - These are the most abundant type of granulocytes found in the peripheral blood and about 90% of circulating granulocytes are neutrophils. They are motile and phagocytic in nature. Mature neutrophils have multi lobed nuclei and granular cytoplasm. They are about 10 micrometers in diameter and live approximately five days. One litre of human blood contains about five billion neutrophils. Mature neutrophils are smaller than monocytes. The granules of neutrophils are different. The large denser azurophilic granules contain peroxidase, lysozyme and various hydrolytic enzymes and the smaller granules contain collagenase, lactoferrin and lysozyme. The collective function of the granules helps in digestion and elimination of pathogen phagocytised by the cell. The chemotactic action of cytokines at the site of inflammation initiates marginalization and extravasculation or diapedisis in neutrophils to attract near to the site of infection

Once neutrophils have received the appropriate signals, they take about thirty minutes to leave the blood and reach the site of infection. Once they reach the site of inflammation they do not return to the blood; they turn into pus cells and die. Production of neutrophils increases in response to many infections and during severe infection neutrophil precursors called myelocytes and promyelocytes are released in to the circulation. In medical terminology the raise of neutrophils is known as leucocytosis.

> **Marginalization:** Cells flowing in the circulation move nearer to the endothelial lining (margin) of blood vessels to squeeze out.
>
> **Extravasculation or Diapedisis:** Emigration of cells through the gaps of endothelial cells of blood vessel.

Eosinophils: Eosinophols with bilobed nucleus and granular cytoplasm are motile phagocytes. They occupy about 2-5% of total blood leucocytes in normal healthy individuals. They are acidophilic in nature and stain with acid dye eosin. Like neutrophils they also exhibit extravasation and phagocytosis during inflammation reactions. Basically they help in the eradication of big parasites such as round worms, pin worms etc., because their granules contain a unique toxic basic protein and cationic protein (e.g. cathepsin) and the receptors that bind to IgE are used to help in this task. In addition to that they help in the removal of immune complexes through phagocytosis and regulate functions of other immune cell (e.g. CD_4^+ T cells, dendritic cells, B cells, mast cells, neutrophils, and basophils functions). In healthy individuals raise of eosinophils is a general immunological response to intestinal parasites. Unlike neutrophils the granules of eosinophils are membrane bound. An appropriate stimulus induces fusion of cytoplasmic granules with plasma membrane to release their toxic protein contents and histamine in the surroundings of parasite, when the parasite is too big for phagocytosis. The released substances of eosinophils bind to the membrane of the parasite to kill and eliminate. In general atopic persons show high levels of eosinophils (Refer Chapter 14 for further details of Hyper sensitivity). Eosinophils respond to chemotactic factors released by basophils and mast cells. In healthy individuals secretions of eosinophils suppress the activity of mast cell secretions to regulate the immunological response.

Basophils: - Basophils are one of the least abundant cells in blood (comprise less than 0.2% of total leucocytes count). Unlike neutrophils and eosinophils they are non phagocytic in nature. They contain granules that are receptive to basic stains hence they were named as basophils. They work by releasing their pharmacologically active substances such as histamine, sertonine, heparin, peroxidase, platelet activating factor etc. When basophils are induced they release histamine; this contributes to the inflammatory response that helps in fighting with invading organisms. In general the released substances of basophils result in Type I hypersensitivity/ allergic reactions. Basophils have receptors that allow binding of IgE, IgG, complement, and histamine. Since they have receptors for Fc region of Ig E antibodies the IgE antibodies produced against an allergen bind to basophils. Interaction of antigen with the basophil bound IgE antibody induces release of basophil contents, histamine in the released substances causes dilation and increased permeability of capillaries close to the basophil. Another substance called prostaglandins contributes to an increased blood flow to the site of infection. Both of these mechanisms allow blood clotting elements to be delivered at the infected area, which prevents further spread of pathogens. Increased permeability of the blood also allows more phagocyte migration to the site of infection so that they can devour the microbes.

ACCESSORY CELLS

(1) Mast cells: - Mast cells are found in almost all parts of the body along with the endothelial cells of the blood vessels as well as mucosal cells. Unlike other blood cells they are sessile and differentiation of mast cells from precursor cells takes place in tissues. They are about 10-30μ m in diameter with a polymorphic nucleus. Even though they are absent in circulation they are quite similar to basophils in various aspects, such as morphology, function, surface receptors etc. On the basis of origin and activities mast cells can be differentiated in to two different groups. One is mucosal mast cell group (MMC) and the other is connective tissue mast cells (CTMC). Mucosal mast cells are derivative of thymus derived precursors but connective tissue mast cells arise from bone marrow. Since high affinity receptors for IgE antibodies are present on the surface of mast cells, the IgE antibodies secreted against specific allergen bind to the mast cells and induce mast cell secretions on antigen binding. These chemicals are harmful to the parasite and also serve as signals to other immune cells to come and join in the reaction. The action of mast cells and the effect of their secretions are similar to the action of basophils. In addition to T cells, B cells, Phagocytes, immune system engages mast cells also in defense. The basic function of mast cells is to give protection against large external parasites entering through the skin, respiratory or intestinal tract.

Antigen presenting cells/ Dendritic cells: Antigen presenting cells are a heterogeneous population of leucocytes. Through antigen presentation they play a key role in the immunological reactions. They are found primarily in the skin, lymphnodes, spleen and thymus. They are derived from bone marrow. The migration of dendritic cells (DCs) to lymph nodes (LNs) is pivotal to the establishment of the immune response. In response to danger signals, precursors are rapidly mobilized into the circulation. Chemokine receptors present on the dendritic cells help in their movement towards their precise regions. They hold nonspecific antigen uptake receptors. When they get activated with the antigen, they start migrating towards the T cells for presenting the antigen. When they reach the T cells, they present the processed antigen to the T cell for further action.

To cover long areas antigen presenting dendritic cells holds long cytoplasmic protrusions, like dendrites of nerve cells. Because of dendrites like protrusions they were referred as dendritic cells. Dendritic cells capture the antigens in the tissue by phagocytosis and migrate to various lymphoid organs to present the antigen to lymphocytes for immunological reactions. The dendrities or the filamentous process may help in engulfing and presenting activity, making them better antigen presenting cells than macrophages and B cells. The high levels of MHC class II molecules on the surface of dendritic cells enhance their efficiency. In addition to antigen presentation the activated dendritic cells secrete different cytokines including IL-7 and IL-12. IL - 7 induces CD_4 and CD_8 T cell proliferation and B cell differentiation.

Antigen presenting cells have common progenitor cells together with the monocyte macrophage lineage because both express the medullary antigen CD33 and CD35.

On the basis of tissue location dendritic cells are classified as follows.

(1) Langerhans Cells: -These are found in the epidermal layer of the skin, where they are thought to act as sentinels for the detection of invading pathogens. Interaction with pathogens induces their migration to lymphoid regions to prime T cell immunity.

(2) Interdigitating Cells: - The antigen presenting cells, interdigitating the T lymphocytes are localized in T cell dependent paracortex areas of lymph node and thymus.

(3) Follicular dendritic cells (FDCs): - Follicular dendritic cells (FDCs) are the stromal cells located in the germinal centers of spleen and lymph node. They lack MHC class II molecules, but show protrusions like dendrites of nerve cells. The dendrites in the network bind immune complexes in a periodicity that is pivotal in the binding of immune complexes to B cells in the germinal centers. This binding initiates a specific antibody response to antigens.

Follicular dendritic cells (FDCs) have important functions in the selection of memory B lymphocytes during germinal center reactions (GCR). They present native antigens to potential memory cells, of which only B cells with high affinity receptors (BCR) can bind. These B lymphocytes survive, whereas non binding B cells undergo apoptosis (cell death).

FDCs are present in follicles of any secondary lymphoid organ and belong to the stromal cells of these organs. They contain large amounts of MHC class II molecules (Refer Chapter 11 for further information). In addition to MHC class II molecules they have various surface bound adhesion molecules and co stimulatory molecules to execute their function perfectly.

The development of FDCs is not restricted to secondary lymphoid organs, but it is a matter of local conditions that drives a precursor cell type into FDC-maturation. A precursor of FDCs has presently not been identified, but phenotypic marker studies, in vitro experiments with fibroblast-like cell lines and recent data on mesenchymal precursor cells from the peripheral blood suggest a close relation to fibroblast-like cells.

(4) Interstitial dendritic cells: -They are found in most of the organs like heart liver kidney and gastrointestinal tract. They are efficient in presenting soluble antigens. Circulating antigen antibody complexes fasten to the receptors on follicular dendritic cells, there by helping in activation of B cells in lymph nodes.

Platelets: - These are small granular a nucleated cells, derived from mega karyocytes. Usually, they are about 3μm in diameter and about 150,000 to 350,000 platelets in a micro litre of blood. Besides their role in blood clotting they are involved in hyper sensitivity and inflammatory reactions. In addition to receptors for factor VIII they express MHC class I molecules, they express IgG receptors and low affinity receptors for Ig E on their surface. Following injury platelets aggregate and adhere to damaged vascular epithelial cells and release their secretions. Histamine and serotonin of the released substances cause inflammatory response.

In people with a low platelet count, bleeding is more likely to occur, even after a slight injury. When the platelet count is below 20,000 (very low), massive bleeding may occur even when there is no injury. Aspirin, nonsteroidal anti-inflammatory drugs (NSAIDs), and antihistamines may interfere with how platelets function, although the platelet count remains normal.

Monocytes or Mononuclear phagocytes: -They are the largest mono nucleated cells found in the blood stream. They are produced from hemopoitic stem cells in bone marrow. Their size ranges from 10-20μm in diameter. They circulate in blood stream for about 8 hours and migrate to tissue spaces to differentiate in to tissue specific macrophages. Phagocytic activity of monocytes increases when they differentiate into macrophages. They are dispersed through out the body. After differentiation some of the macrophages become fixed to reside in certain tissues and some become motile. The fixed macrophages show amoeboid movement in the tissue to engulf foreign particles. In addition they acquire certain characters specific for their surrounding tissue. With reference to surrounding tissue, the fixed macrophages are named differently. They are as follows.

Liver-Kuffer cells, Connective tissue –Histocytes, Bone-Osteoclasts, Kidney-Mesangial cells, Brain-microglial cells.

Blood monocytes are also heterogenous and two main subsets have been described in human blood. These are the classical CD_{14}^{++} monocytes and the pro-inflammatory $CD_{14}^{++}CD_{16}^{++}$ monocytes. The latter cells are characterized by their high level production of the pro-inflammatory cytokine TNF and by their propensity to preferentially develop into potent dendritic cells.

Monocytes and macrophages play important role in immune defence, inflammation and tissue remodeling. They do so by phagocytosis, antigen processing and presentation and by cytokine production. Certain factors such as C3b fraction of compliment system, IgG binding with surface receptors, released cytokines of T_H cells; bacterial surface components etc. enhance the phagocytic activity of macrophages. Since they are capable of chemotaxis, they get attracted towards the pathogen or antigen antibody complex through chemotaxis.

4

T LYMPHOCYTES

T Lymphocytes are the most common cells of immune system, that matures in the thymus and are responsible for cell-mediated immunity. The letter T sands for thymus, the primary lymphoid gland that helps in their differentiation and development. A group of cells known as "progenitor T cells", from the pleuripotent stem cells of bone marrow migrate to thymus to become an immunologically competent cells.They develop in thymus and expand their number by cell division to generate a large population of immature thymocytes and get differentiated into immunecompitent "T Lymphocytes" under the influence of thymic hormones. Since progenitor T cells are not self renewing they are constantly supplied from bone marrow. The migration of haematopoietic stem cells to the thymus may be due to the chemotactic substances released by thymic epithelial cells.

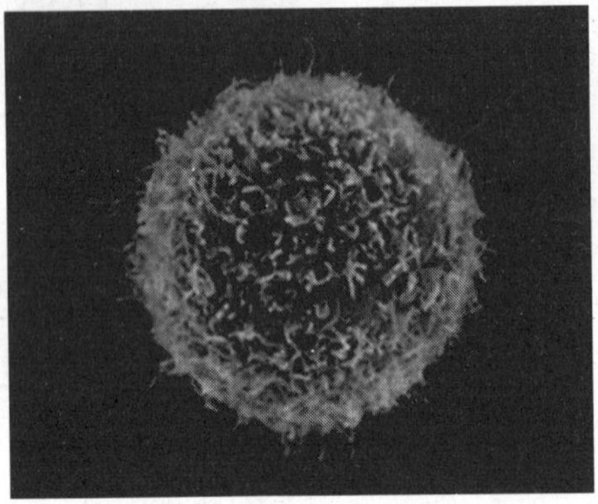

Fig. 4.1

Differentiation and maturation of T Lymphocytes reflects a change in nature and distribution of surface markers. Since progenitor T cells do not express characteristic surface markers of T cells, the surface markers and receptors of developing T cells provide a powerful tool for studying the differentiation process. In early developmental stages the thymocytes express neither CD_4 nor CD_8 surface markers, and are therefore referred as double negative ($CD_4^-CD_8^-$) cells. During maturation the genes of T cell receptors get rearranged leading to a change in surface markers. At this point the alpha chain of TCR undergoes rearrangement. The successful rearrangement of this chain serves as a signal for these cells to undergo further proliferation. During this time, both CD_4 and CD_8 start to be expressed. Thus these cells are referred to as "double positive cells (CD_4^+ CD_8^+)". At this point the beta chain of the TCR undergoes rearrangement and the cells undergo the processes of Positive and Negative selection. The highly variable genetic rearrangement in the Tcell receptor (TCR) genes during their development helps to generate millions of different TCRs. T cells with different TCRs, help the body's immune system to respond to almost any protein of an invader. Since the functional immune system requires T Lymphocytes expressing receptors that are major histocompatibility complex restricted but tolerant to self-antigens, the developing T cells under go the selection of T Lymphocytes expressing receptors that are major histocompatibility complex restricted but tolerant to self-antigens.

The Positive and Negative selection process in the thymus results in the death of about 98% of thymocytes or T cells within the thymus before their release from the thymus to reach the functional sites - peripheral/secondary lymphoid regions.

POSITIVE SELECTION:

Since TCR's recognize antigen only in the context of MHCs, T cells must be tuned to recognize host MHC first. During positive selection double positive T cells that can recognize self MHCs are selected for proliferation and those T cells that do not recognize self MHC die via apoptosis. The cells undergoing positive selection initially express both CD_4 and CD_8 co receptors. Positive selection also assures that the right TCR selection will go with the appropriate CD_4 or CD_8. For example, TCRs specific for MHC II need to retain CD_4, and lose CD_8. If the reverse occurs, they will die via apoptosis.

The thymocyte's fate is also determined during positive selection. Double positive cells (CD_4^+/CD_8^+) that are positively selected on MHC class II molecules eventually become CD_4^+ cells, while cells positively selected on MHC class I molecules mature into CD_8^+ cells.

NEGATIVE SELECTION:

T cells that are strongly activated by self MHC plus self peptides are eliminated through negative selection in the thymus. If they escape this elimination, they may subsequently react against self antigens, and cause autoimmune disease.

The single positive cells with CD_4^+ or CD_8^+ survived after positive and negative selection, then release from thymus to reach peripheral or secondary lymphoid tissues through circulation.

CD - Clusters of differentiation: The label CD stands for "cluster of differentiation". It is a historical term that was coined to define cell-surface molecules that are recognized by a given set of monoclonal antibodies. This cluster of differentiation then received a number, for example CD_1, CD_2 etc., which stands only for the order of discovery. In general, each CD is associated with one or more function.

The CD nomenclature was proposed and established in the 1st International Workshop and Conference on Human Leukocyte Differentiation Antigens (HLDA), held in Paris in 1982. This system was intended for the classification of the many monoclonal antibodies (mAbs) generated by different laboratories around the world against epitopes on the surface molecules of leukocytes (white blood cells). Since then, its use has expanded to many other cell types, and more than 320 CD unique clusters and subclusters have been identified.

SURFACE MARKERS AND RECEPTORS OF MATURE T CELLS

The mature T cells display thousands of heterodimer surface receptors known as T cell receptors (TCRs).

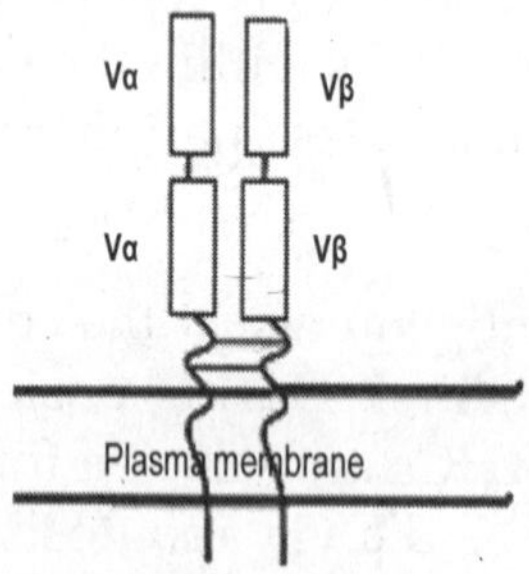

Fig. 4.2 T cell Receptor

Based on the surface receptors T cells are differentiated into two types. They are:

(1) Alpha/beta (α/β) T cells: The antigen receptors are made up of two transmembrane polypeptides designated alpha and beta. Like antibodies each polypeptide chain has an N terminal variable region with 3 hypervariable or complementary determining regions (CDRs). The CDRs of the two chains cooperate to form a single binding site for the epitope. The epitope seen by T cells consists of an antigenic peptide inserted into a groove formed by a major histocompatibility complex (MHC) molecule. Typically the two supervariable CDR3s bind to the peptide while the less variable CDR1s and CDR2s bind to the MHC molecule.

(2) Gamma/delta (γ/δ) T cells: A small percentage of the T cells in the blood use a TCR consisting of a heterodimer of two other types of transmembrane polypeptides: gamma and delta. They differ from their alpha/beta cousins in several ways:

1. Their TCR is encoded by different gene segments.

2. Their TCR binds to antigens that can be (1) intact proteins (just as antibodies do) as well as a variety of other types of organic molecules (often containing phosphorus atoms). (2) not "presented" within class I or class II histocompatibility molecules; (3) not presented by "professional" antigen presenting cells (APCs) like dendritic cells.

3. Most of these T cells have neither CD_8 nor CD_4 on their surface. This makes sense because they have no need to recognize class I and class II histocompatibility molecules.

4. Gamma/Delta T cells, like alpha/beta T cells, develop in the thymus. However, they migrate from there into body tissues, especially epithelia (e.g., intestine, skin, lining of the vagina), and don't recirculate between blood and lymph nodes (they represent no more than 5% of the T cells in the blood and are even rarer in lymph nodes). They encounter antigens on the surface of the epithelial cells that surround them rather than relying on the APCs found in lymph nodes.

The function of this subset of T cells is still a mystery. Since they are situated at the interfaces between the external and internal worlds, they may represent a first line of defense against invading pathogens. Their response does seem to be quicker than that of γδ T cells. Curiously, many of the antigens to which γδ T cells respond are found not only on certain types of invaders (e.g., Mycobacterium tuberculosis, the agent of tuberculosis) but also in host cells that are under attack by pathogens.

Certain common receptors present on T cells:

Erythrocyte receptors (E receptors): These receptors help in distinguishing T cells from B cells. For unknown reasons the T cells of man and other animal T cells processes this polypeptide receptors. This helps in the formation of rosettes of foreign erythrocytes. Their physiological role is probably that of a negative signal receptor.

(3) Compliment receptors: T cells process receptors for activated components of compliment system, that probably expressed after activation followed by antigen interaction.

(4) Ia Protein Receptor: This receptor recognizes immune associated proteins (Ia proteins) and help in coordination with B cell and macrophages.

(5) Histamine receptor (H2): T cells process H_2 histamine receptors. They help in regulation of T cell activity. Binding of histamine with this receptor reduces T cell activity.

(6) IL-1 and IL-2 receptors: The IL-1 interleukin produced by macrophages combine with IL-1 receptor to initiate T cell response. The IL-2 interleukin secreted by activated T cells binds again to IL-2 receptor of the T cell for autocrine and paracrine signaling to the T cells.

(7) Ti Receptor: It is a basic antigen receptor with two transmembrane glycoprotein chains α (50 kD) and β (45 kD) joined by disulphide bond. In certain situations the Ti may have a third γ chain of 55kD. γδ heterodimer is expressed on about 5% of cells. TCR with γδ are known as TCR1 and TCR with αβ glycoproteins are known as TCR2 receptors.

(8) CD3 receptor: It is a non covalent complex of 3 types of chains γ (25 kD) γ δ (20 kD) and ε (20 kD). All the three chains are essential for T cell function, CD_3 peptide chains are involved in signal transduction after interaction with antibody. CD_3 with TCR produces the TCR CD_3 complex an "ion channel" for the entry of Ca+ into the T cell.

(9) CD_4 marker: This marker is found on T helper cells. It is a 60 kD glycoprotein and is involved in interaction of the T cell with MHC class II molecules of antigen presenting cells (APC). This acts as a receptor for HIV virus.

(10) HIV CD4 marker: It is a glycoprotein marker formed on T_C and T_S cells. It is involved in interaction of the T_C cells with class I molecules present on infected cells or Tumour cells.

TYPES OF T CELLS AND THEIR FUNCTION

The sub populations of T cells with functional difference can be identified by means of surface markers (CD markers) or antigens. Approximately 60 - 65% of mature T cells that leave the thymus display CD_2^+, CD_3^+, CD_4^+ and CD_8^- markers on their surface and are generally referred as CD_4 cells or TH cells or T helper cells. These cells play a major role in the initiation of immunological reactions. In the remaining cells 30-35% poses CD_2^+, CD_3^+, CD_4^- and CD_8^+ markers and they are referred as CD_8 cells or "cytotoxic T cells" or T_C cells that act as effector cells in immunological reaction. A small group of cells express neither CD_4^+ nor CD_8^+ but express CD_2^+, CD_3^+ markers. Function of these cells is yet to be studied.

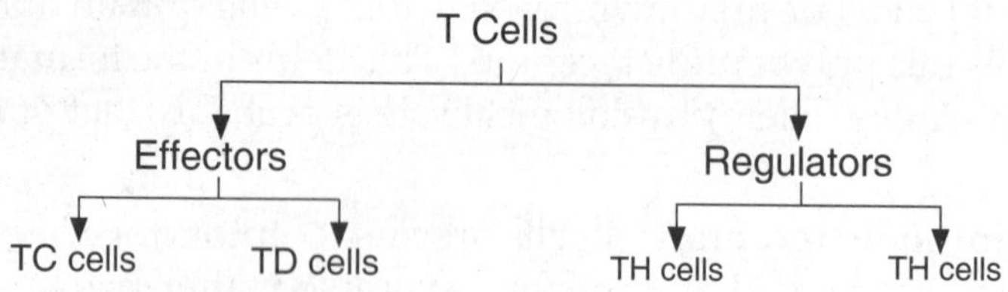

Fig. 4.3

A small fraction of CD_4 cells are referred as "Delayed T cells or DT_H or T_D cells" due to their delay in expression of their activity. They serve as non specific effectors of inflammation. In the same way certain CD_8^+ cell populations help in regulation of immunological reactions and they were referred as "T suppressor cells" or T_S cells. Both T_C cells and T_D cells are considered as effectors cells and they show memory response. T_H and T_S cells are considered as regulators of immunological function. CD_4^+, CD_8^+ populations are MHC restricted (Ref MHC). In contrast the CD_4^- and CD_8^- cells are very few in number and they are not MHC restricted.

T Helper cells or TH cells: T_H cells a distinct subset of T-cells can be identified through their expression of the CD_4 co receptor. They have no cytotoxic or phagocytic activity but are vital for immune response. They are essential in determining B cell antibody class switching, in the activation and growth of cytotoxic T cells, and in maximizing bactericidal activity of phagocytes such as macrophages. Since they initiate the immune response and induce activity of the other cells of immune system they were named as T helper cells. Their response is initiated by the interaction between the T-cell receptor (TCR) and peptide major histocompatibility complex class II (pMHC II). T_H cell activation leads to the induction of a number of pathways that can result in immunoglobulin class switching and antibody production, macrophage action through direct interaction and by means of the release of soluble factors. The T_H cell response delimited by two distinct pathways involves two different subtypes of T_H cells- the T_{H1} and T_{H2} cells. In most cases, T_{H1} cells are targeted towards intracellular pathogens such as bacteria and parasites via the activation of macrophages, while T_{H2} cells invoke antibody production in B cells, to neutralise extra cellular pathogens and toxins. Once activated, the T_H cells divide rapidly and release cytokines to enhance or regulate immune response.

Cytotoxic T cells or T_C cells:

Cytotoxic T cells also known as T_C, Cytotoxic Tlymphocyte, T-Killer cell, cytolytic T cell, CD_8^+ T-cells or killer T cell are effector cells. They play a major role in cell mediated immunity, to destroy virally infected cells, tumour cells, and tissue grafts. T_C cells express CD_8 glycoprotein on their surface and are associated with MHC class I. Antigen presenting cells degrade the viral proteins into peptides and present to the Tc cells as pMHC I. The affinity between CD_8 and the MHC molecule helps in keeping the T_C cell and the target cell bound closely together during antigen-specific activation. The Tc cells response in most cases is targetted towards intracellular pathogens such as viruses, bacteria and tumour related antigens that exist in the cytosol, or contiguous nuclear compartment. Tc cells activation leads to direct killing of target cell through induction of apoptotic signals by means of the released cytotoxic granules and lymphokines.

T suppressor or T_S Cells:

T suppressor cells are crucial for the maintenance of immunological tolerance. Their major role is to shut down T cell mediated immunity at the end of an immune reaction and suppress auto-reactive T cells that escaped the process of negative selection in the thymus. Two major classes of CD_4^+ regulatory T_S cells have been described; they are the naturally occurring T_S cells and the adaptive T_S cells. Naturally occurring T_S cells are also known as CD_4^+ CD_{25}^+ $FoxP_3^+$ T_S cells. They arise in the thymus, whereas the adaptive T_S cells also known as Tr_1 cells or TH_3 cells. They may originate during a normal immune response. Naturally occurring T_S cells can be distinguished from other T cells by the presence of an intracellular molecule called FoxP3. Mutations of the FOXP3 gene can prevent regulatory T cell development, causing the fatal autoimmune disease IPEX.

Delayed T cells or TD cells: - This cell type is not individually well characterized; on the basis of surface markers. They are probably Th1 cells, functioning to produce a delayed type hypersensitivity reaction. The quality of cytokines they secrete is different. Subsequent exposures to the antigen induce the effector phase of TD cells. The TD cell secretions are responsible for the recruitment and activation of macrophages and other nonspecific inflammatory cells. Generally TD cells response occurs after 24 hours of secondary contact with the antigen, hence they were known as delayed T cells or TD cells.

Activation of mature T cells:-

The naïve CD_4^+ and CD_8^+ T cells leave thymus and enter the circulation as resting cells in the G0 stage of the cell cycle. The naïve T cells have condensed chromatin with little cytoplasm. They circulate continuously between the blood and lymph system (once in 24 hours) till they encounter an antigen in the secondary lymphoid organs. Since 1 in 10^5 naïve T cell can bind with the new antigen the continuous circulation of naïve T cells increase the chances of interaction of appropriate T cell with the new antigen.

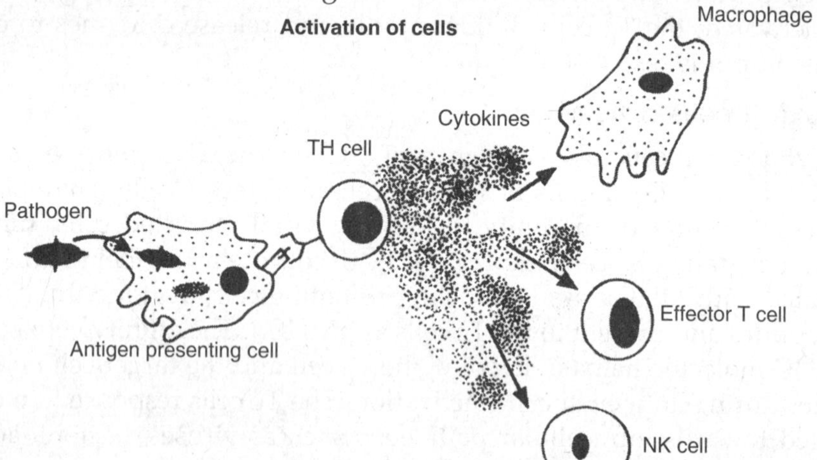

Fig. 4.4

If the naïve T cells interact with suitable antigens through antigen presenting cells, they get differentiated in to effector T cells. The differentiation is initiated by interaction of T cells TCR, CDs (receptors) complex, with a processed antigen bound to the surface MHC class II molecules of antigen presenting cells. Co stimulatory factor B_7 on antigen presenting cells is necessary for activation of naïve T cells. Since it is absent on their surface resting macrophages and B cells, they fail to activate naïve T cells. Some times T cells fail to respond even after interacting with the antigen. The non responsiveness of T cells after interaction with antigen MHC class II complex is known as "clonal anergy". This is due to the unavailability of naïve T cells to undergo clonal expansion in the absence of co stimulatory signal produced by the interaction of TCR, CDs complex on TH cells with B_7 on antigen presenting cells. Apart from this, the cytokines released by the antigen presenting cells also involve in the activation process. A series of membrane and cytoplasmic events take place during differentiation and proliferation. The composition of cell membrane also changes resulting in the development of new receptors such as high affinity IL-2 and gain of specific functional characters. Antigen interaction with naïve T cell provides the first activating signal and interleukin -1 (Refer interleukins) secreted by antigen presenting cell serves as second signal for T cell activation.

Within half an hour of activation a number of transcription factors were expressed by activated T cells and release various cytokines within 1 to 2 hours of activation. A co stimulatory signal produced by the CD_{28} present on TH cells and B_7 present on antigen presenting cells support and enhances the differentiation process of naïve T cell. Interaction of naïve T cells and antigen provides the first activating signal and interleukin -1 secreted by antigen presenting cell serves as second signal in activation of naïve T cells. Activated T cells secrete various cytokines such as interleukin -2 (IL- 2), to promote differentiation of both B and T cells. Interleukin 2 (IL-2) provides an autocrine signal to induce repeated cell divisions ((2 to 3 times a day for 4-5 days) for clonal expansions.

Some of the differentiated naïve T cells remain in the body as memory cells without involving in immunological activity. Unlike effector cells they have long life span and provide quick secondary response to subsequent challenge with the same antigen. Even though memory cells are in G_0 phase of life cycle like naïve T cells, they get activated easily by macrophages, dendritic cells, and B cells.

CELL MEDIATED IMMUNITY (CMI):

T cells are responsible for large number of functions that collectively result in cell mediated immunity (CMI). It is most effective in removing virus-infected cells, and also participates in defending against fungi, protozoans, cancers, and intracellular bacteria. It also plays a major role in transplant rejection. Antigen-specific cytotoxic T-lymphocytes, macrophages, natural killer cells (NK) and various cytokines released in response to an antigen are involved in CMI. Cellular immunity protects the body by:

1. Activating antigen-specific cytotoxic T-lymphocytes (CTLs) that are able to destroy body cells displaying epitopes of foreign antigen on their surface, such as virus-infected cells, cells with intracellular bacteria, and cancer cells displaying tumor antigens.

2. Activating macrophages and NK cells and facilitating them to destroy intracellular pathogens.

3. Stimulating cells to secrete a variety of cytokines that influence the function of other cells involved in adaptive immune responses and innate immune responses.

T_H cells are involved in the selection of the effector mechanism to be directed against the selected target antigens. Since activation of inappropriate mechanism results in enhanced susceptibility to the pathogens rather than protection, selection of effector mechanism is very important.

Even though cell mediated immunity strongly suggests the T cell dependent action, certain cell mediated immune reactions are T cell independent. Of course no cell mediated immune response is likely to occur in the total absence of T cells and antibodies. Hence depending upon the involvement of T cells and antibodies cell mediated immunity can be classified in to (1) T cell independent (2) T cell dependent (3) antibody independent and (4) Antibody dependent cell mediated immunity.

T cell independent CMI: Certain phagocytic NK cells kill and remove pathogens like bacteria and virus in the absence of T cells. The chemotactic factors released by the activated compliment system (Refer compliment system) or the cytokines released by the macrophages following activation through binding through antibodies draw phagocytic cells towards the pathogens and enhance their characteristic function. For example TNFα released by the macrophages in response to the microbial components enhance the microbicidal activity of remaining macrophages, neutrophils, NK cells and K cells. In addition to that TNFα cause marginalzation and diapedisis of phagocytes to infiltrate the area of inflammation and phagocytose the pathogens. The total reaction is T cell independent, different cells of immune system excluding T cells provide this immediate but non specific protection. This T cell independent CMI reaction may dependent on antibodies or may be independent of antibodies. With reference to the role of antibodies it can be further divided in to antibody independent and antibody dependent T cell independent CMI.

(a) T cell independent, antibody dependent CMI: Certain cells like K cells; eosinophils etc., have receptors for Fc region of antibodies. Through these receptors they fasten themselves to the antibody bound pathogens and kill the target cells by their cytotoxic action. Since antibodies are mediating this CMI reactions, this CMI is referred as "T cell independent antibody dependent CMI" and the immune cells involved in this reaction are considered as cytotoxic cells.

(b)T cell and antibody independent CMI: Cells like natural killer cells and macrophages can kill the pathogen without the participation of antibodies. In this reaction enzymes of compliment system or the cytokines released by macrophages induce the cytotoxic action.

T cell dependent CMI: Intracellular pathogens were removed by T cell dependent CMI. The effector T lymphocytes -TC, TD are responsible for this kind of CMI. Activated cytotoxic T cells bind to the target cell through MHC class I molecules present on the cell surface and cause lysis of the target cell.

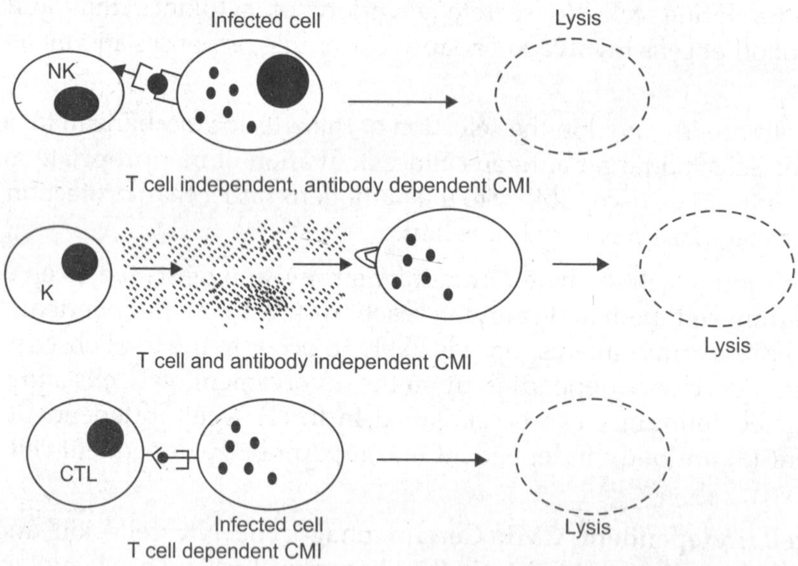

Fig. 4.5

THE MECHANISM OF CELL MEDIATED IMMUNITY: -

The mechanism of cell mediated immunity includes

(1) Activation of antigen-specific cytotoxic T-lymphocytes that is able to induce apoptosis in body cells displaying epitopes of foreign antigen on their surface such as cells with intracellular bacteria, virus-infected cells and cancer cells displaying tumor antigens.

(2) Activating macrophages and natural killer cells, enabling them to destroy intracellular pathogens.

(3) Stimulating cells to secrete a variety of cytokines that influence the function of other cells involved in immune responses.

Irrespective of the type of cells involved in CMI reaction, the complete mechanism of cell mediated immunity proceeds in three phases.

(a) Binding of the cytotoxic cells to the target cells (b) Release of cytokines (c) Lysis of the target cell.

(a) Binding of the cytotoxic cells to the target cells: Close binding of the cytotoxic cells with the target cells is essential to execute the action of lysis. The cytotoxic cells bind to the target either through antibody or MHC class I molecules or by the receptors.

(b) Release of cytokines: Following binding with the target cells, the cytotoxic cells release their secretions. The secretions (cytokines) contain perforin and other enzymes that can cause apoptosis like reactions in target cells.

(c) Lysis of the target cell: The perforin enzyme present in released cytokines binds to the cell in the presence of Ca+, and develops trans membrane channels (pores). The remaining cytotoxic products pass through the pores and cause fragmentation of nucleus, followed by disintegration of cell in to small membrane bound vesicles. TNFα of released cytokines play an important role in killing tumor cells. It acts via receptors and the susceptible cell dies after 3 - 4 hours. Subsequent to killing the target cell, the cytotoxic cell remains active and continues its lytic activity to kill some more target cells. They protect themselves from the action of released lytic enzymes by means of *proteoglycan* present in them. It prevents pore forming activity of released lytic enzymes.

Role of Macrophages in CMI: Since microbicidal activity is one of the properties of macrophages, they provide rapid protection prior to T and B cell mediated activities, but their activity is non specific and multidirectional. In addition to CMI they take part in initiation of T cell activity by processing and presenting the engulfed antigen to T_H cells. Macrophages and their products are important not only for immune response and inflammation but also for repair of damaged tissues.

Pathology related with CMI: Cell mediated immunity is intended to protect the body from the invading pathogens but under certain circumstances the protective action or hyper action of CMI results in pathological conditions. For example excessive release of cytokines particularly TNFα can lead to shock syndromes, hemorrhagic necrosis and necrosis within the sites of cell mediated response. The developed pathology during the CMI action may obstruct the function of the near by tissue. Some times it may lead to fatal action for instance granuloma developed adjacent to the nerve cells may block nerve function. If granuloma develops in brain or retina it may result in certain functional abnormalities. Autoimmune diseases such as rheumatoid arthritis, psoriasis, multiple sclerosis etc. are due to chronic tissue damage caused by CMI.

DEFICIENCY OF "T CELLS": Since cell-mediated immunity is mediated by T-lymphocytes (T-cells) and their effector response and interactions with other immune cells, any defect in T cells production results in impaired protection to viral and other intracellular parasitic pathogens. The reason for deficiency may be inherited or due to abnormality in thymus functions. Even though B cell levels are normal, T cell deficiency cause impaired immune response.

Even though rare, several inherited T-cell disorders such as Ataxia telangiectasia, Chronic mucocutaneous candidiasis, DiGeorge syndrome, Severe combined immunodeficiency (SCID), Wiskott-Aldrich syndrome (WAS), Adenosine deaminase deficiency and Purine nucleoside phosphorylase deficiency have been identified.

TREATMENT: In severe inherited T-cell defects, such as severe combined immunodeficiency, bone marrow or stem cell transplantation or gene therapy may help in protecting the patient. If the defect is owing to functional defects of thymus, possible treatment is neither transplantation of thymic epithelial cells, or thymic hormone replacement to boost T cell production.

5

B LYMPHOCYTES

Bruce Glick's experiments on chicks specify that, lymphocytes derived from bursa of fabricus are responsible for humoral immunity. The cells derived from bursa are referred as "B Lymphocytes" to specify the region of their development. Since bursa is absent in mammals and other vertebrates bursa equivalent regions involved in B lymphocytes production are identified in bone marrow. Rabbits are an exception; their B cells develop in the appendix-sacculus rotundus. Generation of B cells starts from the embryo stage and continues through out life. In early stages of embryo development B cells production takes place in yolk sack and liver. In later stages bone marrow starts the production of B cells and continues through out the life.

Development of B cells: Development of B cells occur in several stages, each stage represents some rearrangement in the genome content at the antibody loci, to produce unique immunoglobulins from each individual B cell and the change is known as 'class switch' on the whole, differentiation of B cells can be studied in two segments, one is antigen independent and the other is antigen dependent.

(1) Antigen independent development of B cells: The haematopoietic stem cells of bone marrow first differentiate into "Progenitor B cells" or "Pro B cells" and the progenitor B cells with transmembrane tyrosine phosphate (CD 45R marker) move to bursa or bursa equivalent areas of bone marrow and multiply to increase their number. The stromal cells of bone marrow provide suitable environment for the differentiation of pro B cells into "Precursor B cells (pre-B cells)". The interaction of stromal cells and their secretions with C kit receptors of pro-B cells play a crucial role in initiation of differentiation process. The differentiated pro B cells start expressing IL-7 receptors (interleukin-7) on their surface. The interleukin-7 (IL-7) secreted by surrounding stromal cells enhances maturation process and detachment of matured B cells from the surrounding cells. By the time of their release, each B cell carry membrane bound immunoglobulins with unique binding sites or paratopes. Rearrangement and random recombination in immunoglobulin or antibody gene, during maturation of B cells is responsible for the production of immunoglobulins with unique binding site or paratopes from each B cell of a group (Refer genetical basis of immunoglobulin diversity for further details).

The initial rearrangements that occur in the genome of the antibody loci are designed to produce a functional Ig heavy chain. Once a progenitor B cell has made a productive rearrangement for μ heavy chain (IgM is the first immunoglobulin to be produced by B cells) they synthesize the heavy chain and retains it in the cytoplasm. The pre B cells with diffuse heavy chains of IgM immunoglobulin class are large in size. The cytoplasmic μ heavy chain later joins with "surrogate light chain" to become expressed at the surface as the "pre-B receptor. Surrogate light chains resemble actual light chains but are alike on every pre-B cell. When Pre-B cells express membrane μ heavy chains with surrogate light chains they divide rapidly and are referred as "Lymphoblast cells".

Lymphoblast cells then cease dividing and become small resting pre-B cells, at which point they cease expression of the surrogate light chains and express the heavy chain alone in the cytoplasm. When the cells become small again, they start to rearrange the light-chain (L-chain) genes. If a productive light chain rearrangement is made, it is expressed with μ heavy chains on the surface of the cell. The cell with surface bound immunoglobulin loose BCR, CD25 markers of pre B cells and are called as "immature B cell". Immature B cells produce a δ heavy chain in addition to μ heavy chain, by a mechanism of alternative mRNA splicing, and express on their surface along with IgM. The B cells with immunoglobulins that can bind with self antigens die before reaching the secondary lymphoid organs through negative selection. It is estimated that about 80-90 per cent of the B cells produced by the bone marrow die before they enter in to the circulation. B cells that acquired membrane bound IgM and IgD leave the bone marrow and pass to secondary lymphoid organs via blood. Rearrangement in genetic material of immunoglobulins during maturation process helps in the expression of immunoglobulins that can suit the limitless array of antigens.

Alternative splicing (or differential splicing) is a process by which the exons of the RNA produced by transcription of a gene (a primary gene transcript or pre-mRNA) are reconnected in multiple ways during RNA splicing. The resulting different mRNAs may be translated into different protein isoforms; thus, a single gene may code for multiple proteins.

The surface markers of B cells also changes along with the genetical changes of the developing B cells. The pro B cells express C kit receptor, CD45R, CD19, CD 43, and CD24 markers on the surface to support their differentiation activity. During metamorphosis from pro B to pre B cells, C kit & CD43 receptors disappear with the gradual development of new CD25, 1L-2 and pre BCR receptors. The pre B cells become immature B cells by loosing pre BCR, CD25 markers and express surface immunoglobulin IgM. The immature B cells become mature B cells by the addition of IgD immunoglobulin on their surface.

(2) Antigen dependent B cell development: Mature and immuno competent B cells in secondary lymphoid organs prior to antigenic interaction are referred as "naïve B lymphocytes" and they are in G_0 of their cell cycle. Since the membrane bound immunoglobulin in each B cell is unique in its binding site (paratope) interactions of naïve B lymphocytes with appropriate antigens result in differentiation and proliferation of B cells to produce clones of antibody synthesizing plasma cells and memory cells. Plasma cells secrete different immunoglobulin isotypes, through class switching in Ab gene loci (See genetical basis of immunoglobulin diversity for clarification). In the absence of antigen interaction naive B cells die within a few days (about 3-8 days) through apoptosis. The antigens giving stimulation to B cells may be thymus dependent or thymus independent. The response to thymus independent antigen is generally weak and results in the production of IgM type of antibodies without forming any memory cells. Thymus dependent antigens are responsible for humoral immunity.

C-kit receptor or cytokine kit receptor or CD117 is also called KIT, is a cytokine receptor expressed on the surface of hematopoietic stem cells as well as other cell types. This receptor binds to stem cell factor (a substance that causes certain types of cells to grow). Altered forms of this receptor may be associated with certain cancer cells.

CD45 is also called "common leukocyte antigen". It is a protein tyrosine phosphatase (PTP) located in hematopoietic cells except erythrocytes and platelets. Protein tyrosine kinases constitute a family of receptors and enzymes that catalyze the dephosphorylation of phosphor tyrosine residues. It has several isoforms and the hematopoietic cells express one or more of the isoforms. The specified expression of the CD45 isoforms can be seen in various stages of differentiation of normal haematopoietic cells; some isoforms of CD45 are CD45RO, CD45RA, and CD45RB.

B cell activation by "T - independent" antigens:-

The thymus independent antigens (TI Ags) are of two types Type I and Type II.

(a) Type I : Type I thymus independent antigens act as mitogens (an agent that triggers mitosis). Some lipopolysaccharides of bacterial cell wall show mitogenic property and act as polyclonal B cell activators regardless of antigenic specificity. They can activate both mature and immature B cells. Since their activity is independent of T cells, they were considered as true T cell independent antigens. T cell independent antigens are usually polymorphic with repeated identical epitopes. They can stimulate B cells directly by cross linking with surface immunoglobulins. Antibodies produced as a result of interaction of Type I antigens and B cells are generally of IgM type, these antibodies show low affinity due to a little class switching. Generally Type I antigens induce weaker or no memory cells. The interaction of antigen with B cell surface immunoglobulin receptors induces a cascade of reactions in cell membrane, nucleus and cytoplasm. The cell membrane undergoes depolarization leading to the entry of Ca^{+} from extra cellular environment to initiate membrane associated pathways to form secondary messenger substances, such as inositol triphosphate (ITP), diacyl glycerol (DAS) and cyclic GMP (cGMP). The secondary messenger substances activate protein kinases that promote the division of activated B cells. During this stage the B cells express several receptors such as receptors for interleukins (IL's), Fc receptors, CD19, CD21, CD22, CD23, B cell growth factor receptors (BCGF's), receptor for B cell differentiation factor (BCDF's) etc. to respond to several cytokines. The binding of cytokines to their respective receptors of B cells help in regulation of activity in B cells, to match with the requirement of the immune system. Even through T cell independent antigens activity suggests their independence of T cells, certain T cells concretions are essential for proper functioning of B cells. In the absence of B cell growth factors (BCGFS) released by T cells, B cells continue to repeat multiplication only. BCGF binding to B cells is necessary to produce antibody secreting plasma cells.

(b) TYPE -2 : Unlike type I thymus independent antigens they are not B cell mitogens. They activate only mature B cells and depend on cytokines derived from T_H cells for competent B cell explosion and class switching to isotopes such as IgG, IgA and IgE.

B cell activation by T dependent antigens: Most of the antigens that stimulate humoral immunity are T dependent. Antigens presenting cells and T cells are essential forT dependent antigens to activate B cells. Antigen presenting cells engulf and process the antigen to presents it in a suitable form for activation of T cells. The processed antigens are presented to the naïve T cells through MHC class II and co stimulatory molecule B7.

The T_H cells on interaction with antigen secret different lymphokines that induce activation, differentiation and proliferation of naïve B cells. Differentiation and proliferation of B cells leads to the production of a colony that can secrete antibodies for the antigen responsible for its activation. Some of the cells from the colony become short lived plasma cells that in turn secrete antigen specific antibodies/immunoglobulin and the remaining become memory cells with long life span for future defense against the same antigens.

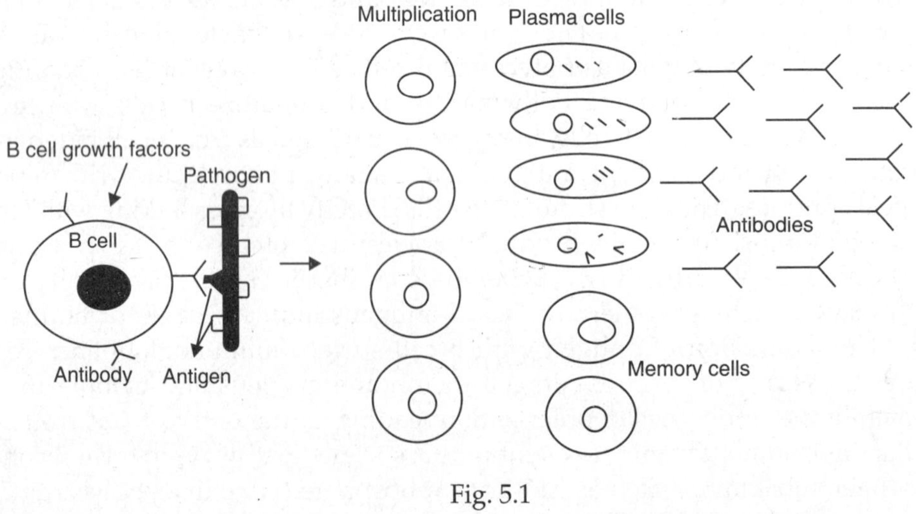

Fig. 5.1

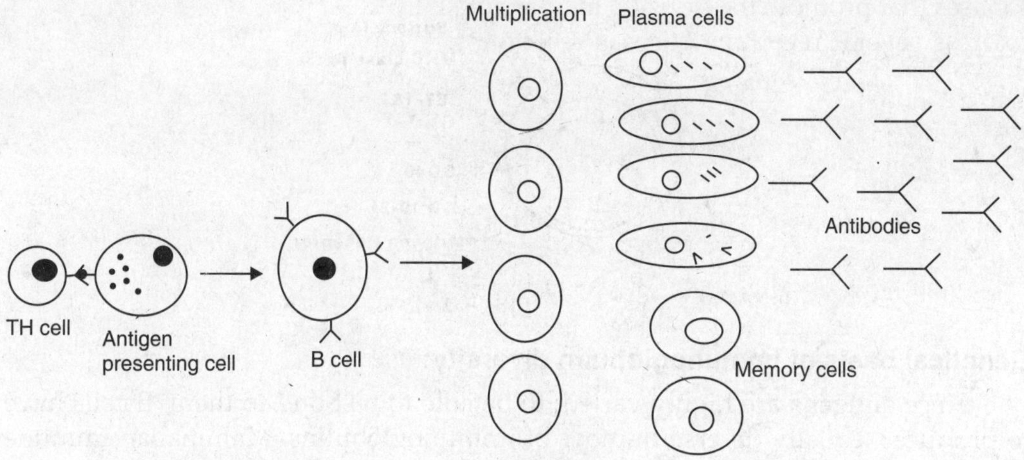

Fig. 5.2

Hematopoietic stem cell

↓ Bursa/Bursa equivalent region

Pro B cells with CD 45R marker

↓ Interleukin-7

Procursor B cells

↓ Genomic rearrangements

Large Pre B cells with cytoplasmic μ heavy chain

↓ Sur rogate light chain

Lymphoblast cells with surface m chain

↓ Multiplication

Small resting pre-B cells

↓ Lose of BCR, CD25 markers

Immature B cell

↓ Addition of IgD on their surface

Mature B cells with surface IgM, IgD

↓ Secondary lymphoid organs

B lymphocytes (G0 phase of their cell cycle)

↓ Ag interaction

Differentiation and proliferation

↓

Plasma cells + Memory cells

Fig. 5.3. Differentiation of B cells

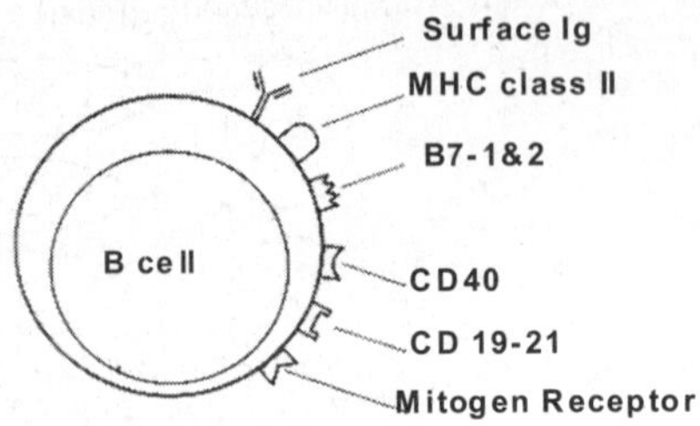

Fig. 5.4

Genetical basis of immunoglobulin diversity:

Since antigens are highly varied, to be able to respond to them, B cells have to produce equally diverse number of immunoglobulins. Mammalian immune system has evolved unique genetic mechanisms that enable it to generate an almost unlimited number of Immunoglobulins and there will be an antigen-binding site to fit almost any potential antigenic determinant, even though with low affinity. The genes encoding immunoglobulins are composed of multiple gene segments, which are cut-and-pasted together in each B cell to form a functional Ig gene through a process called V(D)J recombination, or gene rearrangement.

The light and heavy chains of imunoglobulins are encoded by separate multigene families situated on different chromosomes. Each of the multigene family contains a series of coding sequences called gene segments. The gene segments in light-chain family are L (leader), V (Variable), J (Junctional), and C (Constant). The gene segments of the heavy-chain family contain the same families and an additional group called the D (Diversity) region. In non-lymphocytes, which do not undergo rearrangement, the gene segments are clustered in 2 or 3 groups. For example, at the Ig heavy chain locus, there is a cluster of about 50 V gene segments, a second cluster of 27 D gene segments, and third cluster of 6 J segments. During B cell development, a random gene segments from each cluster is joined to form a continuous V-D-J gene. Each V gene segment is separated from the next by a noncoding sequence called an intron. Each gene segment (V, D, and J) has an adjacent Recombination Signal Sequence (RSS). These are recognized by two proteins encoded by two Recombination Activating Genes RAG-1 and RAG-2. The RAG1 and RAG2 proteins cut through both strands of DNA at the RSS forming double-stranded breaks (DSBs). The regular machinery for repairing double-stranded breaks (by nonhomologous end-joining) then swings into action. The cut ends are stitched together (ligated) to form:

1. A coding joint (D-J or V-DJ for heavy chains; V-J for light chains)

2. A signal joint (usually a loop of DNA deleting all the intervening DNA initially presents between the 2 gene segments chosen).

D-J joining occurs first then the combined DJ segment is joined to a V segment (as shown in the figure).

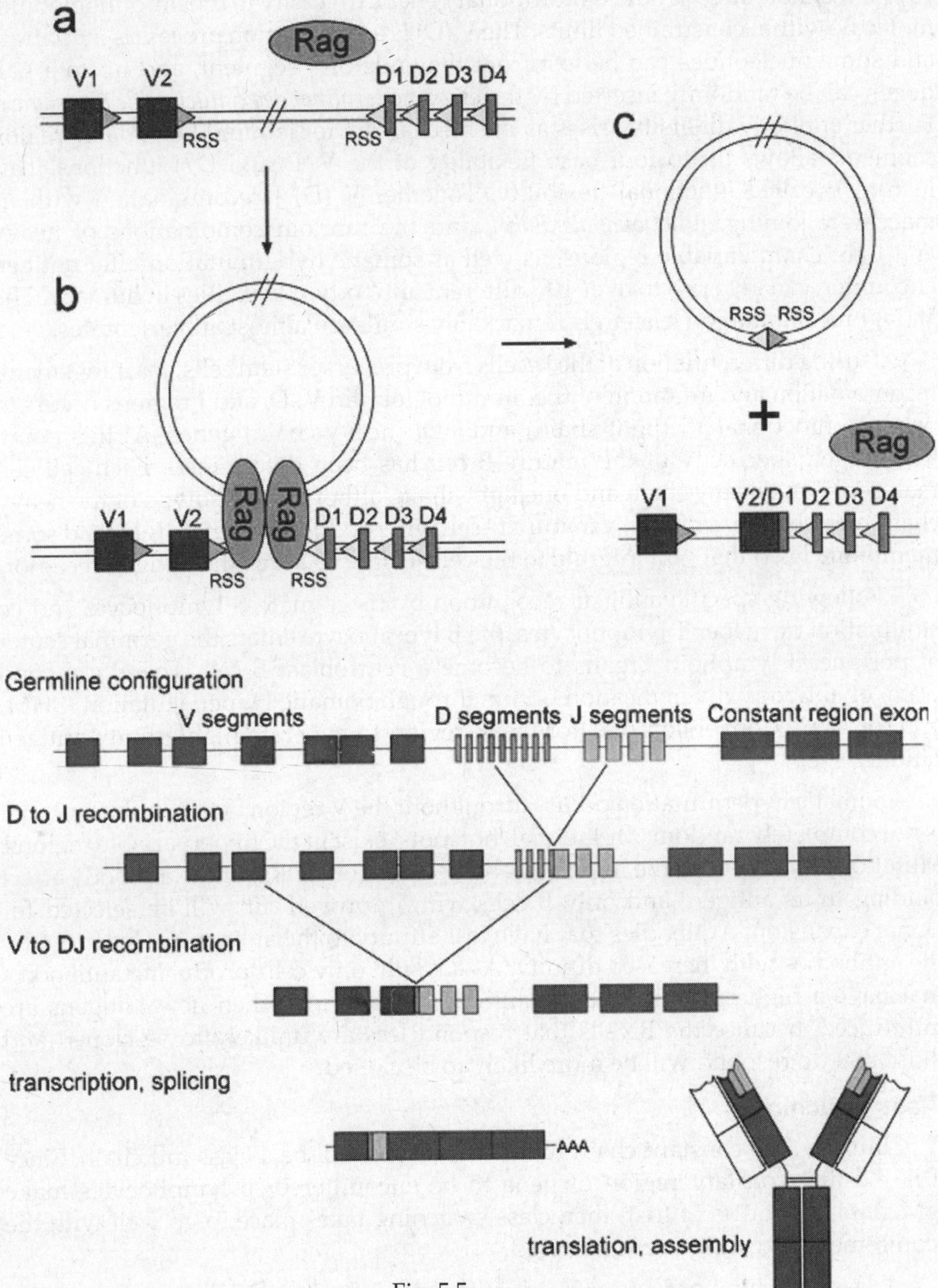

Fig. 5.5

Random assortment of multigene family segments in this way makes the largest contribution to the diversity of antibodies.

Normal genetic recombination is very accurate, but a special design in the V (D)

J system deliberately produces additional genetic diversity in the immunoglobulin molecule within constrained limits. The V (D) J recombination process is inaccurate and some nucleotides can be lost from the ends of a segment, and up to a half dozen can be randomly inserted by the enzyme *terminal deoxynucleotide transferase*. Further antibody diversity arises as the mechanism for joining the variable region segments allows up to four-base flexibility at the V/D and D/J junctions. This feature is called junctional flexibility. Together V (D) J recombination with its inaccurate joining, *junctional flexibility* and the random combinations of heavy and light chain variable regions, as well as somatic hypermutation after antigen encounter, can give rise to over 10^{11} different antibody specificities in humans. The V (D) J recombination system is remarkably similar in almost all vertebrates.

During differentiation of the B-cells from precursor stem cells, rearrangement, recombination and mutation of the immunoglobulin V, D, and J regions occurs to produce functional VJ (light chain) and VDJ (heavy chain) genes. At this point, the antigen specificity of the mature B-cell has been determined. Each cell can make only one heavy chain and one light chain, although the isotype of the heavy chain may change. Initially, a mature B-cell will produce primarily IgD (and some membrane IgM) that will migrate to the cell surface to act as the antigen receptor.

Following specific antigen recognition by its cognate B lymphocyte and co stimulation by helper T lymphocytes, the B lymphocyte enters the germinal center of peripheral lymphoid organs to become a centroblast B cell. There, a second wave of antibody diversification occurs through Somatic Hyper Mutation (SHM) and/or Gene Conversion (GC) of the V region to generate high-affinity antigen binding site.

Somatic hypermutation occurs throughout the V region of the antibody, but it is not completely random. Mutational 'hotspots' exist in the hypervariable regions. Mutations that occur in the hypervariable regions (or CDRs) of the antibody affect binding to its antigen, and only B cells with improved 'fit' will be selected for clonal expansion. Antibodies that have lost affinity to the antigen are balanced by the antibodies with increased affinity. As a result, only cells producing antibodies that have a higher affinity for the antigen are selected when new antigens are introduced, because the B cells that respond less are unlikely to be cloned and those that do respond will be more likely to be cloned.

Class switching:

Initially, the constant chain that is expressed will be a class mu chain. Since μ is the first constant region of gene to be encountered, B lymphocytes make IgM class antibodies at first, then class switching takes place to go well with the requirement and antigen encountered.

Class switching or Isotype production is a biological process occurring after activation of the B cell. This mechanism allows the cell to produce different classes of antibodies (IgA, IgE, or IgG). The different classes of antibodies, and their effector functions, are defined by the constant (C) regions of the immunoglobulin heavy chain. Each isotype is adapted for a distinct function, therefore, after activation, an antibody with IgG, IgA, or IgE effector function might be required to effectively eliminate an antigen. Class switching allows different daughter cells from the same activated B cell to produce antibodies of different isotypes. Only the constant region of the antibody heavy chain changes during class switching. The variable regions, and therefore antigen specificity, remain unchanged. Thus the progeny of a single B cell can produce antibodies, all specific for the same antigen, but with the ability to produce the effector function appropriate for each antigenic challenge. Class switching is triggered by cytokines; hence the isotype generated depends on the cytokines present in the B cell environment.

Class switching occurs in the heavy chain gene locus by a mechanism called class switch recombination (CSR). This mechanism relies on conserved nucleotide motifs, called switch (S) regions, found in DNA upstream of each constant region gene (except in the δ-chain). The DNA strand as shown in the figure is broken by the activity of a series of enzymes at two selected S-regions. The variable domain exon is rejoined through a process called non-homologous end joining NHEJ) to the desired constant region (γ, α or ε). This process results in an immunoglobulin gene that encodes an antibody of a different isotype.

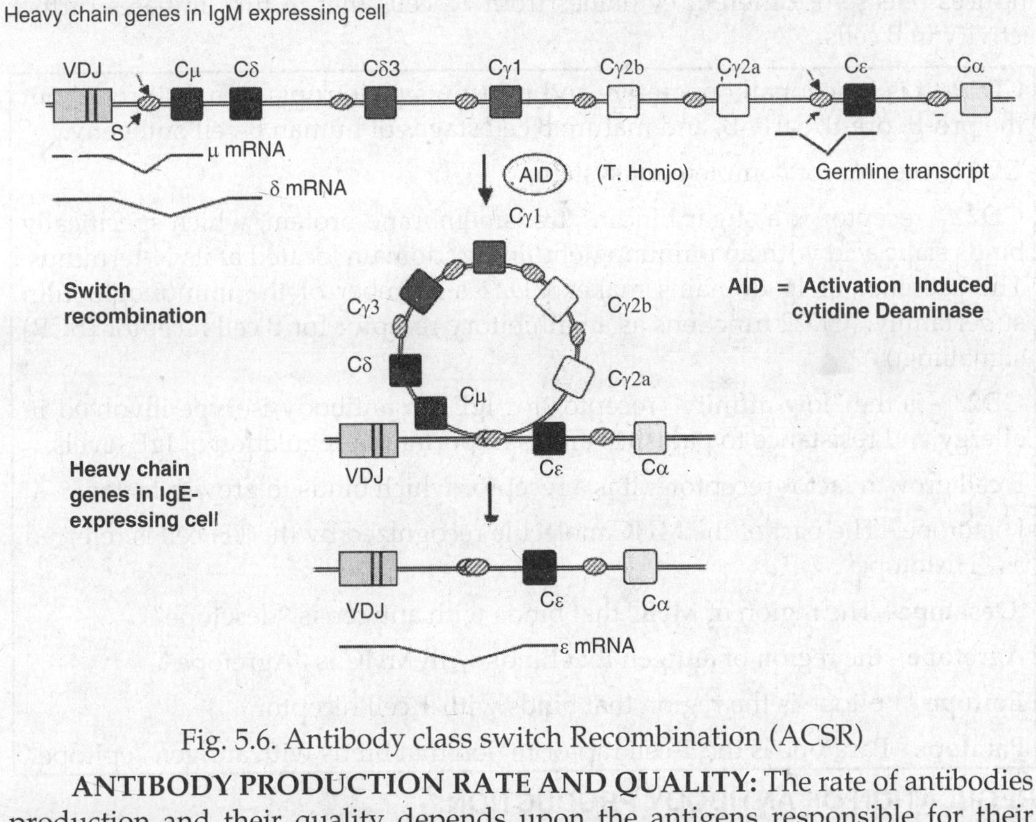

Fig. 5.6. Antibody class switch Recombination (ACSR)

ANTIBODY PRODUCTION RATE AND QUALITY: The rate of antibodies production and their quality depends upon the antigens responsible for their production. High concentration of new antigens initiates early differentiation and proliferation of B cells. When the concentration of antigens is low, the B cells differentiation is also fairly low but the antibodies produced by the plasma cells show high affinity towards their antigens. The time availability in the differentiation process might allow the proper rearrangement of genes responsible for the production of variable domains to generate high affinity (highly specific) binding regions in antibodies.

ROLE OF TH CELLS IN B CELL ACTIVATION AND FUNCTION: Even though certain T cell independent antigens are capable of activating B cells, without T cells cooperation B cells cannot induce an effective and competent response. B and T_H cells interaction is essential for proper activation and optimal function of B cells. Binding of antigen with surface immunoglobulin of mature B cells initiates changes in membrane bound class II MHC molecules, and B_7 molecules, that start appearing in large number to have better chances of T_H cell interaction. Through MHC class II molecules, B cells present the processed antigen peptide to T_H cells, like an antigen presenting cell. The surface B_7 molecule supports the reactions. Generally antigen presentation through B cells occurs when antigen concentration is low and the macrophages, dendrite cells fail to catch and present them to T_H cells. Exposure of antigenic peptide over MHC class II molecules of B cells initiates T_H cells interaction with B cells through them. The T_H cells interaction with B cells induces release of different cytokines from T_H cells that in turn initiates further activity in B cells.

CD19- It is functionally operative and transmits pleiotropic signals throughout the pro-B, pre-B, early B, and mature B cell stages of human B-cell ontogeny.

CD21-receptor for complement system,

CD22 - receptor is a sugar binding transmembrane protein, which specifically binds sialic acid with an immunoglobulin (Ig) domain located at its N-terminus. The presence of Ig domains makes CD22 a member of the immunoglobulin superfamily. (CD22 functions as an inhibitory receptor for B cell receptor (BCR) signalling.)

CD23 - is the "low affinity" receptor for IgE, an antibody isotype involved in allergy and resistance to parasites and is important in regulation of IgE levels.

B cell growth factor receptor – it is a receptor which binds to growth factor.

Histotope - The part of the MHC molecule recognized by the TH cell is referred as "Histotope".

Desetope - The region of MHC that binds with antigen is "desetope"

Agretope - the region of antigen that binds with MHC is "Agretope".

Epitope - Epitope is the region that binds with T cell receptor.

Paratope - Paratope is the T cell raptor region that binds with antigen "epitope"

REGULATION OF ANTIBODY PRODUCTION: -

In a biological system regulation of any activity is equally important to intiation of the action. In the same way regulation of antibody production is also important to keep the body in heathy and normal condition. Feedback mechanism, cross linking of receptors, and idiotypic net works are some of the mechanisms through which antibody production is regulated .

Feedback Mechanism: Activation of B cells by antigen leads to production of antibody specific for those antigens. Subsequently, the antibody produced binds to the antigen and reduces the concentration of that specific antigen. Eventually, antigens are completely removed and no further stimulation of the production of antibodies to that particular antigen occurs. As long as free antigens are present, stimulation to B cells continues to produce the antibodies.

Feedback Mechanism

Antigen → Activation of B cells → production of antibody → Antigen and antibody complex

Removal of antigen → No Antigen → No stimulation of B cells → No antibody production

Cross linking of receptors: Antibodies released in response to antigenic stimulation binds to their specific antigens and reduce the chances of antigen binding and further induction of antibody production without affecting immunological response to other antigens. This suppresses antibody production for that specific antigen. An antigen that is complexed with antibody has differential effects on immune responses. At low Ab/Ag ratios, suppression of antibody production can occur. Under these conditions, immune complexes can bind to both membrane bound Ig and FcRs of the B cells. This suppresses antibody production. In contrast, at high Ab/Ag ratios, immune responses can be stimulated. This occurs through binding to FcRs on APCs that leads to activation of T helper cells and subsequent enhancement of immune responses.

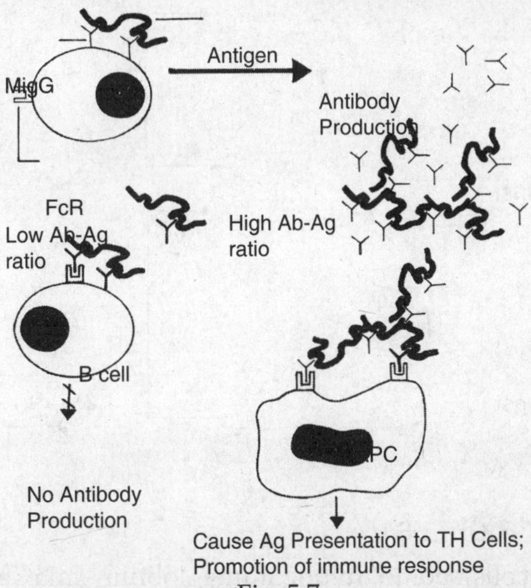

Fig. 5.7

Idiotypic net works: The antibodies produced (Ab -1) not only react with the antigen, but also serve as antigens for the immune system. This triggers the production of a second level of antibodies (Ab-2). The second level antibodies react with Ab-1 and induce production of antibodies (Ab -3). The process continues for several generations. The antibodies formed against the Ab formed by the immune system it self s are known as idiotype antibodies. At each step, the concentration of antibodies available to provoke formation of idiotype antibodies is less than in the preceding step. As a result, a level is eventually reached at which there is insufficient antibodies to provide and antigenic signal.

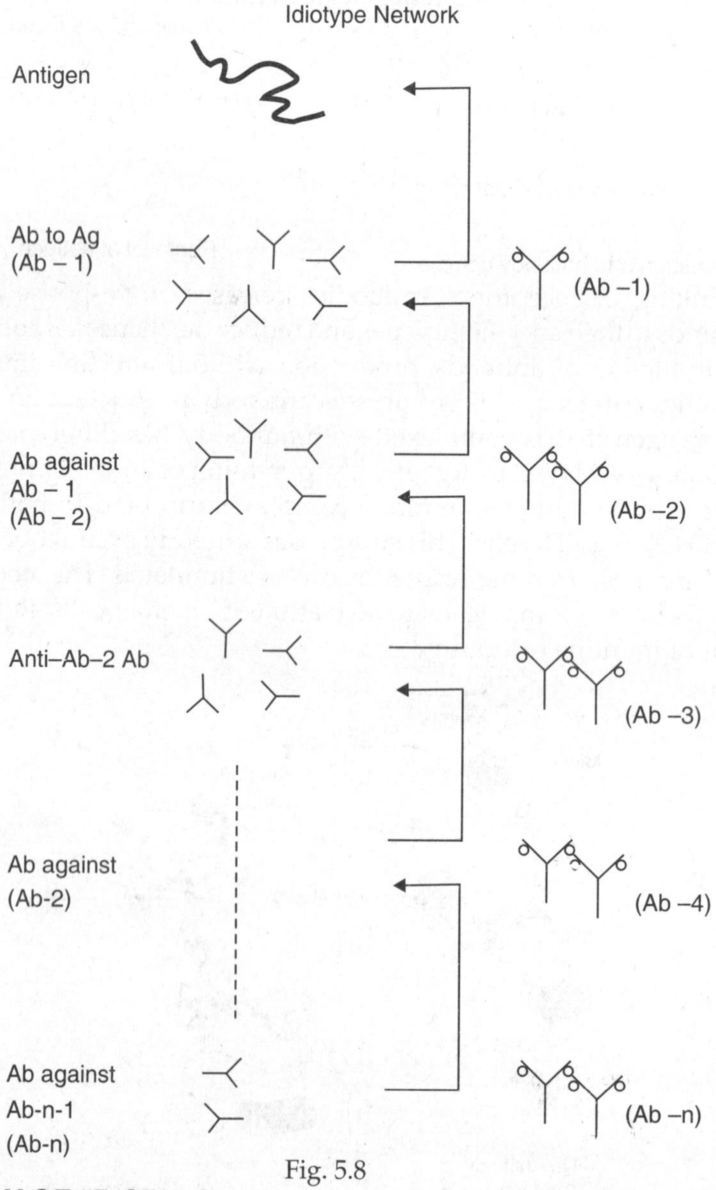

Fig. 5.8

DEFICIENCY OF "B CELLS":

DeficiencyofBcellsleadsto"hypogammaglobulinemia",agammaglobulinemia etc. diseases associated with antibody deficiency. Generally immune system in children starts producing antibodies by the time the maternal immunoglobulins acquired through placenta and breast milk exhausts. But some children fail to produce antibodies due to deficiency of B cells.

Since all antibodies are secreted by B-lymphocytes (B-cells), any disease that harms the development or function of B-cells reflects in the production of immunoglobulins. Even though immunesystem is functional, people with immunoglobulin deficiency syndromes become ill more often, because most of the invading microbes for example *streptococci, meningococci, and Haemophilus influenzae* escape attack by immune cells through encapsulation. Since immunoglobulins are capable of binding to the encapsulate microbes, their survival becomes difficult in people with normal immunoglobulin production. This kind of protection is lost in people with B cell deficiency. Patients with immunoglobulin deficiencies may also show a bad response to the attenuated version of the polio virus vaccine. They are also prone to some viral infections, including echovirus, enterovirus, and hepatitis B.

Two types of immunodeficiency diseases (1) Primary congenital and (2) secondary acquired immunodeficiency are found associated with B cells deficiency.

Primary congenital: Congenital immunodeficiency is present at the time of birth, and is the result of genetic defects. Even though more than 70 different types of congenital immunodeficiency disorders have been identified, they rarely occur. Congenital immunodeficiencies may occur as a result of defects in B lymphocytes, T lymphocytes, or both. But primary congenital immunoglobulin deficiency syndromes are the most prevalent type of immunodeficiency disorders occurring due to defective B-cells or antibodies. They account for 50% of all primary immune deficiencies. Following are some of the examples for congenital immunodeficiency disorders.

(1) Bruton's agammaglobulinemia, also known as X-linked agammaglobulinemia is an inherited disease. The defect is associated with the X chromosome; as a result this disease is seen more frequently in males than females. The defect results in a failure of B-cells to mature and secrete immunoglobulins.

(2) Selective IgA deficiency is an inherited disease that occurs 1 in 700 of population. It is due to failure of B-cells to switch from making IgM, the early antibody, to IgA. Although the number of B-cells is normal, and can make all other classes of antibodies, the amount of IgA produced is limited. This results in more infections of mucosal surfaces, such as nose, throat, lungs, and intestines. Since this deficiency is asymptomatic, it can be identified only by chance.

(3) Ig heavy chain deletion is a genetic disorder in which, part of the antibody molecule is not produced. It results in the loss of several antibody classes and subclasses including most IgG antibodies and all IgA and IgE anti-bodies.

(4) Selective IgG subclasses deficiency is a group of genetic disease. Due to defects in B cell maturation, the process of class switching fails to take place in Ab gene, ensuing failure in the mechanism to produce some of the subclasses of IgG.

(5) IgG deficiency with hyper-IgM is a disease that results when the B-cell fails to switch from IgM making to IgG. This disease is the result of a genetic mutation.

Secondary acquired disorders: Secondary acquired disorders occur in normally healthy individuals due to certain under lying diseases including HIV infection or failure to thrive. But it often occurs as a complication of other conditions and diseases. For example, the most common causes of acquired immunodeficiency are malnutrition, some types of cancer, and infections. Once the disease is treated, the immunodeficiency is reversed. For example

(1) Transient hypo gamma globulenemia of infancy is a temporary disease of unknown cause. Hypogammaglobulinemia is characterized by low levels of gamma globulins (antibodies) in the blood. During the disease period, patients have decreased levels of IgG and IgA antibodies.

(2) Common Variable Immunodeficiency (CVI) can develop at any age of an individual. The underlying cause for CVI is not known, but it is clear that there is a defect in the T cell – B cell cooperation that is needed for B cells to differentiate into plasma cells. This results in very low levels of antibody in the circulation but a normal B cell count. The imbalance of T cell and B cell function can result in a loss of self tolerance ensuing autoimmune disease.

CONSEQUENCE OF IMMUNOGLOBULIN DEFICIENCIES:

Complications of antibody deficiency include acute infections, due to unusual organisms such as mycoplasmas, and long term complications such as bronchiectasis, fungal infections, granulomas, lymphoma, recurrent sinusitis, giardia, cryptosporidia, colitis, gastric carcinoma, hepatitis, autoimmune haemolytic anaemia, immune thrombocytopenic purpura, acute enteroviral meningoencephalitis etc.

INVESTIGATIONS REQUIRED

1. Serum immunoglobulin concentrations, including IgG subclasses.
2. When serum immunoglobulin concentrations are greatly depressed, confirmatory tests are not always necessary.
3. Functional antibody responses to immunisations, common bacteria and red cell antigens may be required.
4. Plasma B lymphocyte sub-populations concerned with antibody production.

TREATMENT

1. Prompt antibiotic treatment, constant prophylaxis.
2. Regular supply of immunoglobulins intravenously.
3. Subcutaneous immunoglobulin supply is an alternative to intravenous administration.
4. Higher doses may be needed in patients with known lung damage.
5. Side effects (which include headache, nausea, chills, and fever) can be reduced by lowering the rate of infusion.

6

IMMUNOGLOBULINS

A group of glycoprotein molecules present in serum and body fluids of vertebrates are referred as immunoglobulins or Igs in short due to their involvement in immunological reactions and globular structure. Immunoglobulins constitute about 20% of total plasma proteins and are responsible for humoral immunity. The plasma cells derived from activated B cells produce immunoglobulins to interact with foreign antigens. When an immunoglobulin binds with an antigen it is referred as antibody. Even though all immunoglobulins are glycoproteins, all glycoproteins are not immunoglobulins. In a biological system glycoproteins perform various functions. Cells use immunoglobulins (Ig) as multifunctional tools, to mediate interaction of antigens with effectors of cell mediated and humoral immunity.

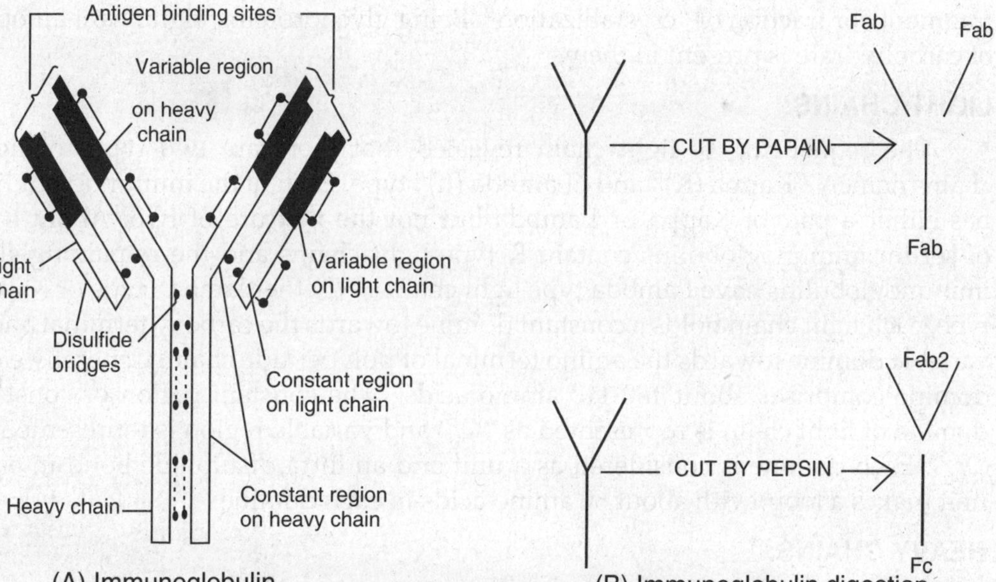

(A) Immunoglobulin (B) Immunoglobulin digestion

Fig. 6.1 Immunoglobulin

FUNDAMENTAL STRUCTURE OF IMMUNOGLOBULIN:

Experiments conducted by Rodney Porter and Gerold Edleman between

1950 to 1960 revealed the structure of immunoglobulin and both the scientists shared Nobel prize in 1972 for their efforts. Their experiment revealed that the immunoglobulins are made up of two identical pairs of polypeptides chains as shown in the figure, one pair is short and the other pair is long. Based on the molecular weights, the polypeptide chains of short pair are referred as "light (L) chains" and the polypeptide chains of long pair are referred as "Heavy (H) chains" Light chains are composed of 220 amino acid residues, while heavy chains are composed of 440-550 amino acids. Both the chains contain several homologous units the "domines" with 110 amino acid residues. An intra chain disulphide bond in each domine forms a loop of about 60 amino acids. The amino acid sequences in domines towards the carboxyl end are constant and are known as "constant domines". But the amino acid sequences are not constant in the domine present near to the amino (NH_2) terminal of polypeptide chain and are known as "variable domines". The four polypeptide chains are held together by covalent disulfide (-S-S-) bonds and the immunoglobulin molecule gets Y or T shape. At the junction of the Y or T shaped structure a flexible region known as "hinge region" is present to facilitate the function of immunoglobulin. As shown in the figure, the two arms from the hinge region with variable domains are capable of binding with antigens hence they are referred as "Fraction of antigen binding" regions or "Fab" regions in short. The other region that is joined to the two arms of Y or T structure does not possess antigen binding capacity. The immunoglobulin, on brief treatment with lytic enzymes, such as papain and pepsin generates two or three pieces, with or without Fab regions. The single piece without Fab region under goes crystallization during cold storage. Hence this part is referred as "Fc fragment" or fraction of "crystallization". Being glycoproteins, significant amount of carbohydrate is present in them.

LIGHT CHAINS:

The sequencing of light chain revealed that there are two types of light chains namely "Kappa (K)" and "Lambda (L)" type. Each of the immunoglobulins has either a pair of Kappa or Lambda but not the mixture of two. About 60% of serum immunoglobulins contain K type light chains and the remaining 40% immunoglobulins have Lambda type light chains. Whether lambda type or Kappa type, each light chain holds a constant domine towards the carboxy terminal and a variable domine towards the amino terminal of polypeptide chain. Generally each domine comprises about 100-110 amino acids. The constant region or constant domine of light chain is represented as "C_L" and variable region is represented as "V_L". Each domine is considered as a unit and an intra disulphide bond in each unit makes a loop, with about 60 amino acids in each domine.

HEAVY CHAINS:

Analysis of heavy chain sequence shows presence of three or four constant domines towards carboxy terminal and a single variable domine towards amino terminal regions of polypeptide chains. Like that of light polypeptide chain, each domine contain an intra disulphide bond. The constant domines are referred as CH_1, CH_2, CH_3 etc. and the variable domine is referred as VH domine. Each variable domine enclose about four hyper variable sites or hotspots. The hyper variable sites are also known as complementarity determining regions (CDRS). The constant domines participate in various biological functions in accordance with the amino acid sequence. The CH1 constant domine next to the variable domine serve to extend and bend the variable domine in various angles to interact with antigens. There are five types of heavy chains, designated by Greek letters namely α (alpha), δ (delta), ε (epsilon), δ (gamma) and μ (mu). With reference to the type of heavy chain, immunoglobulins are referred as immunoglobulin A (IgA), immunoglobulin D (IgD) immunoglobulin E (IgE), immunoglobulin G (IgG) and immunoglobulin M (IgM) respectively.

HYPER VARIABLE REGIONS OR HOT SPOTS:

The amino acids sequence in certain regions of variable domines of both light and heavy chains are highly variable, and they are generally referred as hotspots or hyper variable regions. The light chain variable domine include three such hyper variable regions, they are between the positions of 24 to 34, 50 to 56 and 89 to 97 amino acid moieties. In heavy chains there are four such hyper variable regions between 1 to 23, 35 to 49, 57 to 88, 98 to107 amino acid moieties. The hyper variable regions brought together to form antigen binding site or the "paratope". The chemistry and shape of the paratope is complementary to the epitope of antigen, like the key of a lock. Since epitopes are highly variable in different antigens and even a single antigen processes variable epitopes at the same time, the hyper variability of variable domine in immunoglobulins helps in the production of suitable paratopes to bind with the antigens. As the paratope is very specific for each epitope, the variation in paratope region is responsible for the heterogeneity among the same type of immunoglobulins. For example immunoglobulin G produced in response to different antigens show variation in their variable regions or binding sites only. The immunoglobulin produced in response to a particular antigen will not bind with the other antigen due to mismatch of their paratope with epitope regions.

HINGE REGION:

Hinge region is an extend peptide sequence between CH_1 and CH_2 domines of heavy chain. It is rich in cysteine and proline amino acids, extremely variable in amino acid sequence, and has no resemblance to any other immunoglobulin region. It provides flexibility to the antigen binding part of immunoglobulin. Because of high proline content, hinge region is highly vulnerable to lytic enzymes such as papain and pepsin. The cystein residues in this region help in establishing the disulphide bond with opposite heavy chain. The number of disulphide bonds depends on the length of hinge region; generally they range from 1-13. Hinge region is absent in immunoglobulins of mu (μ) type and epsilon (ε) type. Instead of hinge they have additional constant domine that functions like that of a hinge region.

DISULPHIDE BONDS:

Disulfide bond is a single covalent bond derived from the coupling of thiol (SH) groups. In proteins they are formed between the thiol groups of cysteine residues. The linkage is also called as an "S-S-bond" or "disulfide bridge". Disulfide bonds play an important role in the folding and stability of some proteins usually secreted to the extra cellular medium. The disulfide bond stabilizes the folded form of a protein in several ways: 1) It holds two portions of the protein together, biasing the protein towards the folded topology. 2) The disulfide bond may form the nucleus of a hydrophobic core of the folded protein, i.e., local hydrophobic residues may condense around the disulfide bond and onto each other through hydrophobic interactions. Light and heavy chains of immunoglobulins join together by means of inter disulphide bonds in hinge region. The number of disulphide bonds in hinge depends upon the length of the hinge region. In addition to inter disulphide bonds, each domine of light and heavy chains contain an intra disulfide bond. The total number of these bonds depends upon the number of domains in the polypeptide chains of the immunoglobulin molecule. The cystein residues help in the formation of inter and intra disulphide bonds. Disulphide bonds present in different parts of immunoglobulins help in stabilization of the structure. Even in the absence of disulphide bonds, under appropriate conditions the heavy and light chain pairs associate spontaneously to form a biologically active immunoglobulin molecule.

CARBOHYDRATE MOIETY:

Virtually all immunoglobulins contain significant amounts of carbohydrate in CH_2 region. There is however, a considerable quantitative and qualitative variation, even among molecules from the same species and of the same class. The carbohydrate component of the immunoglobulin is an oligosaccharide with variable mono-saccharide units. It may include simple mannose rich units as in IgM or complex N- acetyl lactosamine rich units as in IgG. In IgG, the carbohydrate portion is about 2.5% of the total molecule and it is equally divided between the two gamma heavy chains. It is linked through amino acids, aspartic acid and threonine residues in the polypeptide chain. Mostly there will be no glycosylation in Fab fragments; therefore glycosylation generally has no effect on antigen binding property of antibody. It, however, does influence effector's function controlled by Fc fragment.

The biological role of the carbohydrate in immunoglobulins is yet unknown. It is postulated that it may play a role in the passage of immunoglobulins through biological membranes during their secretion from the cell or their passage through the placental barrier, and also in certain other biological functions of the immunoglobulins.

CLASIFICATION OF IMMUNOGLOBULIN:

The immunoglobulins can be divided into five different classes, based on differences in the amino acid sequences in the constant region of the heavy chains. The genetic variations or differences in the constant region determine the three-dimensional structure of the molecule. All immunoglobulins within a given class contain similar heavy chains. The classes of immunoglobulins can de divided into subclasses based on small differences in the amino acid sequences of constant regions in heavy chains. All immunoglobulins within a subclass have similar amino acid sequences in the constant regions of heavy chains. In placental mammals e.g. man there are nine classes that migrate in five different groups in electrophoresis; each one consist of two light and two heavy protein chains, and each group has distinguishing structural and functional properties .They are known as IgA (α-alpha), IgD (δ - delta), IgE (ε - epsilon), IgG (γ - gamma) and IgM (μ - mu). Immunoglobulin class switching can be used to change the class of the heavy chain, but not of the light chain.

TYPES OF IMMUNOGLOBULINS:

IMMUNOGLOBULIN "A" (IgA)

Immunoglobulin A type is the most important immunoglobulin fundamentally in mucosa immunity and lactation. They are predominantly seen in seromucosal secretions such as saliva, nasal fluids, sweat, colostrum, and cretin of respiratory, gastrointestinal, urinogenital tract etc., to act at different levels. They help in preventing the attachment of pathogens to the walls, and neutralizing the activity of some viruses, both inside and outside epithelium cells. Since they are resistant to degradation by enzymes, secretary IgA can survive in harsh environments such as the digestive and respiratory tracts, to provide protection against microbes that multiply in body secretions. They constitute about 10-15% of total immunoglobulins. The daily production of secretary IgA is greater than that of any other immunoglobulin class. Every day human mucosa produces 5 to 15gms of secretary IgAs. IgAs are poor activators of the complement system, and opsonises faintly.

In general IgA molecules are monomers in their basic structure with 8-10% of carbohydrate content. Each IgA monomer molecule encompass two identical heavy chains of alpha type and two identical light chains of kappa or lambda just as other immunoglobulins do. The molecular weight of IgA monomer is 1, 50,000 Daltons or 150 kD, sedimentation coefficient is 6.85, and half life is 6-8 days. Since IgA molecules express morphological diversity in different locations, the secretary IgA is much larger than serum IgA. Formation of dimmers during secretion through a J chain makes the secretary IgA molecules larger than the plasma IgAs (J chain is a cysteine rich polypeptide with a molecular mass of 15kD). Prior to secretion, IgA produced by plasma cells in the lamina propria (adjacent to mucosal surfaces) bound to poly Ig receptors present on the basolateral membranes of mucosal epithelial cells. IgAs bound to this receptor are internalized through receptor mediated endocytosis, the poly Ig receptors cleave from membrane and becomes secretary component to release in to the lumen as IgA polymer. The secretary component masks protease susceptible regions of hinge region to prevent cleavage of IgA molecules in protease rich mucosal environment. Since IgA molecules are helping in the protection of mucosal membrane, IgA immunoglobulins are referred as "antiseptic paint of mucosal membrane". IgA immunoglobulins secreted along with breast milk provide protection to the gastro intestinal tract of new born babies. Hence the health secret of breast fed babies is presence of IgA immunoglobulins in breast milk. In blood circulation IgA interacts with an Fc receptor called Fcα RI (or CD89) expressed on immune effector cells, to initiate inflammatory reactions. Ligation of Fc α RI by IgA containing immune complexes induces various immunological responses such as antibody-dependent cell-mediated cytotoxicity (ADCC), degranulation of eosinophils and basophils, phagocytosis by monocytes, macrophages, neutrophils and eosinophils etc.

Two sub classes of IgA molecules namely IgA1 and IgA2 exist in mammals. IgA2 is completely devoid of inter chain disulphide bonds and the four polypeptide chains are held together by non covalent linkages. IgA1 is found in serum and made by bone marrow B cells. IgA2 is made by B cells located in the mucosae and has been found to secrete into colostrum, breast milk, tears and saliva.

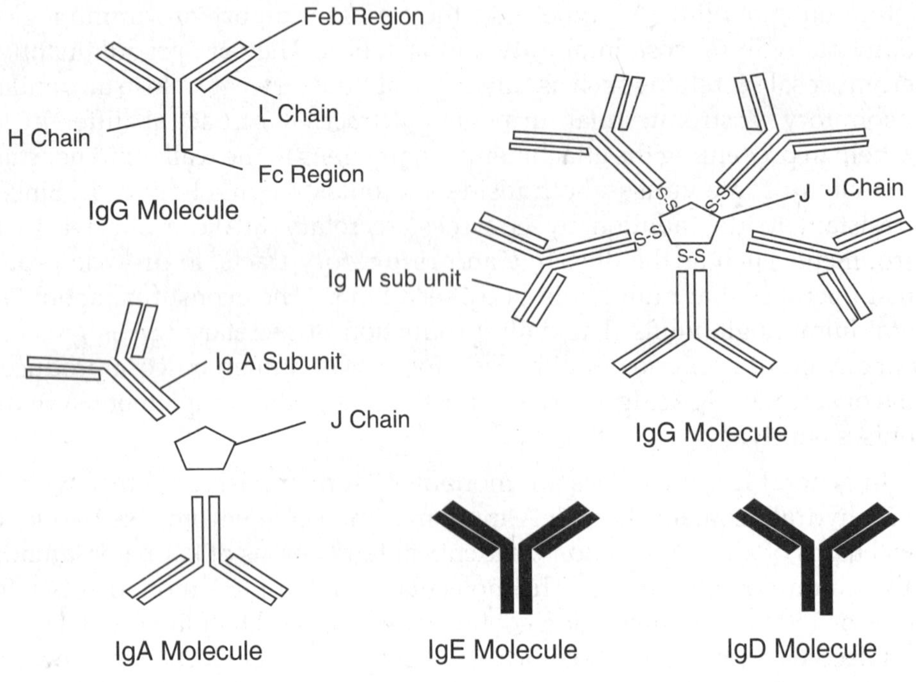

Fig. 6.2

IMMUNOGLOBULIN "G" (IgG)

IgG is the major and most abundant immunoglobulin type in normal human serum. It constitutes about 70-75% of the total immunoglobulins and is about 8-16 mg/ml in serum. The heavy chains in this immunoglobulin are of gama (γ) type and the light chains are either kappa or lambda type. Molecular Weight of IgG is about 1,46,000 daltons with 2 to 3% of carbohydrate content. Sedimentation co efficient of IgG is 7S. In general IgG is the major immunoglobulin secreted in secondary response. The structure of IgG reflects the basic structure of immunoglobulin. When compared to the other immunoglobulins rate of production of IgG is high (about 33 mg/ Kg body weight/day) and their half life is about 23 days. IgG is the only immnunoglobulin type that can cross the placental barrier to reach the fetus. Along with IgA secreted in the breast milk, residual IgG absorbed through the placenta provides immunity to the neonate prior to the establishment of its own immune system. The passive protection provided by the maternal immunoglbulins remains up to 6 months soon after birth.

IgG antibodies are predominantly involved in the secondary antibody response, (the main antibody involved in primary response is IgM), thus IgG immunoglobulins presence generally corresponds to maturation of antibody response. IgG can bind to many types of pathogens, such as viruses, bacteria, fungi etc. and provides protection against them through agglutination and immobilization, complement activation (classical pathway), opsonization for phagocytosis and neutralization of their toxins.

In humans the IgG class of immunoglobulins can be divided into four subclasses based on minor variations in the amino acid sequences of heavy chains. They are named as IgG_1, IgG_2, IgG_3 and IgG_4 with reference to their abundance in serum. Quantitatively, the relative serum concentrations of the human IgG subclasses are as follows $IgG_1 > IgG_2 > IgG_3 > IgG_4$. The four subclasses show more than 95% homology in the amino acid sequences of the constant domains but, show most conspicuous differences in the amino acid composition and structure of the 'hinge region. The hinge region of IgG_1 encompasses amino acids 216-231 and since it is freely flexible, the Fab fragments can rotate about their axes of symmetry and move within a sphere centered at the first of two inter-heavy chain disulfide bridges. IgG_2 has a shorter hinge than IgG_1, with 12 amino acid residues and four disulfide bridges. The hinge region of IgG_2 lacks a glycine residue; it is relatively short and contains a rigid poly-proline double helix, stabilized by extra inter-heavy chain disulfide bridges. These properties restrict the flexibility of the IgG_2 molecule. IgG_3 differs from the other subclasses by its unique extended hinge region (about four times as long as the IgG_1 hinge), containing 62 amino acids (including 21 prolines and 11 cysteines), forming an inflexible poly-proline double helix. In IgG_3 the Fab fragments are relatively far away from the Fc fragment, giving the molecule a greater flexibility. The elongated hinge in IgG_3 is also responsible for its higher molecular weight compared to the other subclasses. The hinge region of IgG_4 is shorter than that of IgG1 and its flexibility is intermediate between that of IgG_1 and IgG_2. All the subclasses except IgG_2 can cross placenta and provide protection to the baby.

The structural differences between the IgG subclasses are also reflected in their susceptibility to proteolytic enzymes, such as papain, plasmin trypsin and pepsin. IgG_3 is very susceptible to cleavage by these enzymes, whereas IgG_2 is relatively resistant. IgG_1 and IgG_4 exhibit an intermediary sensitivity, depending upon the enzyme used. As a consequence of the structural differences, the four IgG subclasses show differences in some of their physicochemical characteristics and biological properties also.

Table: 6.1

Physicochemical properties of human IgG subclasses

	IgG_1	IgG_2	IgG_3	IgG_4
Heavy chain type	gamma 1	gamma 1	gamma 1	gamma 1
Molecular mass (kD)	140	146	170	146
Amino acids in hinge region	15	12	62	12
Inter-heavy chain disulfide bonds (in hinge region)	2	4	11	2
Susceptibility to proteolytic enzymes	++	+/–	+++	+

Table: 6.2

Biological properties of human IgG subclasses

	IgG1	IgG2	IgG3	IgG4
Adult serum level	4.9-11.4	1.5-6.4	0.201.10	0.08-1.40
Range (g/I) (mean, g/I)	(6.98)	(3.8)	(0.51)	146
Proportion of total IgG (%)	43-75	16-48	1.7-7.5	12
Half-life (days)	21	21	7	2
Placental transfer	+	–	+	+

IMMUNOGLOBULIN M (IGM)

It is the most primitive immunoglobulin and is present in almost all vertebrates. It is about 5 to 10% in total serum immunoglobulins. In general IgM is the first immune globulin class synthesized by babies and is produced in primary response. In germline cells, the gene segment encoding the μ constant region of the heavy chain is positioned first among other constant region gene segments. For this reason mature B cells express IgM in initial stage. Immunoglobulin M is the largest antibody in human circulatory system and is often referred as macroglobulin because of its high molecular weight (950000 kD). It is secreted as a penatamere, each monomer of IgM have two antigen binding sites. The monomers are held together by means of disulphide bonds in Fc regions and a "J chain" (a poly peptide chain) linked by disulphide bonds to the Fc region in two different monomers stabilizes the polymer. The pentameric structure of IgM gives 10 antigen binding sites and the binding sites are projected towards periphery of the molecule. Even though its valence (binding capacity) is 10, it binds with only 5 antigens or less than that. IgM molecules are very efficient in binding with multidimensional antigens and activating complement system (activation of complement system requires its binding with two FC region of antibody). The half life period of IgM is 5 days and their synthetic rate is 5-8 mg/Kg body weight /day. Due to short life span their concentration in serum is very low (about 15mg/m1). The carbohydrate content in IgM is about 10-25% and sedimentation coefficient is 19S for pentamer, 7S for monomer.

IgM immunoglobulins cannot cross placenta, but fetus can synthesize IgM immunoglobulins. IgM detection in new born indicates congenital infections such as *syphilis, rubella, toxoplasmosis* etc. Most of the natural antibodies (eg blood group Abs) are of the IgM type. Due to its heavy size IgM remains in blood and provides very good defense against infectious agents entered in to the blood. Since IgM is large in size, it cannot diffuse out from blood vessels; hence it is found in very low quantities in interstetium.

IMMUNOGLOBULIN E (IgE)

Immunoglobulin E is typically the scarce isotype and is found only in mammals. It was discovered in 1966 by Teruka and Kimishige Ishizaka. IgE is a monomer showing basic structure but, with out hinge region. Instead of hinge region IgE has an additional domain CH_4. Molecular weight of IgE is 190000 Dts, and half life period is 2-3 days. The average serum concentration of IgEs is 0.3mg/kg body weight. IgE concentration is very high (about 50mg/100ml of serum) in atopic persons (people prone to allergy). The normal rate of synthesis of IgE is 2-3mg/kg body weight /day. Carbohydrate content occupies about 12% of total molecular weight. Unlike other immunoglobulins IgE is a heat labile molecule with a sedimentation coefficient of 8 S. IgE binds to FC receptors of basophils and tissue mast cells. Cross linkage of receptor bound IgE with an antigen induces release of pharmacological substance from the basophiles and mast cells. The released pharmacological substances initiate allergic reaction. Hence raise in serum IgE concentration indicates allergic conditions. Even in normal individuals intestinal helminthes parasites induce raise of serum IgE levels, this rise suggests IgE role in protection against the parasites.

IMMUNOGLOBULIN D (IgD)

IgD is the major antigen receptor isotype on the surface of most peripheral B cells, where it is co expressed with IgM. It is a unique immunoglobulin with molecular weight of 185,000 Dts. It represents about 0.25% of the total serum immunoglobulins (average serum level is 0.03mg/ml) and has a half-life of 2-3 days, similar to that of IgE. Its synthesis rate is at least 10 times lower than that of IgA, IgM, and IgG. The IgD molecule has a long "hinge" region that appears to make the fragment very susceptible to proteolytic degradation with production of Fab and Fc fragments and also renders the molecule flexible, thus enhancing antigen binding. Carbohydrates occupy about 12% of total molecular weight. The sedimentation coefficient of IgD is 7S and rate of synthesis is 0.4mg/kg body weight/day.

Mature B cells express a membrane bound immunoglobulin and it is thought to function in the activation of B cells after binding with antigens. Serum IgD and membrane-bound IgD are antigenically similar, but they differ in susceptibility to proteolysis by plasmin (A proteolytic enzyme that is formed from plasminogen in blood plasma dissolves the fibrin in blood clots.). Instead of being secreted in large amounts, after antigen binding to the B-cell receptor, the secreted form of chain is shut off. The B cells enter the pathways of plasma cells (which do not have IgD except for IgD-secreting plasma cells, where the μ gene is deleted) or of memory cells in secondary lymphoid organs.

Table: 6.3

Properties of Different Types of Human Immunoglobulins

Characteristics	IgG	IgA	IgM	IgD	IgE
Svedberg units	6-7S	6-11S	19 S	6.1 S	8.2 S
Molecular weight	150 kd	160 kd	900 kd	185 kd	200 kd
Carbohydrate percentage	3	8	12	13	12
Percent total Ig concentration	75-85	10-15	5-10	1	0.002

GENERAL FUNCTIONS OF IMMUNOGLOBULINS:

Immunoglobulins play a key role in humoral immunity; they defend the body either through direct attack or indirect means (by complement fixation of inflammation).

DEFENCE THROUGH INDIRECT ATTACK

In direct attack antibodies obstruct the movement of foreign agents. Binding of antibodies with the antigenic sites of the invading foreign agents either agglutinates or precipitates them and the resulting product- the antigen-antibody complex is removed by the other immune cells through phogocytosis or cytolysis. Some of the toxins released in the body get neutralized as a result of antibody binding to the toxins molecules and later removed through phagocytes. Binding of antibody to the antigen makes them vulnerable to phagocytes and the process that makes antigen vulnerable is known as opsonization. The binding of antibody to the antigen may alter the surface properties of pathogen and the pathogen fails to escape phagocytosis. Binding of antigen with IgE immunoglobulins bound to the mast cells initiates hypersensitive reactions (Refer Chapter 14 for details of hypersensitivity).

DEFENCE THROUGH DIRECT ATTACK

Immunoglobulins bound to the antigens activate the complement system, resulting in the formation of membrane associated complex (MAC) that destroys the foreign agent; added to that they initiate inflammation reactions (Refer Chapter 13 for details of Inflammation) to optimize the defense mechanism.

EPITOPES (ANTIGENIC DETERMINANTS) IN IMMUNOGLOBULINS:

Like all other proteins and glycoprotein molecules, immunoglobulins too have antigenic sites to induce antibody production against them. The antigenic determinants of imunoglobulins can be broadly divided into 3 types such as isotypes, allotypes and idiotypes.

ISOTYPES: - Isotypes are antigenic determinants that characterize classes and subclasses of heavy chains and types and subtypes of light chains. The prefix "Iso" means same in all members of a species. Some individuals with immunodeficiency may lack one or more isotypes but normal individuals have all isotypes. Therefore if antibody of an individual is injected to another individual of the same species, it is not immunogenic but if injected to individual of other species it is immunogenic, because individuals of different species have different amino acid sequences in their constant domines, this difference in amino acid sequences of constant domines makes antibody species specific and antigenic in individuals of other species. Antibodies to isotypes are used for the quantification of Ig classes and subclasses in various diseases, in the characterization of B cell leukemia and in the diagnosis of various immunodeficiency diseases.

ALLOTYPE: - Even though all members of a species inherit same set of genes for immunoglobulins, multiple alleles exist for same set of the genes, and encode slight variations in amino acid sequence leading to the development of allotypic determinants. Even a single amino acid difference can give rise to an allotypic determinant. In short, allotypes are immunoglobulins with sequence differences between alleles of a subclass. Development of allotypic determinants occur only in few individuals of a species. Allotypic determinants induce production of antibodies against them, if injected in to other individuals of the same species with out that particular set of alleles in their genome. Some times even paternal allotypic determinants of fetus induce antibodies production in mother's body. The immunoglobulin allotypes are one of the characteristics used in legal cases involving paternity. Since they are detectable in blood stains and semen they are useful in forensic medicine.

IDIOTYPE: - The paratope region of an immunoglobulin (variable domine of an antibody) is a good immunogenic part in immunoglobulins. Idiotypes are the antigenic determinants created by the hypervariable regions, localized on the Fab fragment of the immunoglobulin molecules and the anti-idiotypic antibodies are those directed against the hypervariable regions of an antibody. In many instances the actual antigenic determinant (i.e. idiotype) may include some of the framework residues near the hypervariable region. Immune responses may be regulated by anti-idiotypic antibodies directed against our own antigenic determinants. In some cases anti-idiotypic antibodies can be used to stimulate B cells to make antibodies that can act as a vaccine. This approach is being tried to immunize against highly dangerous pathogens that cannot be safely used as a vaccine. Idiotypes are useful markers for a particular variable region

MONOCLONAL ANTIBODIES

The term "monoclonal" pertains to a single clone of cells - a single cell and the progeny of that cell; the antibodies produced by the single clone of cells are known as "monoclonal antibodies". B cells following antigenic stimulation proliferate and give clones that are capable of producing homologous antibodies with a paratope that can bind with the epitope of antigen responsible for its creation. The homologous antibodies produced by the cells of a single clone are referred as monoclonal antibodies. Since a single antigen posses number of antigenic determinants or epitopes it can initiate proliferation and differentiation of a variety of B cell clones, that in turn produce heterogenous group of antibodies in normal conditions. Hence collecting monoclonal antibodies from biological system is almost impossible. However to be useful as a tool, molecular biologists need substantial amounts of a single antibody (and that antibody alone) for research, diagnostic and therapeutic purpose. In 1975 Georges Kohler and Cesar Milstein in 1975 developed an in vitro method for the production of monoclonal antibodies by fusing a normal antibody producing B cell with myeloma cell. The hybrid cell formed by the fusion of B cell and myeloma cell is refered as "hybridoma cell" and it becomes a powerful and versatile research tool. In 1984 the scientists were honored with Nobel Prize for their work. In 1988 Greg Winter and his team pioneered the techniques to humanize monoclonal antibodies.

PRODUCTION OF A HYBRIDOMA CELL:

A hybridoma cell can be produced in laboratories by fusing myeloma cells, with the B cells extracted from spleen of a mouse that has been immunized with the desired antigen. Use of a selective medium with Hypoxanthine, Aminopterin, and Thymidine helps in retaining and multiplying hybridoma cells. Aminopterin (a folic acid analogue) inhibits Dihydrofolate reductase, (DHFR), hence the cells in culture media fail to use the de novo pathway to synthesize purines and fully dependent on the salvage pathway for their survival. Since myeloma cells have lost the ability to synthesize hypoxanthine-guanine-phosphoribosyl transferase (HGPRT), an enzyme is necessary for the salvage synthesis of nucleic acids. Even through myloma cells are immortal loss of ability to synthesize HGPRT makes them die in the culture media. When the myloma cell fuses with spleen cells, the myloma cell acquires HGPRT from the spleen cell partner and becomes immortal hybridoma cell in the media. Fusion of myeloma cell with B cell can be done by using polyethylene glycol, a virus or through electroporation.

Limited life span of normal spleen cells, inability of myloma cells to synthesize HGPRT helps removal of unfused spleen cells and myloma cells from culture media, leaving only the immortal hybridoma cell. This mixture of cells is then diluted and clones are grown from single parent cells and can be maintained indefinitely either in vitro (that is, in culture vessels) or in vivo; i.e., growing in mice. The antibodies secreted by the different clones must be tested for their ability to bind to the antigen by using ELISA or Antigen Microarray Assay or immuno-dot blot assays to select the most productive and stable clone. Production in cell culture (in vitro method) is usually preferred, as the in vivo method is considered unethical.

PURIFICATION OF MONOCLONAL ANTIBODIES: While extracting antibodies from the monoclones maintained either in vitro or in vivo methods, certain contaminants such as growth factors, hormones, transferrins etc. of culture media, or host antibodies, proteases, nucleases, nucleic acids etc. also may be extracted. Hence the sample is first conditioned, or prepared for purification. Cells, cell debris, lipids, and clotted material are first removed, typically by filtration with a 0.45μm filter and condensed by ultra filtration or dialysis. Since most of the charged impurities are usually anions such as nucleic acids and endotoxins, they are often separated by ion exchange chromatography.

SALVAGE PATHWAY: A salvage pathway is a pathway in which nucleotides (purines and pyrimidines) are synthesized from intermediates in the degradative pathway for nucleotides. They are used to recover bases and nucleosides that are formed during degradation of RNA and DNA. This is important in some organs because some tissues cannot undergo de novo synthesis. The salvaged bases and nucleosides can then be converted back into nucleotides.

DE NOVO SYNTHESIS: It refers to the synthesis of complex molecules from simple molecules such as sugars or amino acids, as opposed to their being recycled after partial degradation. For example, nucleotides are not needed in the diet as they can be constructed from small precursor molecules such as formate and aspartate

Monoclonal Antibody Production

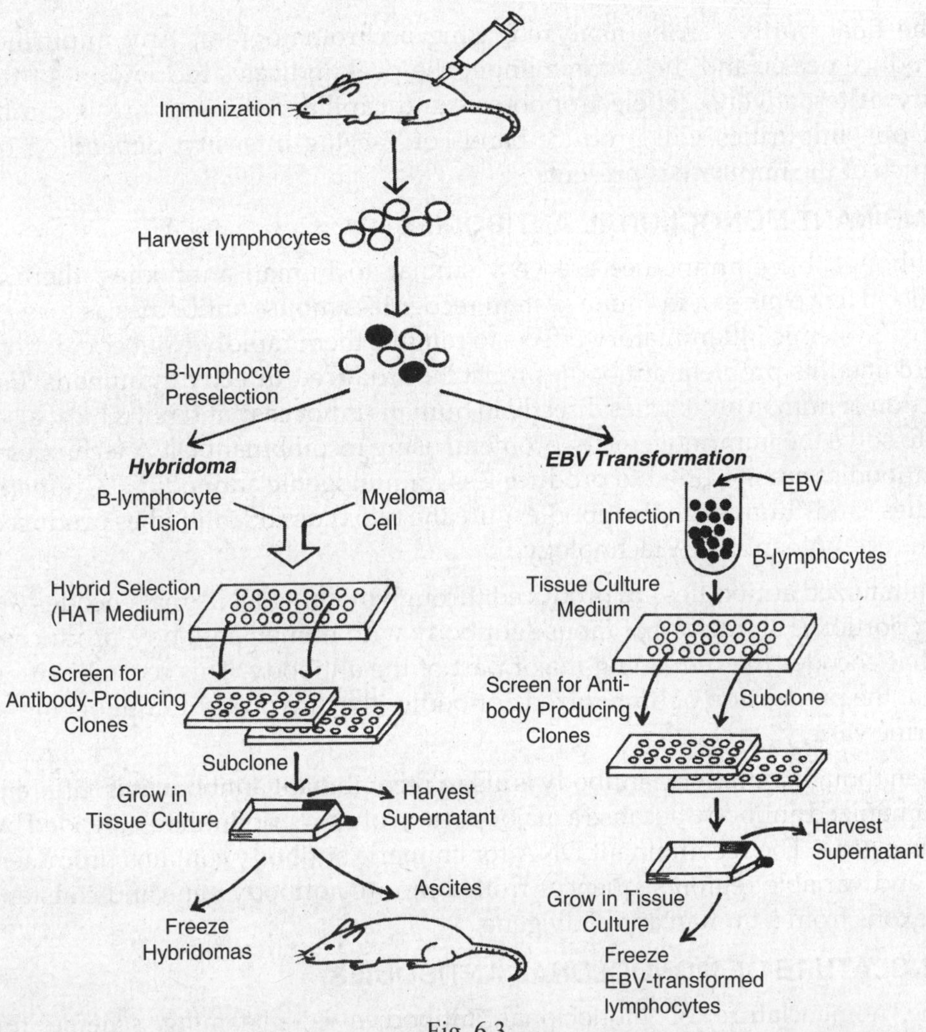

Fig. 6.3

POLYETHYLENE GLYCOL is a family of long chain polymers made up of ethylene glycol subunits. It allows a slowed clearance of the carried protein from the blood. This makes for a longer acting medicinal effect and reduces toxicity, and it allows longer dosing intervals.

To achieve maximum purity in a single step, affinity purification can be performed, using the antigen to provide exquisite specificity for the antibody. In this method, the antigen used to generate the antibody is covalently attached to an agarose support. If the antigen is a peptide, it is commonly synthesized with a terminal cysteine which allows selective attachment to a carrier protein, such as keyhole limpet haemocyanin (KLH) during development and helps in purification. The antibody-containing media is then incubated with the immobilized antigen, either in batch or the antibody is passed through a column, where it selectively binds and can be retained while impurities are washed away. An elution with a low pH buffer or a gentler, high salt elution buffer is then used to recover purified antibody from the support.

The final purity can be analyzed using a chromatogram. Any impurities will produce peaks, and the volume under the peak indicates the amount of the impurity. Alternatively, gel electrophoresis and capillary electrophoresis can be carried out. Impurities will produce bands of varying intensity, depending on how much of the impurity is present.

RECOMBINANT MONOCLONAL ANTIBODIES

Although mice antibodies are very similar to human antibodies, there is difference. Hence human immune system recognizes mouse antibodies as foreign and cause systemic inflammatory effects to remove them rapidly from circulation. To overcome this problem antibodies must be produced directly in humans, but production of human antibodies directly in humans is not easy and not ethical also. Hence to solve the immunogenicity problem, using recombinant DNA technology mice antibodies are modified to produce less immunogenic antibodies. "Chimeric antibodies" and "humanized antibodies" are the two types of antibodies produced through recombinant DNA technology.

Humanized antibodies are produced through merging DNA that encodes the binding portion (Fab region) of mouse antibody with human antibody-producing DNA that encodes the remaining major part of the antibody. This recombination results in the production of humanized antibodies that are not as immunogenic as the murine variety.

Even though a chimeric antibody is also a recombinant antibody it is different from humanized antibody because a major portion of chimeric antibody is coded by the mouse gene. The recombinant DNA for chimeric antibody contains promoter, leader, and variable region sequences from a mouse antibody gene and constant region exons from a human antibody gene.

NOMENCLATURE OF MONOCLONAL ANTIBODIES

The nomenclature of monoclonal antibodies is a naming scheme for conveying generic, or nonproprietary, names to a group of medicines prepared with antibodies. This scheme is used for both the World Health Organization's International Nonproprietary Names and the United States Adopted Names. In general, suffixes are used to identify a class of medicines; all monoclonal antibody pharmaceuticals end with the suffix "mab". However, different infixes are used depending on the structure and function of the medicine.

INFIX FOR ORIGIN / SOURCE:

The infix preceding the -mab suffix denotes the animal origin of the antibodies. Although the original monoclonal antibodies are produced in mice (infix, -o-), these antibodies are recognized as foreign by human immune systems and may be rapidly cleared, provoke an allergic reaction, or both. Therefore, parts of the antibody may be replaced with human sequences. If the constant region is replaced with the human form, it is termed chimeric and the infix used is -xi-. Part of the variable regions may also be substituted, in which case it is termed "humanized" and the infix used is -zu-. Antibodies originating in humans use -u-.

INFIX FOR TARGET:

The infix preceding the source of the antibodies refers to medicine's target. Most of these consist of a consonant, vowel, then another consonant. For ease of pronunciation and to avoid awkwardness, the final consonant is dropped if the following infix begins with a consonant (such as -zu- or -xi-). Examples of these include –ci (r) - for the circulatory system and -tu(m)- for miscellaneous tumors (cancers).

PREFIX AND SECOND WORD

The prefix carries no special meaning and should be unique for each medicine. A second word may be added if there is another substance attached or linked. For example Abciximab is a commonly used medication to prevent platelets from clumping together. It can be broken down into ab - + - ci (r) - + -xi- + -mab. Therefore, it is a chimeric monoclonal antibody used on the cardiovascular system. Another example is the breast cancer medication trastuzumab, which can be broken down into tras- + -tu(m)- + -zu- + -mab. Therefore, it is a humanized monoclonal antibody used against a tumor.

MONOCLONAL ANTIBODY THERAPY

Since the early description of monoclonal antibodies by Kohler and Milstein in 1975 there has been considerable interest in their adoption for human sero therapy. In 1895 Hericourt and Richet described the first trials in which cancer cells were injected into animals to raise an antiserum for treating the patient. Their results seemed very promising and several patients with different types of advanced cancer are treated, each receiving an individual, tailor-made antiserum. None of them was cured, but they showed significant improvements in their symptoms. It was discovered that an antiserum contains a mixture of many different antibodies, each one directed against a different antigens on cancer cells. Many of these antigens are also present on normal tissue cells and so the antibodies against them could be harmful. Hybridoma technique developed by Georges Kohler Cesar Milstein and Niels Kaj Jerne for the production of monoclonal antibodies allowed their development in the mid 1970s. Chimeric, humanised and fully humanised mAb can now be made by recombinant engineering.

Specificity against antigen made monoclonal antibodies (mAbs) made them blockbuster potential drugs. The specificity of monoclonal antibodies has tremendous clinical value and makes them very attractive therapeutics. The focus, which was once dominated by their use in oncology, has now broadened to encompass additional disease areas. About a quarter of all biotech drugs in development are mAb, and around 30 products are in use or being investigated. Licensed products are available for inhibition of alloimmune and autoimmune reactivity, and for antitumour, antiplatelet, or antiviral therapy.

Monoclonal antibodies are now a major component of the pharmaceutical pipeline. Of the estimated 370 biotechnology-based drugs in development in 2000, approximately 70 are mAbs, second only to therapeutic vaccines. There are currently 132 mAb products in development. Majority of the products are either humanized (42%) mAbs or fully human (28%) mAbs. A healthy future is anticipated for novel mAbs based therapies.

Certain monoclonal antibodies have been introduced into human medicine for controlling various problems are as follows:

To suppress the immune system:

Muromonab-CD3 (OKT3) and two humanized anti-CD3 monoclonals are used in transplantation treatments to prevent acute rejection of organ.

Infliximab is useful in controlling certain inflammatory diseases such as rheumatoid arthritis.

Omalizumab showed positive effects against allergic asthma by preventing IgE's attachment to mast cells. Daclizumab is useful to prevent acute rejection of transplanted kidneys.

To kill or inhibit malignant cells

Rituximab is used to treat B-cell lymphomas.

Trastuzumab is the only monoclonal so far that seems to be effective against solid tumors.

Angiogenesis Inhibitors

Vitaxin. Bevacizumab has shown some promise in shrinking solid tumors without harmful side effects by inhibiting angiogenesis.

Abciximab is helpful in preventing reclogging of the coronary arteries in patients who have undergone angioplasty.

PROBLEMS WITH MONOCLONAL THERAPY

Problems with monoclonal therapy Antibody immunogenicity remains one of the inherent therapeutic limitations associated with administration of murine monoclonals to human subjects. In most instances, single injections of the murine monoclonal antibodies elicit an immune response in 50 to 80% of patients. Human anti-mouse antibodies (HAMA) are generally detected within 14 days of administration. In practice, repeated administration of the monoclonal antibodies increases the HAMA response significantly, therefore, therapeutic efficacy of murine monoclonals is limited to the first and at most, the second dose administration. Even though monoclonal antibodies rose in humans lessen the immunogenicity problem, most of the attempts that have been made are unsuccessful and need several attempts to make them immunized.

Some of the rare, but more serious side effects of monoclonal antibody therapy include:

Infusion reactions usually occur while treatment or soon after and in very few cases, it may lead to death. Low levels of red blood cells, white blood cells and platelets may develop leading to serious complications. Certain monoclonal antibodies may root cardiac problems, including heart failure and a small risk of heart attack. Serious sores can also occur on the tissue that lines cheeks and gums (mucosa). Some of the monoclonal antibody drugs designed to stop cancer, through blocking angiogenesis may cause bleeding.

7

ANTIGENS

Any thing that makes the immune system produce a response is referred as "antigen". Antigens may be living foreign bodies such as viruses, bacteria, and fungi that cause disease and infection or non living agents such as dust, chemicals, pollen grains, or food proteins that can cause allergic reactions in the host. All antigens may not be foreign bodies; they may be produced in the body itself. For example, cancer cell antigens that are produced inside by the body.

The intensity or strength of immunological response that an antigen can generate is referred as "immunogenecity". The nature and strength of immune response is not identical for all the antigens. Generally proteins and polysaccharides are potent immunogens. Nucleic acids and synthetic polypeptides are also immunogenic but not strong immunogens. Certain substances such as nylon, plastic, or Teflon that rarely display antigenic properties are referred as "tolerogens". A tolerogen can become an immunogen if there is any alteration in its molecular form. Hence immunogenecity of an antigen depends on certain physico chemical properties of the antigen molecules. Factors that generally influence immunogenisity of an antigen are as follows.

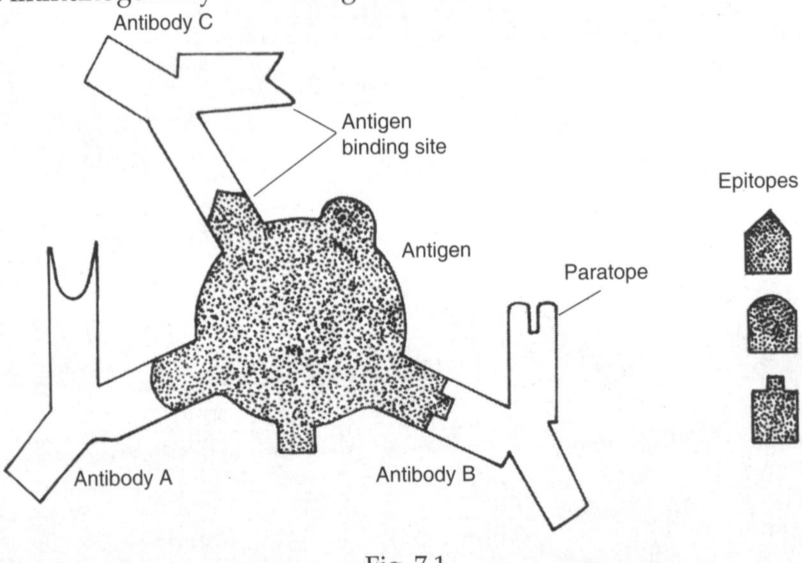

Fig. 7.1

(1) CHEMICAL COMPOSITION AND HETEROGENITY: Chemical composition and heterogenity of antigens play an important role in immunogenecity. Generally proteins are good immunogens because of their high internal molecular complexity and heterogeneity. A homopolymer polypeptide chain of any amino acid, even though big in size, fails to induce immune response due to lack of heterogeneity. Addition of different amino acids at different sites of the same homopolymer makes it immunogenic. Since the structural complexity of a protein is different at different levels of formation, the immunogenecity of a protein during its formation and after its formation are different. Study of synthetic lysine and glutamic acid co-polymers suggest that a minimum of substance with 30000-40000 Daltons molecular weight is required to be immunogenic, but when tyrosine is added to this synthetic co-polymer, a molecule of even 10000-20000 Daltons molecular weight is sufficient to be immunogenic. The increased complexity of the co-polymers by the addition of other amino acids helps to raise its immunogenecity.

(2) SIZE:- Generally the size of the antigen molecule influences the immunogenecity. Substances with a molecular weight of about 100000 Daltons show best immunogenecity and substances less than 5000 to 10000 Daltons are poor immunogens. For example large molecules such as hemocyanin (6000.000 dt) and thyroglobulin (9669000 dt) show excellent immunogenecity. The proteins like insulin, histone etc. with low molecular weight fails to produce proper immunological response when exposed to immune system.

(3) FOREIGNNESS: The very important and essential character required for any substance to be immunogenic is its foreignness. Since immune system is designed to react with foreign molecules, antigens from related species are less antigenic than that of unrelated species. The phylogenetic distance between two species generates disparity between antigens, but there is same exception to contain molecules such as collagen, and cytochrome C, because they are highly conserved throughout evolution and therefore display very little immunogenecity across diverse species lines

(4)SUSCEPTIBILITYTOANTIGENPROCESSINGANDPRESENTATION: Antigen presentation to T_H cells through antigen presenting cells after processing is essential for both humoral and cell mediated immune responses. Hence molecules that cannot be processed and presented to the T cells become poor immunogens. In this aspect, large insoluble molecules are more immunogenic than smaller ones because larger molecules are easily identified and phagocytosed by antigen presenting cells for processing and presentation.

(5) DEGRADABILITY AND SOLUBILITY: The substance that is not soluble in body fluids fails to induce immune response. If the substance is soluble in body fluids there is a possibility of exposure of hidden epitopes to induce immune response. For example pneumococcal polysaccharides are greater immunogens in mice but not in rabbits, because the pneumococal molecules are highly soluble in mice body fluids but not in rabbits.

ORIGIN OF ANTIGENS:

With reference to the source from which they have been produced, antigens are broadly named as exogenous and endogenous antigens.

(1) EXOGENOUS ANTIGENS: Exogenous antigens are the antigens that enter into the host from the outside, through inhalation, ingestion, or injection. Exogenous antigens include particles considered foreign within the organism. For example, allergens (such as pollen), proteins from transplanted tissues and organs, and parts of microorganisms (such as coat, capsule, cell wall, flagella, fimbria, or toxin of bacteria, viruses, etc.) can serve as antigens. These exogenous antigens are taken up by endocytosis or phagocytosis into the antigen presenting cells (APCs), and degraded into fragments. The fragments are then presented on the surface of APCs by class II histocompatibility molecules to T helper cells (CD_4^+ or T_H). The T helper cells then get activated and release cytokines. The cytokines then activate cytotoxic T lymphocytes (CTL), antibodies secreting B lymphocytes, macrophages and other cells.

Generally microorganisms, pollen, drugs and pollutants are considered as exogenous antigens. The disease causing pathogens induce immune response after entering into the host body. Host may develop resistance after the first attack of certain pathogens, for example the virus responsible for small pox and chicken pox induce resistance in the host due to the formation of memory cells developed after the first exposure. But certain pathogens such as virus responsible for common cold, bacteria causing Pharyngitis etc. fail to induce resistance due to various reasons. Frequent alterations in pathogen epitopes due to mutations is one of the reason.

(2) ENDOGENOUS ANTIGENS: Endogenous antigens are antigens that have been generated within the body. They include xenogenic (heterologus), autologus, idiotypic or allogenic antigens and autoantigens.

Xenogenic antigen: These are also known as "hetero antigens". It is an antigen common to members of one species but not to members of other species. Generally immune system does not produce any antibodies against self antigens but the antibodies produced against foreign agents some times react with certain surface molecules of their own cells due to their similarity with the foreign antigen. The surface molecules or antigens that are attacked by self antibodies are known as xenogenic antigens. The cardiolipin antigen, forssman antigen present on cells are some of the xenogenic antigens that show similarity with antigens present on pneumococci and salmonella bacteria.

Cardiolipin antigen and Forssman antigen: Heterogenetic antigens occurring in various unrelated species, mainly in the organs but not in the erythrocytes (guinea pig, horse), but sometimes only in the erythrocytes (eg sheep), and occasionally in both (eg chicken).

Autologous antigens:-Certain auto antigens that were not exposed to immune system during development are recognized as foreign antigens. For example the antigens present on the sperm are not recognized by the immune system as its own, because the development of sperms takes place during adolescence and immune cells never come across the developing sperm cells. In the same way proteins of cornea are also identified as foreign antigens (Refer Chapter 15 for autoimmunity)

Allogenic antigens: Antigens such as blood group antigens, tissue antigens are under the control of genes. Since the genes controlling the antigens are polymorphic in nature the antigens also express polymorphism and are specific for each individual. Exact matching of these antigens between two individual is not possible, due to different combinations of genes. Identical twins alone show exact matching because of genetical similarity. Allogenic antigens are responsible for blood transfusion reactions and graft rejection reactions between individuals of same species.

IMMUNOGENICITY/BIOLOGICAL SYSTEM: Immunogenicity of any antigen depends upon the biological environment in which it has to generate immune response. The immune response to antigen depends on the following factors of the biological system.

(1) Genetic constitution of the recipient: Genetic constitution of the recipient influences the type and intensity of immune response to the antigen. The receptors of T and B cells are under the control of genes. They play a key role in binding with antigens; hence their structural and molecular characteristics (controlled by genes) directly influence the antigen binding. Antigen binding is essential for initiation of immune response. For example people with normal hemoglobin are susceptible to death from malaria, but people with sickle cell trait have a greater chance of surviving malaria and do not suffer adverse consequences, due to the presence of one gene for hemoglobin A and one gene for hemoglobin S. Sickle trait provides a survival advantage over people with normal hemoglobin in regions where malaria is endemic. Hemoglobin C is also believed to protect against malaria Hemoglobin C heterozygotes had significantly fewer episodes of P. falciparum malaria than did controls with only hemoglobin A. The risk of malaria was lower still in subjects who were homozygous for hemoglobin C.

(2) Dose of antigens: An insufficient dose of even an effective immunogen may fail to induce immune response in the host. To produce the immune response the immune system has to identify and recognize the antigen. If the dose of antigen is too low, the chances of encounter of this immunogen with T and B lymphocytes are remote. Non specific phagocytes may remove these antigens from biological system, even before they interact with T and B cells. An excessive dose of antigens also fail to induce a response, because it causes lymphocytes to enter in to a no responsive state. In case of certain antigens a single dose may not be sufficient to induce a strong response. Repeated administrations (booster doses) over a period of time may be required to stimulate strong response.

(3) Route of administration: The encountering lymphocytes in different routes are different and the type of response depends on the type of lymphocytes encountering the antigen. Hence the route of administration influences the immune response. For example cell mediated response can be expected for antigens introduced intra dermaly. If antigens enter the body through respiratory or gastric intestinal tract, Ig1A antibody mediated response can be expected. Because the B cell in those areas are committed to produce Ig1A antibodies. Routes commonly used for immunization depend on the type of antigen. It may be intra muscular subcutaneous, intravenous, intraperitoneal, and intro dermal. In spite of the route of administration most antigens eventually become distributed through out the body by circulation and induce both humoral and cell mediated response.

Sickle cell trait and malaria: Sickle cell trait occur when someone inherits a normal hemoglobin gene from one parent (HbA) and a sickle hemoglobin gene (HbS) from the other (resulting in HbAS). People (particularly children) infected with P. falciparum are more likely to survive the acute illness if they have sickle cell trait. The precise mechanism by which sickle cell trait imparts resistance to malaria is unknown. A number of factors are likely to be involved and contribute in varying degrees to the defense against malaria. Several theories were proposed to explain why people with sickle cell trait have milder cases of malaria. Some are

- The parasite inside the red cell produces acid. In the presence of acid, HbS has a tendency to polymerize which causes the cells to sickle. Since sickled cells are destroyed as the blood circulates through the spleen, the parasites are destroyed as well.
- Deformation of sickle trait erythrocytes would mark these cells as abnormal and target them for destruction by phagocytes. Experiments carried out in vitro with sickle trait red cells showed that under low oxygen tension, cells infected with P. falciparum parasites sickle much more readily than do uninfected cells
- oxygen radical formation in sickle trait erythrocytes retards growth and even kills the P. falciparum parasite
- Malarial parasites do not live long under low oxygen conditions. Since the oxygen concentration is low in the spleen, and since infected red cells tend to get trapped in the spleen, they may be killed there.
- Another thing that happens under low oxygen conditions is that potassium leaks out of HbS-containing cells. The parasite needs high potassium levels to develop. This may be the reason why the parasite fails to thrive in red blood containing Hb S.

Hemoglobin C and malaria: Hemoglobin C heterozygotes had significantly fewer episodes of P. falciparum malaria when compared with only hemoglobin A. The risk of malaria was still lower in subjects who were homozygous for hemoglobin C. Homozygous hemoglobin C produces a mild hemolytic anemia and splenomegaly. The much milder phenotype of the condition relative to homozygous hemoglobin S led the investigators to speculate that without medical intervention for malaria, hemoglobin C would replace hemoglobin S over the next few thousand years as the dominant "antimalarial".

Adjuvant: Response to an immunogen can be enhanced by mixing the antigen with certain adjuvants. Adjuvant is a group of structurally heterogeneous compounds capable of enhancing immunogenity of an antigen. The term adjuvant is derived from Latin. In Latin adjuvant means "to help". Adjuvant help to induce greater, more prolonged antibody production and increased effector cell count. When only small amounts of antigens are available, adjuvant can be mixed to get maximum effect from the minimum antigens. Certain oil emulsions, saponins, aluminums or calcium salts, derivatives of lipopolysaccharides, mycobacteria etc. can be used as adjuvants. Adjutants stimulate nonspecific lymphocyte proliferation and granuloma formation. When an antigen is mixed with alum (as adjuvant) and injected, the adjuvant slowdown the release of antigen from the site of injection so that the effective time of exposure to the antigen is increased. The size of the antigen increases, when it is mixed with an adjuvant. The increase in size of the antigen increases the likelihood of phagocytes. Adjuvant perhaps alters traffic of circulating lymphocytes. In various instance a combination of all the functions of adjuvant might occur. A commonly used adjuvant was initially formulated by Freund. It is "stable water in oil emulsion", which may (complete) or may not (incomplete) contain killed ***Mycobacterium tuberculoses.***

Freund's complete adjuvant (FCA): Freund's complete adjuvant is a water-in-oil emulsion consisting of a mineral oil, an antibody stimulator such as ***Mycobacterium tuberculoses***, and an emulsifying agent such as lanolin or Arlacel A." Muramyl dipeptide is a component of the mycobacterial cell wall; it is capable of activating macrophages. Since activated macrophages are more phagocytic than inactivated macrophages it is more potent than incomplete Freunds adjuvant and used in initial injections. But it is difficult to mix with immunogen and can cause tissue necrosis at the site of injection.

Freunds incomplete adjuvant: This is similar to complete adjuvant but the oily phase does not contain the killed bacteria. The small droplets formed in emulsion helps in slow release of antigen from the site of injection, to prolong the exposure period of antigens to the cells of immune system. Typically used for subsequent boosts after initial injection with FCA.

Antigen presentation and epitope recognition: Recognition of an antigen by immune cells takes place through their epitopes or determinant sites. Immune response follows with the interaction of antigens and lymphocytes. Generally antigens express more than one epitope on their surface and hide some epitopes inside. Exposure of hidden epitopes takes place only when the antigen is processed by antigen presenting cell. The number of antigenic determinants or epitopes per antigen molecule is refereed as the "valence of the antigen". The functional valence number (surface epitopes) is different from the non functioning (hidden epitopes) valence. For example the bovine serum albumin valence is 18 but functional epitopes or functional valence is only 6.

Classification of Antigens

B cells can respond to the surface epitopes of intact antigens but fail to recognize internal epitopes or processed antigens. But T cells respond to small and cleaved peptides (epitopes) that were buried inside the native antigen, if they were presented through MHC class II molecules of antigens presenting cells. With reference to this character antigens are classified as T cell dependent Antigens and T cell independent antigens.

T cell dependent Antigens: The antigens that require T lymphocytes to induce immune response and antibody production are referred as "T cell dependent antigens". Hence T-dependent antigens do not directly stimulate the production of antibody without the help of T cells. Structurally these antigens are characterized by a few copies of many different antigenic determinants. Proteins are T-dependent antigens.

T cell independent antigens: The antigens that are capable of inducing antibody production without T cells help are considered as "T cell independent antigens" (Refer Chapter 5 for B cell activation). The substances of polysaccharide, lipids, and nucleic acids are T cell independent antigens. These antigens are characterized by repetition of the same antigenic determinant.

HAPTENS

Haptens are low-molecular weight molecules with an antigenic determinant but are not antigenic independently. They can elicit an immune response when attached to a large carrier, such as a protein. The term hapten is derived from the Greek haptein, meaning "to fasten." Due to their small size immune cells fail to recognize haptens to produce immune response against them. Many drugs that cause allergic reactions, such as penicillin are haptens. When injected or ingested, penicillin reacts chemically with proteins in the body to form a hapten-carrier complex that can lead to the life-threatening syndrome called anaphylaxis. Other haptens include synthetic substances, such as the organic compounds benzene arsonate or tri nitrophenol, and naturally occurring polysaccharides, such as lactose. Researchers have used haptens to construct synthetic vaccines to immunize people against various infectious organisms. Haptens can induce autoimmune disease. For example hydralazine, a blood pressure lowering drug, occasionally produce drug-induced lupus erythematosus in some individuals.

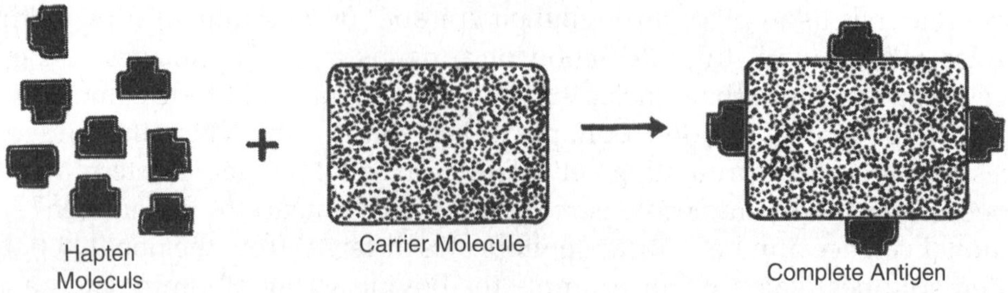

Fig. 7.2

SOME SPECIFIC GROUPS OF ANTIGENS:

Bacterial antigens: - Cell wall, capsule and the flagella of bacteria are antigenic in nature. The cell wall consists of oligosaccharides attached to a lipid and to a series of repeating tri saccharides. The polysaccharide and lipo-protein substances are responsible for antigenesity. The antigenic structure of cell wall varies from species to species. On the basis of the cell wall structure, the genus of bacteria can be classified into different species. The bacterial polysaccharide antigens are referred as "O antigens".

The capsule antigen of bacteria may be a polysaccharide or protein. The capsular antigens of bacteria are referred as "K antigens". The flagella consist of a single protein, the fixed or polymerized flagella protein acts as a good antigen and it is referred as "H antigen". The proteins secreted by bacteria or derived from their autolysis are very good antigens and are highly toxic. The antibodies produced against them are referred as "antitoxins".

Virus antigens: The capsid (protein coat of virus) proteins of virus are good antigens. Since they are not found free in the circulation, the viral antigen may not induce antibody production. The host cell of the virus expresses certain altered surface antigen molecules. Antibody production takes place against the host cell altered surface molecules to eradicate the internal parasite.

Blood group antigens: The antigens present on the surface of red blood cells plays a major role in blood transfusion reactions and Rh factor incompatibility reactions such as "erythroblastosis fetalis".

(Refer Hemato immunology).

Tumor (cancer) antigens: A cell becomes a cancer cell due to accumulation of mutations at random. A number of alterations occur in enzymes, receptors, membrane antigens etc. of the cell during tumorigenesis. Since they have a selective advantage over cells with other mutations, tumor cells can survive. Most chemically or physically induced tumours or tumours produced by virus have "neo-antigens or onco-fetal antigens". Neo-antigens that contribute towards tumor rejection are referred as "tumor associated transplantation antigens (TATA)".

Neo-antigens (or) Onco-fetal antigens: They may appear due to de-repression of genes that were only expressed early in life. Two major onco-fetal antigens are alpha-fetoprotein (AFP) and carcino-embryonic antigen (CEA). AFP is produced only as a secreted protein, whereas CEA is found both on cell membranes and in secreted fluids. Since secreted antigens contribute little toward immunity against tumors, the role of these neo-antigens in immuno-surveillance is questionable.

Tumor associated transplantation antigens (TATA) on virus induced tumors: Different viruses such as SV-40 virus, adenovirus, Rous sarcoma virus, Friend erythroleukemic virus, Moloney Rauscher Gross viruses etc. cause tumors in animals. Virus-induced tumors express characteristic surface antigens of the virus that induced the tumor. They are portions of intracellular molecules expressed on the cell surface as part of the major histocompatibility complex and can be presented in a way, that they can be recognized by T-cells. Expression of these antigens is regardless of tissue origin of the tumor or animal species in which the tumor exists.

Tumor associated transplantation antigens on chemically-induced tumors:

Chemically-induced tumors are different from virally-induced tumors in that they are extremely heterogeneous in their antigenic characteristics. Thus, any two tumors induced by the same chemical, even in the same animal, rarely share common tumor specific antigens (Figure 7.2). These unique antigens on chemically-induced tumors are referred to as tumor specific transplantation antigens (TSTA). They are also called as tumor-specific antigens (TSAs) or Tumor-associated antigens (TAAs).

8

ANTIGEN AND ANTIBODY INTERACTION

Antibodies produced by B cells bind specifically and non-covalently to their exclusive antigens that induced their production. The substance that has been formed as a result of antigen antibody interaction is known as "immune complex" or "antigen antibody complex". Various reversible, non covalent interactions between antigenic determinants and antibody variable regions are responsible for the formation of immune complex. Intermolecular interactions between side chains of epitope subunits and those of the paratope include these non covalent interactions. Immune complex formation is the basis for humoral immunity or antibody mediated immune response.

CHEMICAL BASIS OF ANTIGEN ANTIBODY INTERACTION

When an antibody and its specific antigen come close to each other they interact through the chemical groups established on the surface of epitope and paratope. The bond between them is exclusively noncovalent. The major bonds formed between antigen and antibody is hydrophobic in nature. Many of the nonpolar side chains of proteins are hydrophobic in nature. When antigen antibody molecules come close to each other, these side chains interact and exclude water molecules from the area of interaction. Displacement of water molecules increases the binding force of interacting Ag - Ab molecules and the complex becomes energetically stable. If the non covalent bond between antigen and antibody is mediated through hydrogen bonds, both epitope and paratope share hydrogen. Major hydrogen bonds formed in Ag and Ab interaction are

O-H-O, N-H-N and O-H-N. Even though Van der Waals force between two atoms is very weak, it may become collectively important in immune complex formation.

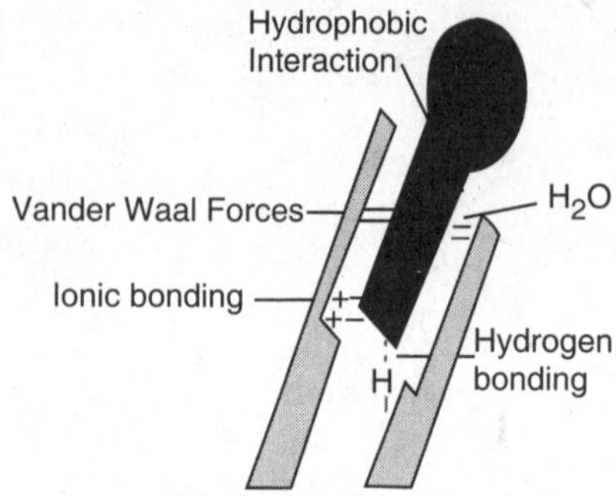

Fig. 8.1

SALIENT FEATURES OF AG-AB REACTIONS

SPECIFICITY OF AG -AB INTERACTION: Like lock and key mechanism, interaction between Ag and Ab is highly specific. Specific antibody can distinguish even minute differences in structure, charge, etc. of an antigens epitope and binds only with its specific Ag. This character of antibody is known as "specificity of antibody". For example Abs produced against blood group B antigens, bind with B antigens only. They never bind with A, or D blood group antigens. Since each antigen enclose different number of epitopes, immune system produces different antibodies to suit each epitope of the antigen. Bacterial species and types can be identified by using this specific nature of antigen antibody reactions.

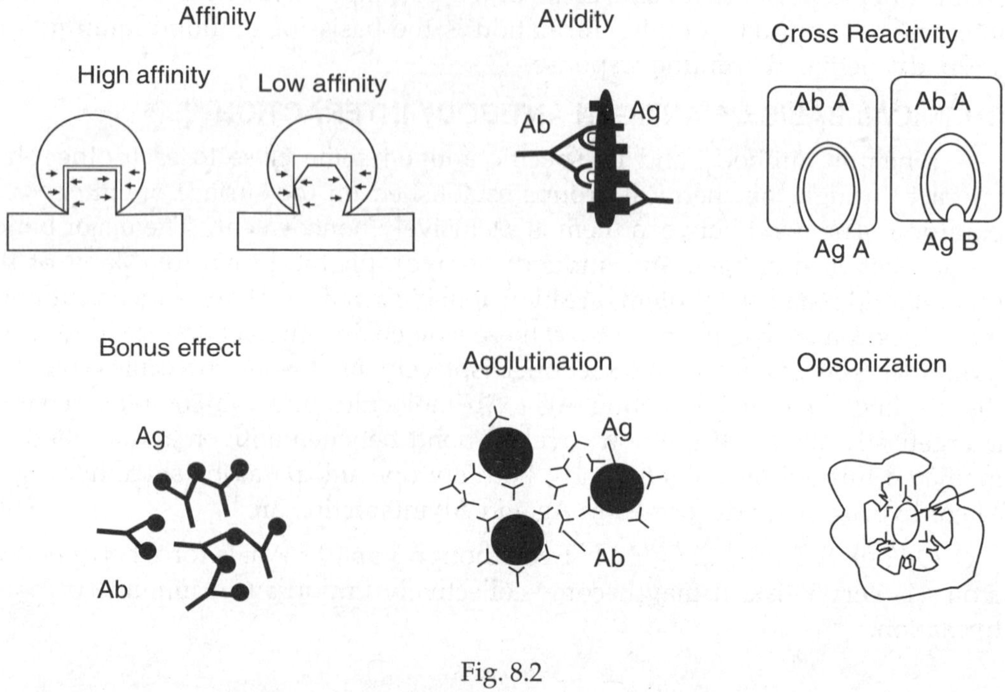

Fig. 8.2

ANTIBODY AFFINITY: It is the strength of the reaction between a single antigenic determinant and a single binding site of antibody. Since the binding between antigen and antibody is mediated by non covalent bonds, it operates over a very small distance. The binding strength depends on distance and compatibility of two substances. Increased distance between the two objects weakens the bonding strength. The sum of the attractive and repulsive forces, such as electrostatic forces, hydrogen bonding, hydrophobic bonding, Van der Waals force etc. operating between the epitope and paratope also influence the affinity. An antibody with high affinity binds tightly with its suitable antigen and the bonding remains for a longer time. If the affinity of Ab is low the bonding strength is also low and the bond remains for a very short time.

In simple terms affinity is the equilibrium constant that describes the strength of antigen-antibody reaction. Most antibodies have a high affinity for their specific antigens. The affinity of an antibody and monovalent antigen can be described by the equation.

$$Ag + Ab \underset{k\text{-}I}{\overset{KI}{\rightleftharpoons}} Ag\text{-}ab$$

Where

KI = Association rate constant.

k-I = Dissociation rate constant.

The ratio of k1/k-1 is the equilibrium constant "ka"

Since ka is the equilibrium constant, it can be calculated from the ratio of the molecular concentration of bound Ag-Ab complex to the molar concentrations of unbound antigen and antibody at equilibrium.

$$Ka = \frac{[Ag - Ab]}{(Ab)(Ag)}$$

Ka depends upon K1, k is expressed in liters / moles/ second

k-1 is expressed in liters /sec

ANTIBODY AVIDITY: Antibody molecules and antigens are multivalent. This multi valency of Abs and Ags tend to increase chances of interaction and also strength of bonding. The overall strength of an antibody binding to multivalent antigen is known as "avidity". For instance, if a multivalent antigen holds repetition of similar epitopes, an antibody having more than one binding site can bind with more than one epitope of the same antigen. Binding of antibody to an antigen at more than one site increases strength of the bond or avidity proportionately. Avidity is influenced by valency of both antibody and antigen. High avidity of antigen and antibody can compensate low affinity.

CROSS REACTIVITY: There is a possibility of presence of similar epitopes on different antigens. Hence antibodies produced for a specific antigen can cross react with antigens having similar epitopes. For example antiserum raised against albumin of hens egg can cross react with the albumin of ducks egg. It is often observed among polysaccharide antigens that contain similar oligosaccharide residues. Cross reaction is the cause for blood transfusion reactions. In blood transfusion, there is no need of pre sensitization to generate rejection reactions against a mismatched blood. The blood group antibodies elicited by microbial antigens are cross reactive in nature and can react with blood group antigens during transplantation. (Refer Chapter 20 for details). Cross reactivity is responsible for various autoimmune diseases also (Refer chapter 15 for details on autoimmunity). Cross reactivity of antibodies, produced against cowpox antigen with variola virus is responsible for the success of Jenner's vaccination trial against small pox.

Cross reactivity character of Abs has been used differently in various diagnostic tests. For example, *Treponema pallidum* (syphilis) infection induces production of antibodies that cross-react with ***cardiolipin*** - a substance found in cardiac muscle. Since it is much easier to obtain pure cardiolipin than pure *Treponemal* antigens, cardiolipin is used in diagnostic test for syphilis (Wassermann test). In the same way antibodies produced against Rickettsia cross-react with antigens from *Proteus*. Since the latter are much easier to obtain, they can be used to test for the former.

Wassermann test – It is a blood test to detect syphilis; a complement fixation test is used to detect antibodies to the syphilis organism treponema; a positive reaction indicates the presence of antibodies and therefore syphilis infection.

ANTIGEN PRECIPITATION: Soluble antigen molecules can be precipitated by antibodies. Antigen interaction enables antibodies to neutralize, opsonize and inactivate toxic substances and pathogens. The soluble antigens that can precipitate Abs are known as "precipitins". Even though Ag-Ab complex formation takes place within minutes, visible precipitates arise more slowly and it depends upon the concentration of Ags and Abs. The precipitin reaction is influenced by the number of paratopes of antibody for the given antigen and by the number of epitopes found on antigen molecule. Antigen with two or more epitopes is essential to produce precipitation reaction in a polyclonal antiserum. If the antigen is allowed to interact with monoclonal antibodies, formation of precipitate is possible only if the antigen express as at least two or more epitopes for the paratopes of monoclonal antibodies.

Precipitation test can be used to check the similarity of soluble antigens.

BONUS EFFECT: The antigen with multivalency or multiple binding sites can react with different antibodies simultaneously. If a single antibody holds two antigens simultaneously the strength of the bond is very weak. But if an antigen is bridged by two or more antibodies at a time the binding strength of Ag-Ab complex increases proportionately. This added strength of Ag- Ab complex is referred as "bonus effect". Increased valency of an antigen and presence of polyclonal antibodies enhances the chance of bonus effect. Generally immune system produces different antibodies at a time to suit different epitopes of an antigen. Presence of antibodies with different paratopes to match with all the epitopes of the antigen enhances the bonding strength of Ag – Ab complex and helps immune system in the removal of foreign agent successfully.

NEUTRALIZATION OF TOXINS: Most of the toxins are antigenic in nature, and induce antibodies production. Binding of Abs to the antigens shields the toxic sites of toxin molecules ensuing neutralization of toxin.

TYPES OF Ag-Ab REACTIONS

1. AGGLUTINATION REACTIONS: Aggregation of cells due to antibody binding is known as "**Agglutination**". The word agglutination is derived from Latin word ***agglutinare***, means "to glue to." In humus, binding of Abs pulls the antigen bearing cells close to each other resulting in the formation of clumps. The antibodies that cause agglutination of cells are called "agglutinins" and the antigens aggregated are called "agglutinates".

MECHANISM OF AGGLUTINATION:

The bivalent or multivalent antibodies can bind with two or more antigens at a time. When Ab binds to more than one antigen present on different cells, the individual antigen molecules brought close to each other, resulting in the formation of clumps. Since IgM antibody has more number of antigen binding sites it is a more effective agglutinin. Agglutination of blood group antigens by IgM antibodies in mismatched blood transfusion is responsible for the blood transfusion reactions. Agglutination test has wide application in clinical field. For example agglutination test is used to test blood groups, and infectious diseases such as typhoid, leptospirosis, malaria, trypanosomiasis, pneumonia etc.

2. PRECIPITATION AND FLOCCULATION REACTION: When an antibody binds to a soluble antigen, the antigen becomes insoluble and it may precipitate or float in the fluids. If Ag – Ab complex precipitates, it is referred as "precipitation reaction". Some times the Ag-Ab complex may float instead of precipitation; in that case the reaction is called as "flocculation reaction" and the Ag-Ab complex is known as "floccule".

MECHANISM OF PRECIPITATION AND FLOCCULATION REACTION:

Depending upon its valency a single antibody can bind to more than two antigens at a time. For example IgM Ab with valency 10 can bind to a maximum of 10 Ags at a time, if it happens to get suitable epitopes in its surroundings. Since IgG antibodies valency is two they can bind to two antigens only. When a single antibody binds to more than one antigen a bridge between the soluble antigens develops and the grouped soluble antigens fail to dissolve in body fluids resulting their precipitation or flocculation.

However, the amount of precipitate and consequently it's' visibility directly depends on the quantities of both antigen and antibody and their ratio. When the Ag, Ab proportion is optimum the precipitate formation shows the maximum level. If the amount of antibody is excess than Ags, precipitation formation is not at maximum level and the serum is not saturated. When antigen is in excess only, small antigen-antibody complexes are able to form and the small complexes are fairly soluble. Since the Ags are excess, the available Abs may not be sufficient to form a lattice, necessary for precipitation or flocculation.

3. COMPLEMENT FIXATION: Antibody binding with antigen is not sufficient to remove the antigen from body. Hence Ag-Ab complex initiates activation and binding of complement system to it. Binding of complement system to Ag-Ab complex is known as complement fixation. The activated complement enzymes continue further immune reaction that finally removes the foreign agent (antigen).

MECHANISM OF COMPLEMENT FIXATION:

Inactive enzymes of complement system get activated in a cascade manner in the presence of Ab- Ag complex, and bind to the pathogen to form membrane associated complex- MAC. (For further details Refer chapter 9). The complement fixation assay can be used to check presence of specific antibody or specific antigen in an individual's serum. It was widely used to diagnose infections, particularly microbial infections and rheumatic diseases that are not easily detected by culture methods. But now new serological methods such as ELISA, PCR and DNA-based methods of pathogen detection are in use for clinical diagnosis.

4. OPSONIZATION: Innate immunity of an individual keeps constant vigil on foreign agents entering in to the body and the accessory cells of immune system phagocytise the foreign agents to save the body from them. However certain antigens escape the phagocytic action through various ways. If antibody binds to such antigen, it becomes susceptible for phagocytosis. This process is known as "Opsonization". The antibody that is making the antigen susceptible for pagocytosis is known as "opsonin".

MECHANISM OF OPSONIZATION:

The antibodies or opsonins bind to the surface antigens of bacteria. The antigen antibody complex in turn initiates complement system (Refer Chapter 9). Phagocytes with receptors for Fc region of antibody moves towards Ag Ab complex through chemotactic action of activated complement system factors C2a, C4a etc. and attach to the bacteria through Fc region of antibody. Either phagocytosis or MAC formation on the surface of bacteria results in lyses and removal of bacteria.

EFFECTS OF Ag – Ab INTERACTION:

Generally antigen antibody interaction is beneficial to the host. It enhances humoral immune response of the host. Binding of antibodies to toxic molecules neutralizes their toxic effect and protects the host from the adverse effect of toxins. Through activation of compliment enzymes and phagocytic cells Ag – Ab complex helps the host in removal of pathogens from the body. In certain conditions such as auto immune diseases Ag - Ab works in a negative manner and cause problem to the host (Refer chapter 15).

HARMFUL ACT OF Ag –Ab COMPLEX:

Immune complex helps the host in various ways, such as activation of complement system, neutralization of toxins, enhancing production of phagocytes etc. But under certain conditions Ag-Ab complex induces pathological effects and results a number of diseases. For example the precipitates or floccules formed are circulated and deposited on epithetical cells of various organs and initiates immune reactions. The immune cells cause damage to their own healthy cells to which the immune complex has been attached.

Diagnostic tests and Ag-Ab complex: Direct measurement of antibodies binding to antigens is the principle, generally used in majority of quantitative serological assays. Since secondary reactions such as agglutination, complement fixation, precipitation etc. can be detected in a variety of ways, majority of diagnostic tests depend on secondary reactions followed by Ag, Ab binding. Some of the popular diagnostic tests are as follows.

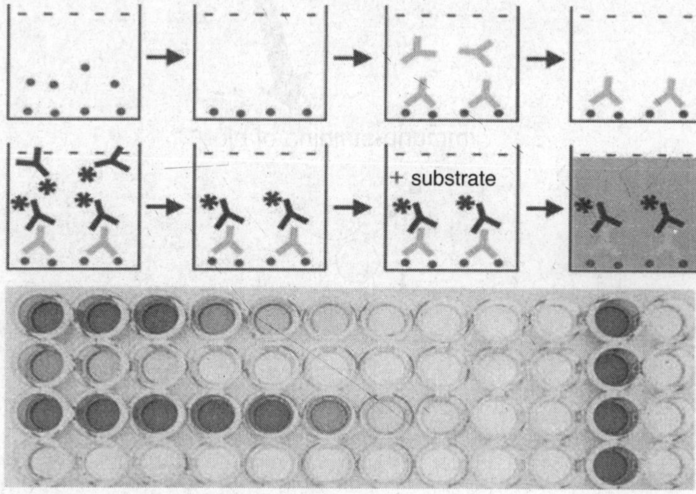

Fig: 8.3

1. ELISA or Enzyme linked immunosorbant assay: ELISA is a widely-used method for measuring the concentration of a particular molecule (e.g, a hormone or drug) in a fluid such as serum or urine. It is also known as "enzyme immunoassay or EIA". It is used as an initial screen for HIV detection. Based on the principle of antigen - antibody interaction, this test allows for easy visualization of results and can be completed without the additional concern of radioactive materials use. The test is performed in a 8 cm x 12 cm plastic plate which contains an 8 x 12 matrix of 96 wells, each of which are about 1 cm high and 0.7 cm in diameter. In HIV test partially purified, antigens are pre-coated onto an ELISA plate. When patient serum with antibodies for pathogen/ HIV is added the antibodies bind to the antigens of pathogen on the plate.

2. Western Blot:

Western blots allow investigators to determine the molecular weight of a protein and to measure relative amounts of the protein present in different samples.

1) Proteins are separated by gel electrophoresis, usually sodium dodecyl sulfate polyacrylamide gel electrophoresis (SDS-PAGE).

2) The proteins are transferred to a sheet of special blotting paper called

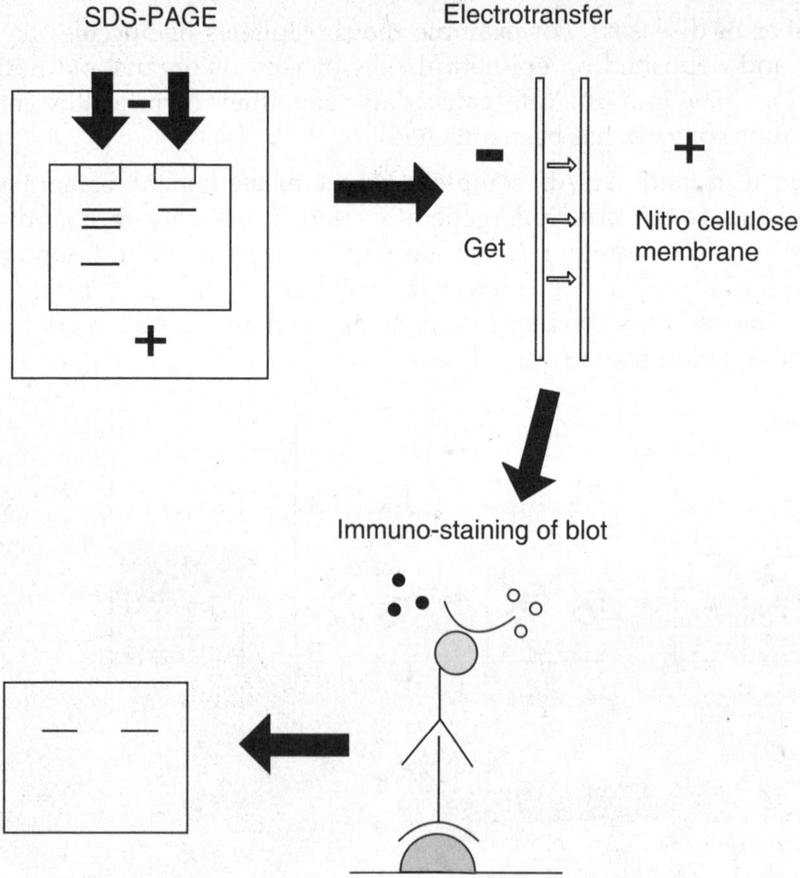

Fig. 8.4

nitrocellulose, though other types of paper, or membranes, can be used. The proteins retain the same pattern of separation they had on the gel.

3) The blot is incubated with a generic protein (such as milk proteins) to bind to any remaining sticky places on the nitrocellulose. An antibody is then added to the solution which is able to bind to its specific protein. The antibody has an enzyme (e.g. alkaline phosphatase or horseradish peroxidase) or dye attached to it which cannot be seen at this time.

4) The location of the antibody is revealed by incubating it with a colorless substrate that the attached enzyme converts to a colored product that can be seen and photographed.

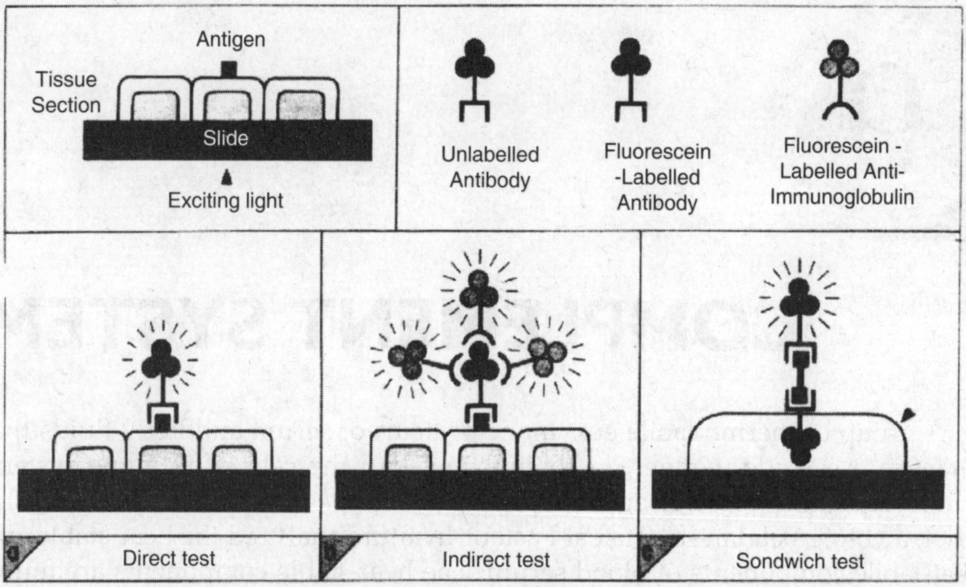

Fig: 8.5

3. Immunofluorescence:

Immunofluorescence is a laboratory technique to identify specific antibodies or antigens. The exact technique may vary depending on the specific antibody that is being investigated and between different laboratories.

In general, cells, tissue, or some other substance is placed onto microscope slides. A small amount of sample containing antibodies (typically serum, a liquid portion of blood) is placed over the cells or tissue, allowing the antibodies that are specific for the particular tissue or cellular antigens to bind.

The serum is washed away, and a second antibody that binds to human antibodies (often made in another animal species such as rabbits or goats) is applied to the slide. This second antibody has a fluorescent dye chemically linked to it. If serum of the person used for test has antibodies that bind to the tissue or cells, a bright fluorescence can be seen by use of a special microscope.

9

COMPLEMENT SYSTEM

A group of thermo labile enzymatic proteins of serum and body fluids that interact in a cascade manner, in conjunction with the cells of immune system, during eradication of foreign agents is known as "*Complement System*". In 1896, Jules Bordet, a young Belgian scientist at Pasteur Institute analyzed the heat-stable and a heat-labile components of blood serum. The heat-stable components are found to provide immunity against specific microorganisms, whereas the heat-labile components are found to be responsible for the non-specific antimicrobial activity and are capable of killing bacteria. He referred these heat-labile components as "alexia". Paul Ehrlich introduced the term "complement" to the same components /enzymes to suit their characteristic function. Since components/enzymes are activated immediately in the presence of pathogens, and not specific to any antigen, they are considered as a part of innate immunity. However, antibody activates some of the complement proteins, so complement activation is also a part of humoral immunity.

Complement enzymes stimulates inflammation, facilitates antigen phagocytosis, and also destroy some cells directly. About 20 serum and membrane enzymes or proteins are identified to have a complementary role in immune response. Most of the complement enzymes are inactive, until they are cleaved by a protease. The cleaved complement enzyme in turn becomes protease to activate the remaining enzymes of the complement system. Thus many components of the complement system serve as the substrate of a prior component and then as an enzyme to activate a subsequent component. Their activity remains for a very short time. If they fail to react with next enzyme they become inactive again. This pattern of sequential activation produces an expanding cascade of activity (reminiscent of the operation of the blood clotting system).

Complement components are numbered 1 to 9 with a prefix C e.g. C1, C2.... C9, in the order in which they are discovered. Fortunately numbering is almost the same as the order in which they function in the activation cascade. C1 is composed of three subcomponents C1q, C1r, and C1s. Components C3 and C5 are involved in the generation of anaphylotoxis and in the promotion of leukocyte chemotaxis, the result of these two activities begin the inflammatory response. C1 and C4 are involved in the neutralization of viruses. The components also combine in various sequences to participate in other biological activities, including antibody-mediated cell lysis, phagocytosis, opsonization and anaphylaxis. The complement system is known to be activated by the immunoglobulins IgM and IgG.

During activation, some complement components split into two parts. The larger fragment of the molecule is usually referred as "b" and the smaller fragment is referred as "a". Fragment b remains attached to the pathogen; while the smaller fragment 'a' having other biological activities diffuse away. The b fragment which participates further in the complement cascade is usually larger than the other fragment "a". Activated complement fragments with enzymatic activity may be indicated by placing a bar over their numbers for e.g. active C3 can be represented as $\overline{C3}$ and inactive complement is indicated as Ci. Convertase is the general name used for a complement enzyme that converts an inactive complement protein into an active one. For example, active C3 convertase converts inactive C3 to active C3a and C3b.

Fragments released from individual components during activation of complement system, operate by a non-cytolytic mechanism through specific receptors present on various cell types. The direction and intensity of the biological response depends on the state of the receptors (affinity and density) and on the function of cells bearing the receptors.

From the functional standpoint, complement receptors can be divided into two types. Receptors of the first type are adherent in nature. The adherent receptors mediate adherence of cells and other particles with membrane bound C3b or C4b fragments and are known as "complement receptors" in short they are represented as CRs. Adherence reaction mediated through the CR receptors on phagocytes lead to stimulation of phagocytosis, activation of metabolism, secretary function and movement of phagocytes towards the site of inflammation. The complement receptors, present on the other cells of the immune system are involved in a variety of immunoregulatory reactions. For example CR1 on erythrocytes may bind circulating immune complexes (that had activated complement) and transport them to the liver where the immune complexes are partially degraded and thus become more soluble.

The second type of receptors reacts with small fragments of components of complement system, such as C4a, C3a, C5a etc., as well as with C1q, Ba, and factor H. Stimulation of these receptors results in various biological reactions such as chemotaxis, anaphylactic reaction, secretion of vasoactive amines, mediators of the inflammatory reactions etc.

Synthesis of components of complement system takes place at various sites of the body. For example Hepatic parenchymal cells synthesize C3, C6, C8 and B components. C1 is synthesized by columnar epithelial cells of gut. C4 and C2 are produced by macrophages in primary organs. Fetal lung, liver and intestine produce C5, and C2. C3, C4, C5, B, D, P are synthesized in intestinal epithelium. The levels of complement enzymes are regulated by genes.

Chromosome 1 contains the genes for C1q, C8, C4b, factor H, CR1, CR2, and DAF, and chromosome 12 contains the genes for C1r and C1s. The gene for C3 has been localised to chromosome 19, factor I to chromosome 4 and C1 (IA) to chromosome 11. Four complement proteins, the C4A isotype, the C4B isotype, C2 and factor B, are encoded by genes within the major histocompatibility complex (MHC) on chromosome 6.

Activation of Complement system takes place through three different pathways; they are "**classical complement pathway**", "**lectin pathway**", and "**alternative complement pathway**". The pathways differ in the manner in which they are activated and ultimately produce a key enzyme called C3 convertase, but all the three pathways share a common terminal reaction, i.e. formation of membrane attack complex (MAC). C3 cleavage in each pathway leads to activation of C5-C9 and MAC formation. MAC causes destruction of target cell. Nucleated cells in general are relatively resistant to lysis by complement system, due to their ability to remove MAC by endocytosis or through repair mechanism.

Complete action of complement enzymes in immune reactions can be studied in three phases.

1. Recognition and activation phase: The first stage is recognition and activation phase. In this phase components of complement system recognize cell bound antibodies or antibody in immune complex and get activated.

2. Enzymatic phase: Enzymatic phase is characterized by amplification of complement enzymes.

3. Attack phase: Attack phase shows the formation of membrane bound complement complex (MAC) for attack on the target cell.

Table : 9.1 COMPLEMENT RECEPTORS

RECEPTOR	LIGANDS	FUNCTIONS
CR1 (CD35)	C3b, C3bi, C4b, C4bi	Opsonization and antigen clearance (phagocytes), Antigen persistence (FDC), Immune complex clearance (RBC),Complement regulation
CR2 (CD21)	C3d, C3dg, C3bi, EBV	B cell activation (B cells, FDC)
CR3,(MAC-1, CD11b/CD18)	C3bi	Adhesion, extravasation, phagocytosis (macrophages, neutrophils)
CR4 (p150.95, CD11c/CD18)	C3b	Adhesion, extravasation, phagocytosis (macrophages, neutrophils)
C1qR	C1q	Immune complex binding to phagocytes, (macrophages, neutrophils)
C5aR	C5a	Adherence, phagocytosis, CR1 and CR3 expression (macrophages, neutrophils)
C3aR, C4aR, C5aR	C3a, C4a, C5a	Mast cell degranulation Smooth muscle contraction

THE CLASSICAL COMPLEMENT PATHWAY

Recognition and activation phase: The classical pathway is the major effector function of the complement system in humoral immune response. Either IgG or IgM antibody bound to antigen triggers the classical pathway. Binding of antibody to antigen exposes "Fc region"- the binding and activating site for the first complement component C1. When at least two Fc regions of antigen bound antibodies are exposed, the C1q sub components of C1 get activated and bind to the exposed sites initiating the cascade of complement activation reactions. C1q is a hexameric molecule comprised of "stalks" and "knobs". It undergoes a conformational change after binding with Fc region. The protruding knobs of the C1q molecule bind to exposed Fc sites of antigen-bound antibody, and initiates activation of the remaining sub components of C1, followed by the cascade of remaining activation reactions. Pairs of activated C1r and C1s molecules associate with one another, to make a shape of figure-8. This figure-8 fits over the knobs of the C1q molecule to make a complete, intact C1 molecule. Activated C1s are responsible for the cleavage of the next two components C4 and C2 involved in the reactions. (Remember, the numbers indicate the order in which the components were discovered, not the order in which they activate in the cascade). C4 is cleaved into two unequal fragments C4a and C4b. The larger C4b molecule attaches to the target membrane nearby while the small C4a molecule floats away.

The free surface of deposited C4b is available to interact with the next complement component C2. Activated C1s again cleave the C2 molecule into two fragments C2a and C2b. C2b fragment binds with the C1, C4b complex and C2b fragment floats away. C4b2b is also known as the C3 convertase, because its role is to convert the next complement component. The C3 convertase of the classical pathway splits C3 into two fragments, C3a and C3b. The convertase has the ability to cleave multiple C3 molecules, forming plenty of C3a and C3b fragments. The C3a fragments float away and have a role in inducing an inflammatory response. The C3b binds to the C4b2b to form C4b2b3b complex or C5 convertase. Like the C3 convertase C5 convertase catalyzes the cleavage of number of C5 complement component molecules into C5a and C5b before it reverts to inactivity. C5a floats away and contributes to inflammation while the C5b fragment binds to the cell surface on which the antigen is present. This binding of C5b to the cell surface is the initial step in the formation of the membrane attack complex (MAC). The period of activation reactions, up to the conversion of inactive C5 into active form are considered as enzymatic phase of complement system. C5a is a powerful chemo attractant of neutrophils and monocytes.

The attack phase

Attachment of C5b to the membrane leads to uncovering of binding sites on C6 and C7. The C6 and C7 components with active sites join C5b on cell membrane resulting in the formation of membrane bound C5b67 complex. This trimolecular membrane bound complex initiates binding of C8 to the cell membrane along with them. The C5b678 complex acts as a receptor for a variable number of membrane-disrupting C9 molecules. The resultant C5b678 and poly-C9 complex is known as "membrane attack complex."(MAC). The MAC polymerizes membrane constituents and creates a trans membrane channel of about 1000A in diameter. The trans membrane pore or lesion results lysis of the target cell.

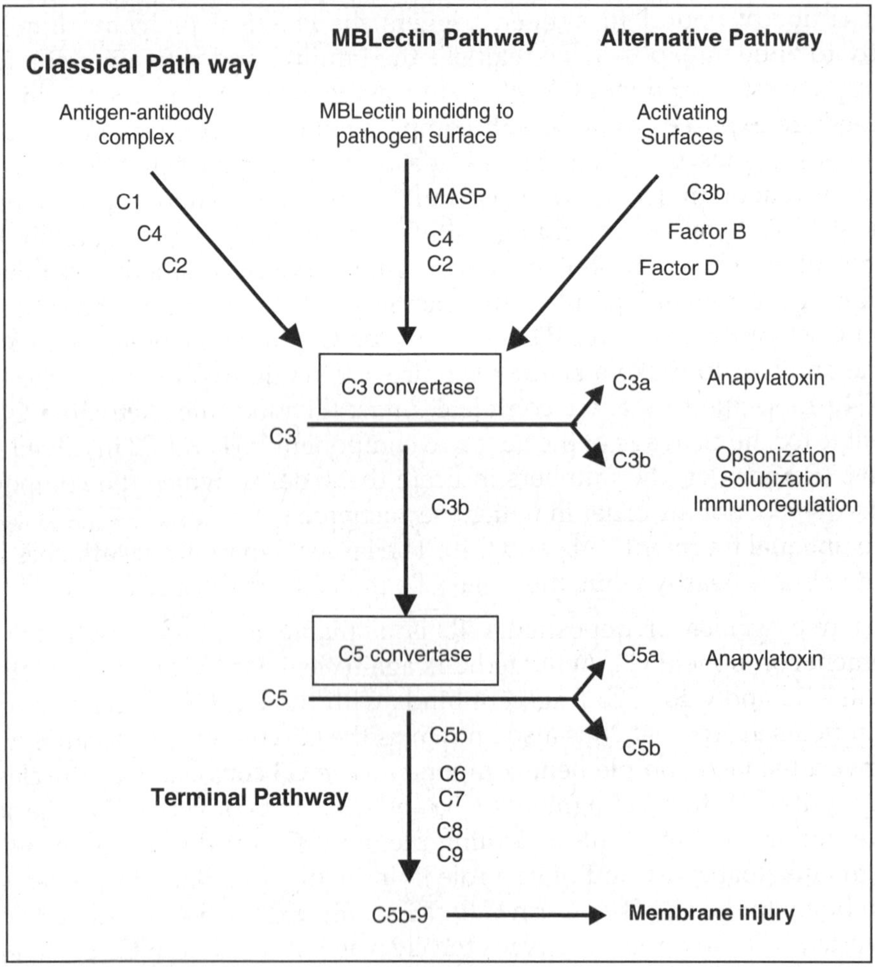

Fig. 9.1

ALTERNATIVE PATHWAY OR PROPERDIN PATHWAY

Alternative pathway is independent of antibodies, surface polysaccharide of certain microbes or antitoxins can activate alternate pathway hence it provides an immediate defense against microbes. This pathway involves about 6 serum proteins C3, B, D, P, H and I. The alternative pathway was discovered by Pillemer in 1954. Alternative pathway is also known as "Properdin path way". The Latin word Properdin (Pro-to prepare, Pedro - to destroy) means to destroy. Properdin path way provides protection against bacteria, flung certain viruses, virus infected cells and tumors.

The Properdin path way skips C1, C4 and C2 components of complement system and start from C3. C3 component breaks down slowly but spontaneously in plasma due to serum and tissue protease activity; hence a small amount of C3b is always present in body fluids. Break down of C3 exposes a highly reactive thiol ester group on C3b fragment. In this condition it may attach to any cell surface. If C3b attaches to any suitable surface and remains active, further cascade action of complement system continues resulting in the formation of MAC. Normal body cells with high levels of membrane sialic acid inactivates C3b even if C3b binds to them, but unlike body cells bacteria with low external sialic acid fails to inactivate C3b and allows further reactions.

Membrane-bound C3b fragments are bound by Factor B which is in turn cleaved by Factor D. From the cleaved B fragments a and b fragment Ba floats away, while Bb stays associated with C3b. The resulting C3bBb molecule acts as C3 convertase in alternative pathway. It rapidly produces more C3b and C3a from C3. C3b covalently attaches to the pathogen surface and acts as an opsonin, while C3a stimulates inflammation. The C3 convertase of the alternative pathway is however not particularly stable. In order to effectively split a relevant number of C3 molecules, the C3 convertase requires the stabilization of another molecule, properdin (a plasma protein), which binds to the C3bBb complex and extends the half-life of its activity. Since C3bBb is stabilized by the plasma protein properdin, the alternative pathway is referred as properdin pathway.

The alternative pathway C3 convertase acts just like the classical pathway enzyme of the same name and cleaves hundreds of C3 molecules into C3a and C3b. The C3b molecule remains attached to form the alternative pathway C5 convertase C3bBb3b. This enzyme cleaves C5 into C5a and C5b. The C5b molecule remains associated with the membrane and associates with C6 through C9 to form the MAC, as described above in classical pathway. Factors H, I and P regulate activity of C3b Bb3b according to the requirement.

THE LECTIN PATHWAY:-

Like Properdin or alternate pathway, Lectin Pathway is independent of Abs. This pathway is activated by mannose binding Lectin (MBL). Mannose binding Lectin is always present in serum and binds to mannose residues on the surface of pathogens. Binding of MBL to the surface of pathogen, induces activation of MBL-associated serine proteases MASP-1, and MASP-2. The MBL with active serine proteases (MBSP) split C4 into C4a, C4b and C2 into C2a, C2b. C4b and C2b then bind together to form the C3-convertase, as in the classical pathway. The remaining cascade action of complement system is similar to classical pathway.

Lectins are sugar-binding proteins which are highly specific for their sugar moieties. They typically play a role in biological recognition phenomena involving cells and proteins. For example, some viruses use lectins to attach themselves to the cells of the host organism during infection.

Ficolins are homologous to MBL and function via MASP in a similar way. In invertebrates without an adaptive immune system, ficolins are expanded and their binding specificities diversified to compensate the lack of pathogen-specific recognition molecules.

REGULATION OF COMPLEMENT ACTIVITY:-

Complement activity is carefully regulated by serum levels of complement components, natural decay of the activated fragments, serum protease inhibitors, and specific complement inhibitors. C1 inhibitor (C1INH) is a plasma protein which dissociates activated C1r and C1s from C1q, limiting the active time of the complex. It blocks spontaneous activation of C1 also.

Several inhibitory proteins such as C4 binding protein (C4Bp), Factor H etc. dissociate the C3 and C5 convertases and promote degradation of C4b and C3b by Factor I. C4Bp and decay accelerating factor (DAF) occupy C2 binding place and prevent C2 binding with C4, an essential step in the activation process of complement system.

Certain enzymes like carboxy peptidases in serum destroy the anaphylactic and chemotactic activities of C3a, C4a and C5a fragments and block formation of MAC on host cells. Factors H, I and P regulate activity of C3bBb according to the requirement. MAC can detach from the target cell and cause damage to the neighbouring healthy cells through its binding. To prevent damage through this mechanism, certain serum proteins known as "S proteins" bind with the detached units to prevent their binding with the healthy cells.

FUNCTIONS OF COMPLEMENT SYSTEM

Complement is not antigen-specific and it is activated immediately in the presence of a pathogen, hence it is considered as a part of innate immunity. Complement stimulates inflammation, facilitates antigen phagocytosis, and lyses of some cells directly. Even though pathways of complement activation are different in different conditions, many of the components participating in the effector functions are same.

The fragments of activated components of complement system are called "opsonins". "Opsonins adhere to micro organisms to promote leukocyte chemo attraction, antigen binding, phagocytosis and activation of macrophage and neutrophil killing mechanisms. Complement fragments also known as "anaphylatoxins" promote an inflammatory response by binding to complement receptors on mast cells and triggering release of histamine. Histamines increases blood vessel permeability and smooth muscle contraction. Complement is also important for neutralization of virus and removal of immune complex.

Complement activation stimulates several antimicrobial activities. The end point is formation of a membrane attack complex (MAC), which inserts into lipid membranes of bacteria or eukaryotic cells and causes osmotic lysis.

Complement binds to specific receptors on various cell types to mediate its inflammatory and opsonic activities. The best characterized of these receptors is CR1, which binds the opsonin fragments C3b and C4b and promotes phagocytosis and clearance of antigen-antibody complexes in combination with antibody binding to FcR.

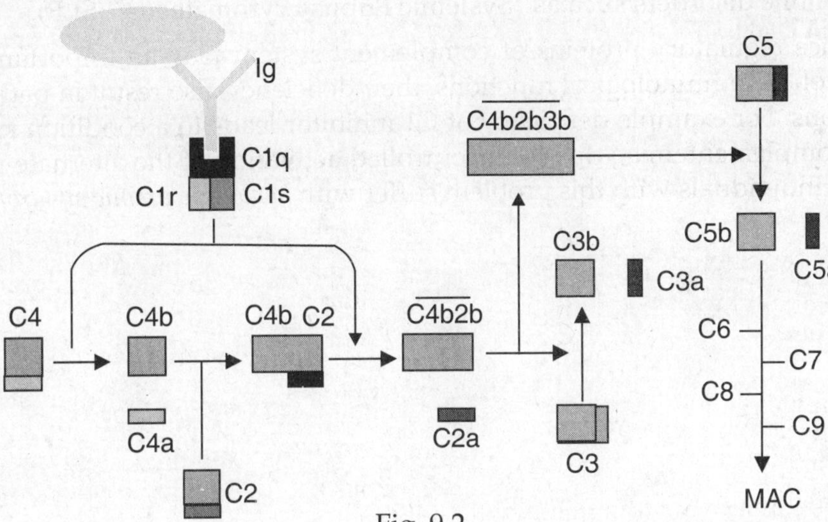

Fig. 9.2

A receptor for C1q also promotes immune complex binding to phagocytes. CR2 (complement 2 receptor) is part of the B cell receptor complex. Binding of antigen-complement complexes to CR2 increases the sensitivity of the B cell to antigen up to a thousand fold. CR3 and CR4 allow monocytes, macrophages, neutrophils, and dendritic cells to adhere to blood vessel walls and move into the tissues (extravasate) at the site of inflammation.

Receptors for the anaphylatoxins signal for mast cell degranulation (releasing histamine) and smooth muscle contraction. C5a receptor also signals macrophages to phagositize complement-coated antigen in the absence of IgG binding to FcR

COMPLEMENT DEFICIENCIES:-

Deficiencies in any of the defense mechanism of host can lead to severe microbial infections. Deficiencies of complement proteins are frequently associated with an immunodeficiency state similar to the condition associated with immunoglobulin deficiency. The individuals suffer with recurrent infections from organisms that are normally susceptible to opsonisation or lysis by complement system.

A variety of hereditary and acquired complement deficiency states have been reported from early 1970s in conjunction with severe bacterial infections and, perhaps more surprisingly in individuals with disease conditions associated with autoimmunity and immune complex formation. Generally deficiencies of complement enzymes are congenital. Properdin deficiency is X-linked, while other genetic defects within the complement system appear to be transmitted as autosomal recessive traits. However hereditary angio-edema is due to heterozygous deficiency or dysfunction of the C1 inhibitor protein. In addition, homozygous C4a and C4b deficiencies may have pathogenetic importance.

Congenital deficiency of C3 component is lethal and results in most hazardous conditions. Deficiency of C6 or C7 components may not show much effect on immunity. Deficiencies of C2, C1r or C4 are commonly associated with autoimmune disorders such as "Systemic Lupus Erythmatosus" (SLE).

Since regulatory proteins of complement system play an important role in regulation of immunological functions, their deficiency also result in pathological conditions. For example deficiency of C1 inhibitor leads to a condition known as "hypocomplementemia" due to uncontrolled activation of the alternate pathway and the individuals with this problem suffer with *hemolytic uremic syndrome*.

10

CYTOKINES

The word "Cytokines" (cyto-cell; and kinos - movement) is derived from Greek which means "cell movement". They are intercellular messengers, responsible for signaling an incredible variety of cell functions, such as embryogenesis, hematopoesis, tissue repair, inflammation, immune reactions etc. In terms of origin and purpose they are a more divers' class of compounds, and are produced by a wide variety of hematopoietic and non-hematopoietic cells. Cytokines are released by cells directly in to the tissue or in to the circulation and can have autocrine, paracrine and endocrine effects.

They act by binding to their specific receptors located in the cell membrane and initiate a signal cascade in the cell that eventually results biochemical and phenotypical changes in the target cell. Even though cytokines perform various functions, generically the term cytokines has been used to refer to the immunemodulating agents such as interleukins, interferons, chemokines, growth factors etc. Cytokines play major role in the development and functioning of both the innate and adaptive immune response.

Cytokines secreted by lymphocytes are referred as lymphokines. Lymphokines are often secreted by lymphocytes that have encountered a pathogen, there by activating and recruiting further immune cells to increase the system's response to the pathogen.

Autocrine effect, influencing the cell that secreted it.

Paracrine, influencing the cells in the immediate vicinity of a cytokine's secretions

Endocrine, influencing the cells at distant regions of the body (carried by blood or plasma)

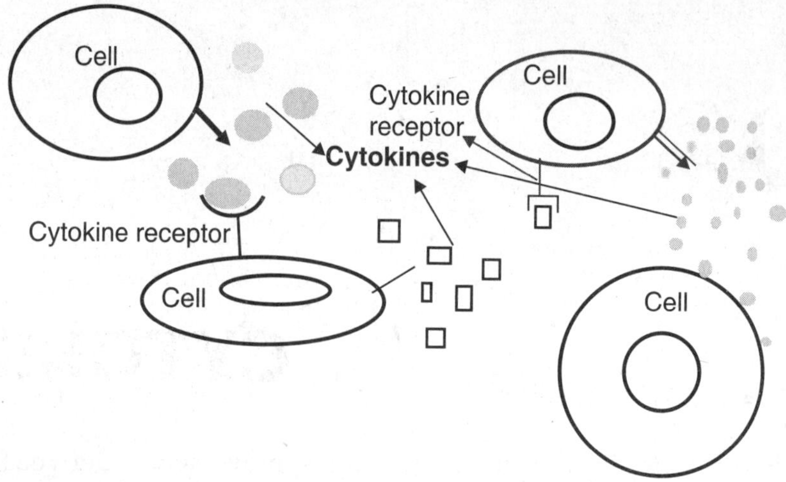

Fig. 10.1

PROPERTIES OF CYTOKINES

(1) The family of cytokines consists mainly of smaller, water-soluble proteins and glycoproteins with a mass between 8 and 30 kDa.

(2) Generally (although not always) they act over short distances and short time spans.

(3) They act by binding to specific membrane receptors, and induce specific gene expression via a second messenger (often tyrosine kinases).

(4) Cytokines are often produced in a cascade, as one cytokine stimulates its target cells to secret additional cytokines.

(5) Cytokines can act "**synergistically**" (two or more cytokines acting together) or "antagonistically" (causing opposing activities).

(6) Certain cytokines are "**redundant**" in their activity, (means similar functions can be stimulated by different cytokines)

(7) Cytokines express "**pleiotropism**" (literally means a single cytokine has many different functional effects on many different cell types, but in fact sometimes even on the same cell).

(8) They act at very low concentrations (typically 10-10 - 10-15 M) and possess very short life span.

(9) They are produced de novo in response to an immune stimulus.

(10) Responses to cytokines include increasing or decreasing expression of membrane proteins (including cytokine receptors), proliferation, and secretion of effector molecules.

(11) Cytokines are released by many cell populations, but the predominant producers are helper T cells (TH) and macrophages.

NOMENCLATURE

In general cytokines are named after their presumed function, or cell secreting it, or their target of action. For instance the term "chemokine" refers to a specific class of cytokines that mediates chemo attraction (chemotaxis) between cells. The word "interleukins" has been used to refer to the cytokines acting as mediators between different leucocytes/lymphocytes. The term "lymphokines", has been used to refer to the cytokines released by lumphocytes.

CLASSIFICATION: Cytokine are classified in two different ways one concerns their structure and the other concerns their function.

CLASSIFICATION BASED ON STRUCTURE:

Structural homology has been able to partially distinguish the cytokines that do not demonstrate a considerable degree of redundancy. Based on structural homology cytokines can be classified into four types:

(1) The four □-helix bundle family: - Members of this type of cytokines have three-dimensional structures with four bundles of □-helices. This family in turn is divided into three sub-families:

(a) The IL-2 subfamily

(b) The interferon (IFN) subfamily

(c) The IL-10 subfamily.

The first of these three subfamilies is the largest. It contains several non-immunological cytokines including erythropoietin (EPO) and thrombopoietin (THPO).

CLASSIFICATION BASED ON FUNCTION:

Classification based on function proves more useful in clinical and experimental practice. Based on the function cytokines are divided in to two types. Cytokines that enhance immunological responses come under type 1. IFN-γ, TGF-β etc. come under this category. Cytokines that favor antibody responses are referred as type -II. IL-4, IL-10, IL-13, etc. are some of the examples for type II.

RECEPTORS FOR CYTOKINES

Cytokines act on their target cells by binding to specific membrane receptors. The receptors and their corresponding cytokines have been divided into several families based on their structure and activities. They are as follows:

1. Hematopoietin family: They generally have two subunits, one is cytokine-specific sub unit and the other one is signal transducing sub unit. Cytokine binding promotes dimerization of the α and β subunits, the dimmer then associate with cytoplasmic tyrosine kinases to phosphorylate proteins which activate mRNA transcription. Receptors for IL-2 through IL-7 and GM-CSF come under this family.

2. Interferon family: These receptors have the conserved cysteine residues, but not the Trp-Ser-X-Trp-Ser sequence, and include the receptors for IFNα, IFNβ, and IFNγ.

3. Tumor Necrosis Factor family: The receptors have four extra cellular domains; they include receptors for soluble TNFα and TNFβ as well as membrane-bound CD40 (important for B cell and macrophage activation) and Fas (that signals the cell to undergo apoptosis).

4. Chemokine family: These receptors have seven transmembrane helices and interact with G protein. This family includes receptors for IL-8, MIP-1. (Some of the chemokine receptors are used by HIV to preferentially enter either macrophages or T cells).

ACTIVITIES OF CYTOKINES

Cytokines are secreted by many cell populations, but the predominant producers are helper T cells (Th) and macrophages. They are often secreted in response to some bacterial infections. While cytokines are essentially chemical messengers, they can help to regulate the quality and intensity of immune system's response. Taking cues from the signals conveyed by the cytokines, the immune system stimulates production of necessary chemicals to fight infection, as well as to suppress spread of harmful bacteria. As signalling compounds cytokines keep cell to cell communication. Since cytokines have both stimulating and suppressing action on lymphocytes and immune response, they induce temporary rise in T-cells production to combat infection, followed by a signal to cease the excess production when the pathogens are brought under control.

Table: 10.1

Selected Immune Cytokines and their Activity

Cytokine	ProducingCell	TargetCell	Function**
GM-CSF	Th cells	progenitor cells	growth and differentiation of monocytes and DC
IL-1 alpha, IL-1 beta	monocytes macrophages B cells DC	Th cells B cells NK cells various	co-stimulation maturation and proliferation activation inflammation, acute phase response, fever
IL -2	Th1 cells	activated T and B cells, NK cells	growth, proliferation, activation
IL-3	Th cells NK cells	stem cells mast cells	growth and differentiation growth and histamine release
IL-4	Th2 cells	activated B cells macrophages T cells	proliferation and differentiationIgG1 and IeG synthesis MHC Class II proliferation
IL-5	Th2 cells	activated B cells	proliferation and differentiation, IgA synthesis
IL-6	Monocytes macrophages Th2 cells stromal cells	activated B cells plasma cells stem cells various	differentiation into plasma cells Antibody secretion differentiation acute phase response
IL-7	marrow stroma thymus stroma	stem cells	differentiation into progenitor B and T cells
IL-8	Macrophages endothelial cells	neutrophils	Chemotaxis
IL-10	Th2 cells	Macrophages B cells	cytokine production activation

IL-12	Macrophages, B cells	activated Tc cells NK cells	differentiation into CTL(with IL-2) activation
IFN- alpha	Leukocytes	various	viral replicationMHC I expression
IFN- beta	Fibroblasts	various	viral replication MHC I expression
IFN- gamma	Th1 cells, Tc cells, NK cells	various Macrophages activated B cells	Viral replication MHC expression Ig class switch to IgG2a
MIP-1 alpha	Macrophages	Th2 cells Macrophages monocytes, T cells	proliferation pathogen elimination chemotaxis
MIP-1 beta	Lymphocytes	monocytes, T cells	Chemotaxis
TGF-beta	T cells, monocytes	monocytes, macrophages activated macrophages Various	Chemotaxis IL-1 synthesis activated B cells IgA synthesis *Proliferation*
TNF alpha	macrophages, mast cells, NK cells	macrophages tumor cells	CAM and cytokines expression Cell death
TNF- beta	Th1 and Tc cells	phagocytes tumor cells	phagocytosis, NO production cell death

INTERLEUKINS

Interleukins (also called lymphokines) are a group of structurally and functionally distinct soluble proteins secreted by different types of leukocytes that are involved in cell-to-cell communication. They regulate both innate and adaptive immune system. Once they are thought to mediate communication between leukocytes, hence they are referred as interleukins (means in between the leukocytes) to specify their function. Currently, it is well-known that in addition to immune cells, interleukins can be produced by many different cell types and an individual interleukin may act on different cell types, eliciting different biological responses, depending on the type of cell.

Interleukins are the primary messengers and directors of the immune system. They can cause cellular proliferation, cell activation, inflammation, physiological changes such as fever and pain, allergies etc. The expression of interleukins is usually strictly regulated, i.e., they are often not secreted constitutively. They are synthesized after cell activation as a consequence of a physiological or non-physiological stimulus. Some interleukins are auto regulatory in their function and regulate their own synthesis or the expression of their own receptors.

The interleukins are abbreviated to IL- followed by their number, eg. IL-1, IL-2, IL-3 etc. (number is given according to their discovery). Receptors of interleukins are represented with a suffix "R" e.g. IL-1R, IL-2R etc. Majority of interleukins are synthesized by helper CD_4^+ T lymphocytes. They promote the development and differentiation of T, B, and hematopoietic cells.

SOME OF INTERLEUKINS ARE AS FOLLOWS:

Interleukin - 1 or IL-1: - This is also known as lymphocyte activating factor, or adherence-promoting factor. It acts both locally and systemically. Monocytes are the main source of secreted IL-1. Activated macrophages from different sources and peripheral neutrophils also produce IL-1. Endothelial cells, fibroblasts, smooth muscle cells, keratinocytes, Langerhans cells of the skin, osteoclasts, astrocytes, epithelial cells of the thymus and the cornea, T-cells, B-cells, NK-cells and many melanoma cell lines also produce IL-1. Antigens, lectins and lymphokines secreted by T cells induce the production of IL-1. IL-1 stimulates B cells proliferation, differentiation and production of immunoglobulins. It also induces lymphokines secretion from T cells. Since it is an endogenous pyrogen it induces fever and increase serum proteins.

There are two functionally almost equivalent forms of IL-1, IL-1alpha (17 kDa, 159 amino acids) and IL-1 beta (17 kDa, 153 amino acids). They are encoded by two different genes. IL-1-beta is the predominant form in humans while IL-1-alpha is predominant in mice.

IL-1 may be of clinical significance due to its activities as a stimulator of T-cells. Since IL-1 is involved in hematopoiesis, acting directly on primitive hematopoietic cells and inducing the synthesis of colony stimulating factors, it may be useful as a stimulator of hematopoiesis either alone or in combination with other substances in clinical exercise.

Interleukin - 2 or IL-2: IL-2 is a protein of 133 amino acids, produced mainly by T-cells expressing the surface antigen CD4 following cell activation by mitogens or allogens. It is a growth factor for all subpopulations of T-lymphocytes and is synthesized as a precursor protein of 153 amino acids with the first 20 amino terminal amino acids functioning as a hydrophobic secretary signal sequence. The biological activities of IL-2 are mediated by a membrane receptor that is expressed almost exclusively on activated, but not on resting, T-cells.

It is an antigen-unspecific proliferation factor for T-cells, thus it allows clonal expansion of activated T-lymphocytes. IL-2 promotes proliferation of activated B-cells also. Due to its effects on T-cells and B-cells IL-2 is a central regulator of immune responses. It also plays a role in anti-inflammatory reactions, in hematopoiesis and in tumor surveillance. Since it supports the proliferation and clonal expansion of T-cells, that specifically attack certain tumor types, IL-2 displays significant anti-tumor activity for a variety of tumors.

Interleukin - 3 or IL-3: IL-3 is produced mainly by T-cells following cell activation by antigens and mitogens. Keratinocytes, NK-cells, mast cells, endothelial cells, and monocytes also initiate production of IL-3 by T-cells. It is synthesized as a precursor containing a hydrophobic secretary signal sequence of 19 amino acids. It functions as a growth factor that establishes link between the immune system and hematopoietic system. It supports proliferation and development of almost all types of hematopoietic progenitor cells. It induce differentiation and proliferation of myeloid progenitor cells such as erythrocytes, granulocytes etc. and release of histamine from mast cells but its biological activities are species-specific. IL-3 is a chemo attractant for eosinophils and also influences the chemotactic behavior of these cells in response to other chemotactically active factors. Substances that inhibit the activation of T-lymphocytes such as glucocorticoids or CsA (Cyclosporin A) also inhibit the production of IL-3.

Interleukin - 4 or IL-4: IL-4 is produced mainly by Th2 cells - the subpopulation of activated T-cells. Another subpopulation Th1 also produces IL-4 to a lesser extent. CD4+ cells, memory cells, mast cells, and macrophages are responsible for the release of IL4. It is a protein of 129 amino acids (20 kDa) and is synthesized as a precursor containing a hydrophobic secretary signal sequence of 24 amino acids. It induces proliferation and differentiation of activated B cells and production of IgE. Hence it plays an important role in allergic response. The biological activities of IL-4 are species-specific. IL-2 and PAF (platelet activating factor) induce the synthesis of IL-4.

Since IL-4 inhibits the production of inflammatory cytokines such as IL-1, IL-6 and TNF-alpha by monocytes and T-cells, it may be of clinical importance in the treatment of inflammatory diseases and autoimmune diseases.

Interleukin –5 or IL-5: It is a specific hematopoietic growth factor produced by T-cells. It is responsible for the growth and differentiation of eosinophils. Cells known to express IL-5 include eosinophils, NK cells, TC2 CD8+ T cells, mast cells, CD45+ CD4+ T cells, gamma delta T cells and IL-1 beta activated endothelial cells. IL-5 is best known for its activity on B cells and eosinophils. Compared to B cells, IL-5 appears to induce the differentiation of activated conventional B cells into Ig-secreting cells. IL-5 also promotes the generation of cytotoxic T-cells from thymocytes. IL-5 has long been associated with several allergic diseases including allergic rhinitis and asthma. IL-5 appears to perform a number of functions on eosinophils. Studies suggest that inflammatory-induced and locally-produced IL-5 and exotaxin may act on the bone marrow in a cooperative manner.

Interleukin - 6 or IL6: IL6 is a protein of 185 amino acids glycosylated at positions 73 and 172. This interleukin acts as both pro and anti-inflammatory cytokine. It is secreted by T cells and macrophages to stimulate immune response to trauma, especially burns or other tissue damage. It is secreted by macrophages, TH2-cells and B cells, targeting activated B cells, plasma cells, hematopoietic stem cells and T cells. IL- 6 influences differentiation of hematopoietic stem cells and induces acute phase reactions, hematopoiesis, inflammation etc. It is capable of inducing the final maturation of B-cells into immunoglobulin-secreting plasma cells, if the cells have been pre-activated by IL4. It stimulates the secretion of antibodies to such a degree that serum IgG1 levels can raise 120 – 400 folds. IL-6 is also a "myokine" (cytokine produced from muscle), and is elevated in response to muscle contraction. Smooth muscle cells in the tunica media of many blood vessels also produce IL-6 as a pro-inflammatory cytokine.

IL-6 is one of the most important mediators of fever and of the acute phase response.

Interleukin - 7or IL7: IL-7 is a hematopoietic growth factor secreted by the stromal cells of the red marrow and thymus. Keratinocytes, dendritic cells, neurons and endothelial cells also produce IL-7. It stimulates the differentiation of pleuripotent hematopoietic stem cells into lymphoid progenitor cells and proliferation of pre-B and pro-B-cells without affecting their differentiation. It also stimulates the proliferation of early and mature activated T-cells and this activity is synergized by suboptimal doses of IL1. IL-7 can be produced locally by intestinal epithelial and epithelial goblet cells, and may serve as a regulatory factor for intestinal mucosal lymphocytes.

The activity of human IL7 is not species-specific. In human peripheral monocytes IL7 induces the synthesis of some inflammatory mediators such as IL1, IL6 and MIP (macrophage inflammatory protein). IL7 also enhances the expression and secretion of IL3 and GM-CSF in activated human T-cells. IL7 down-regulates expression of TGF-beta in macrophages, which has been suggested as an inhibitor of the antitumor immune response.

Interleukin - 8 or IL-8: It is a non-glycosylated protein of 8 kDa, produced by stimulated monocytes and other cell types such as macrophages, fibroblasts, endothelial cells, keratinocytes, melanocytes, hepatocytes, chondrocytes, and number of tumour cell lines. In many cell types the synthesis of IL-8 is strongly stimulated by IL-1 and TNF-alpha. It is one of the major mediators of the inflammatory response and member of chemokine family. It functions as a chemoattractant, and is also a potent angiogenic factor. It differs from all other cytokines in its ability to specifically activate neutrophil granulocytes, In neutrophils IL-8 causes a transient increase in cytosolic calcium levels and the release of enzymes from granules. IL-8 also enhances the metabolism of reactive oxygen species and increases chemotaxis and the enhanced expression of adhesion molecules.

Macrophage-derived IL-8 supports angiogenesis and may play a role in disorders such as rheumatoid arthritis, tumour growth, and wound healing that critically depend on angiogenesis. IL-8 is involved in mediating pain also. Glucocorticoids, IL-4, TGF-beta, inhibitors of 5′ lipoxygenase, and 1, 25 (OH)2 vitamin D3 inhibit the synthesis of IL-8.

Interleukin –9 or IL-9: IL -9 produced by T-cells specifically CD_4^+ cells acts as a regulator for a variety of hematopoietic cells. This cytokine stimulates cell proliferation. Experimental study shows that this cytokine is a determining factor in the pathogenesis of bronchial hyper responsiveness.

Interleukin –10 or IL-10: This cytokine is produced by T-cells and specifically by CD_4^+ helper cells. It acts as a regulator of a variety of hematopoietic cells. This cytokine stimulates cell proliferation and prevents apoptosis. IL-10 displays potent abilities to suppress the antigen presentation capacity of antigen presenting cells. However, it is stimulatory towards certain T cells, mast cells. It stimulates B cell maturation and antibody production also. It is capable of inhibiting synthesis of pro-inflammatory cytokines like IFN-β, IL-2, IL-3, TNFα and GM-CSF.

Interleukin 11 (IL-11): IL-11 is a member of the IL-6-type cytokine family. It is a key regulator of multiple events in hematopoiesis, most notably the stimulation of megakaryocyte maturation. It is also known by the names Adipogenesis inhibitory factor (AGIF) and Oprelvekin. It has been demonstrated to improve platelet recovery after chemotherapy-induced thrombocytopenia, induce acute phase proteins, modulate antigen-antibody responses, participate in the regulation of bone cell proliferation and differentiation. This could be used as a therapeutic for osteoporosis. Besides lymphopoietic/hematopoietic and osteotrophic properties, it has functions in many tissues such as brain, gut and testis. IL-11 stimulates the growth of certain lymphocytes and, stimulates an increase in the cortical thickness and strength of long bones.

Interleukin 12 (IL-12): It is an interleukin that is naturally produced by dendritic cells, macrophages and human B-lymphoblast cells in response to antigenic stimulation. IL-12 is composed of a bundle of four alpha helices. It is a heterodimeric cytokine encoded by two separate genes.

Interleukin 13 (IL-13): It is a cytokine secreted by many cell types especially T helper type 2 (Th2) cells. It is an important mediator of allergic inflammation and disease. IL-13 specifically induces physiological changes in parasitized organs that are required to expel the offending organisms or their products. In addition to its effects on immune cells, it is more importantly implicated as a central mediator of the physiologic changes induced by allergic inflammation in many tissues. The functions of IL-13 overlap considerably with those of IL-4, especially with regard to changes induced on haematopoietic cells, but these effects are probably less important than the more potent role of IL-4.

Although IL-13 is associated primarily with the induction of airway disease, it also has anti-inflammatory properties. Airway matrix metallo proteinases (MMPs), which are protein-degrading enzymes, are required to induce egression of effete parenchymal inflammatory cells into the airway lumen where they are then cleared. Among other factors, IL-13 induces these MMPs as part of a mechanism that protects against excessive allergic inflammation that predisposes one to asphyxiation.

Interleukin-14 (IL-14): It is a cytokine that is also called High molecular weight B-cell growth factor (HMW-BCGF) that controls the growth and proliferation of both normal and cancerous B cells. IL-14 induces B-cell proliferation, inhibits antibody secretion, and expands selected B-cell subgroups. This interleukin is produced mainly by T cells and certain malignant B cells.

Interleukin 15 (IL-15): It is a cytokine with structural similarity to IL-2 that is secreted by mononuclear phagocytes (and some other cells) following infection by viruses. This cytokine induces cell proliferation of natural killer cells; cells of the innate immune system whose principal role is to kill virally infected cells.

IL-15 and interleukin 2 share many biological activities. They are found to bind common hematopoietin receptor subunits, and may compete for the same receptor, and thus negatively regulate each other's activity. The number of CD8+ memory cells is shown to be controlled by a balance between this cytokine and IL2. In the absence of original antigen, IL-15 provides survival signals for memory lymphocytes.

Interleukin 16 (IL-16): It is a cytokine released by a variety of cells (including lymphocytes and some epithelial cells). It is a pleiotropic cytokine that functions as a chemo attractant, a modulator of T cell activation, and an inhibitor of HIV replication. It was previously called lymphocyte chemoattractant factor (LCF). This interleukin has been shown to recruit and activate many other cells expressing the CD4 molecule, including monocytes, eosinophils, and dendritic cells. CD4 is the cell signaling receptor for mature IL-16.

Interleukin-17 (IL-17): It is the starting member of a group of cytokines called the IL-17 family. IL-17A was originally identified as a transcript from a rodent T-cell hybridoma. IL-17 shows high homology to viral IL-17 encoded by an open reading frame of the T lymphotropic rhadinovirus Herpesvirus saimiri. To elicit its functions, IL-17 binds to a type I cell surface receptor called IL-17R of which there are at least three variants IL17RA, IL17RB, and IL17RC.

Interleukin-18 (IL-18): It is pro inflammatory cytokine produced by macrophages and other cells that belongs to the IL-1 super family. IL-18 works together with IL-12 to induce cell-mediated immunity following infection with microbial products like lipopolysaccharide (LPS). After stimulation with IL-18, natural killer (NK) cells and certain T cells release another important cytokine called interferon-γ (IFN-γ) or type II interferon that plays an important role in activating the macrophages or other cells.

Interleukin-19 (IL-19): It is a cytokine that belongs to the IL-10 family of cytokines along with several other interleukins including IL-10, IL-20, IL-22, IL-24, IL-26, and several virus-encoded cytokines. It signals through the same cell surface receptor (IL-20R) that is used by IL-20 and IL-24. The IL-19 gene is expressed in resting monocytes and B cells. It is up-regulated in monocytes following stimulation with granulocyte-macrophage colony-stimulating factor (GM-CSF) or lipopolysaccharide.

Interleukin-20 (IL-20) It is a protein belonging to the IL-10 family of cytokines. IL-20 is produced by activated keratinocytes and monocytes and transmits an intracellular signal through two distinct cell-surface receptor complexes on keratinocytes and other epithelial cells. IL-20 regulates proliferation and differentiation of keratinocytes during inflammation, particularly inflammation associated with the skin. In addition, IL-20 also causes cell expansion of multipotential hematopoietic progenitor cells.

Other groups of cytokines include interferons and chemokines. Interferons inhibit virus replication in infected cells and stimulate MHC expression of antigen-presenting cell also. Chemokines attract leukocytes to infection sites.

Interferons

Interferons are cytokines produced by the cells of the immune system in response to viral infection and other stimuli. They were discovered in 1957 by British bacteriologist Alick Isaacs and Swiss microbiologist Jean Lindenmann. They are named for their ability to interfere with viruses that are replicating in host cell. Interferons are part of the non-specific immune system and are induced at an early stage in viral infection, even before the specific immune system has had time to respond. By inhibiting virus replication within host cells, activating natural killer cells and macrophages and increasing antigen presentation to lymphocytes, they induce resistance of host cells to viral infection. They are produced by all vertebrate animals and possibly by some invertebrates as well. In addition to their anti viral activity, interferons perform immunoregulatory functions such as inhibiting B-cell activation, enhancing T-cell activity, and increasing the cellular-destruction ability of natural killer cells.

Interferons secreted by cells in response to an appropriate stimulus are released into the surrounding medium. Then they bind to receptors on target cells and induce transcription of approximately 20-30 genes in the target cells leading to an anti-viral state in the target cells. Relatively little is known of interferon regulated genes. INTERFEROME is a database of interferon regulated genes and attempts to bridge the gap in knowledge by identifying and integrating information on IRGs

CLASSIFICATION OF INTERFERONS:

These interferons have been classified into two types based on the type of cell that produces the interferon and the functional characteristics of the protein. Four types of interferons have been identified: IFN-α, IFN-β IFN-ω and IFN-γ.

Type I interferons: Interferon type I is a family of products related to genes situated on chromosome 9. Type 1 includes IFN-α, IFN-β IFN-ω molecules that have relatively high antiviral potency. They are produced by macrophages, neutrophils and other somatic cells in response to infection by viruses or bacteria. After they are released, they may bind to their receptors that are expressed on most cell types, resulting in the production of over 30 different proteins in the target cell. Among them, two enzymes RNA-dependent protein kinase (PKR) and 2′-5′ oligoadenylate synthetase (2-5A synthetase) play a critical role in the inhibition of viral replication. Both enzymes can be activated by double-stranded RNA which may be present in some viruses. The activated PKR can phosphorylate a protein (eIF2) in response to new viral infections and inhibit protein synthesis. The 2-5A synthetase produces oligoadenylate that can bind and activate a cellular endonuclease to degrade mRNA. Another cellular enzyme, RNAse L also induced following PKR activation destroys RNA within the cells to further reduce protein synthesis of both viral and host genes. Inhibited protein synthesis destroys both the virus and infected host cells.

eIF-2 is a eukaryotic translation initiation factor that forms an inactive complex with another protein, called eIF2B, to reduce protein synthesis within the cell.

Type II interferon (IFN) also called immune interferon consists of the gamma form (IFN-γ). Its main purpose is to signal the immune system to respond to infectious agents or cancerous growth. IFN-γ is produced in activated TH1 and NK cells, particularly in response to IL-2 and IL-12. Binding of IFN-γ to its receptor increases the expression of class I MHC on all somatic cells and class II MHC on antigen-presenting cells. It also enhances the immunoproteasome activity. Higher

MHC I expression increases presentation of viral peptides to cytotoxic T cells, while the immunoproteasome processes viral peptides for loading onto the MHC I molecule, thereby increasing the recognition and killing of infected cells by T cells. Higher MHC II expression increases presentation of viral peptides to helper T cells; these cells release cytokines that signal to and co-ordinate the activity of other cells of the immune system. IFN-γ may also activate macrophages, neutrophils and NK cells.

Type II interferons induce about 20-30 proteins, and the function of many of these is not fully understood. However, three of the proteins 2′5′ oligo A synthase, ribonuclease and protein kinase playing an important role in the induction of the anti-viral state have been studied intensively. Expression of 2′5′ oligo A synthase results in activation of ribonuclease which can break down mRNA, and expression of the third protein - protein kinase results in inhibition of the initiation step of protein synthesis. These activities target viral protein synthesis, but also result in inhibition of host protein synthesis.

FUNCTIONS OF INTERFERONS:

Interferons increase expression of class I MHC molecules and thus promote recognition by cytotoxic T cells. They can activate NK cells that can kill virus-infected cells. They play an important role in the first line of defense against viral infections. Research work revealed that, these substances could prevent not only viral infections but also suppress the growth of cancers in some laboratory animals.

The gene that codes this cytokine is switched on in an infected cell. The interferon synthesized and secreted to the surroundings warns other viruses. The pre warned cell then produces translation inhibition factor to inhibit viral replication through reduced translation initiation and reduced protein synthesis.

Interferon acts as an inducer and causes increased production of the p53 gene product in virus infected cells. This promotes apoptosis, limiting the ability of the virus to spread.

THERAPEUTIC USES OF INTERFERONS

Interferon has been shown to have therapeutic effect against certain cancers and could supplement or replace chemotherapy drugs that activate p53. But they cause unwanted side effects. In 1980s interferon □ in low doses came into use, to treat hairy-cell leukemia (a rare form of blood cancer). Higher doses are recommended to combat Kaposi sarcoma, which frequently appears in AIDS patients. The alpha interferon form has been approved for treating the viral infections also.

Now interferon therapy in combination with chemotherapy and radiation is in use for many cancers. Interferons (interferon beta-1a and interferon beta-1b) are also used in the treatment and control of multiple sclerosis - an autoimmune disorder. Use of various types of interferons has been approved in the treatment of certain cases of acute and chronic hepatitis. Interferon alpha and beta have been used to treat various viral infections.

Since interferons are species-specific they are scarce and expensive until 1980.

But the advances in genetic engineering (R DNA technology) made it possible to produce interferons on large scale for therapeutic purpose.

SIDE EFFECTS OF INTERFERONS

The most frequent side effects are - increased body temperature, fatigue, headache, muscle pain, convulsion, dizziness, hair thinning, and depression. Erythema, pain and hardness on the spot of injection are also frequently observed. Interferon therapy causes immunosuppression but all the side effects are usually reversible and disappear within a year after the therapy has been stopped.

RESISTANCE OF VIRUS TO INTERFERONS

Unfortunately many viruses have evolved mechanisms to resist interferon activity. Certain viruses evade the interferon's response by blocking downstream signaling events that occur after the cytokine binds to its receptor, by preventing further interferon production, and by inhibiting the functions of proteins that are induced by interferon. Some of the viruses may code proteins that can block interferon binding to cells. The ability of interferon to induce protein production from interferon stimulated genes (ISGs) can also be affected by the viruses. For example production of protein kinase R can be disrupted in cells infected with *Japanese Encephalitis* Virus (JEV) or *flaviviruses*. Some viruses escape the anti-viral activities of interferons by genetic mutation. The resistant virus may escape the influence of interferon by blocking complement activation, interfering in surface expression of MHC or by preventing the host cell committing apoptosis.

CHEMOKINES

Chemokines are chemotactic cytokines which play a crucial role in immune and inflammatory reactions and in viral infection. They are approximately 8 to 11 kilodaltons (kD) in molecular weight and are active over a 1 to 100 ng/ml concentration. Chemokines are produced by a wide variety of cell types. The production of chemokines is induced by exogenous irritants and endogenous mediators such as IL-1, TNF- α , PDGF, and IFN-α .

Their name chemokines is derived from their ability to induce directed chemotaxis in nearby responsive cells. They attract and activate leukocytes and regulate diverse cellular systems and organs ranging from blood vessels to the central nervous system. Some chemokines are considered pro-inflammatory and can be induced during an immune response to promote cells of the immune system to a site of infection, while others are considered homeostatic and are involved in controlling the migration of cells during normal processes of tissue maintenance or development. Chemokines are found in all vertebrates, some viruses and some bacteria, but none have been described for other invertebrates. These proteins exert their biological effects by interacting with G protein-linked transmembrane receptors called chemokine receptors, that are selectively found on the surfaces of their target cells.

Interaction between the chemotactic factor and its corresponding receptor triggers a series of coordinated biochemical events which include changes in the cell transmembrane potential, altered cyclic nucleotide levels and ion flow across the cytoplasmic membrane and increased glucose utilization and oxygen consumption. The composition of membrane phospholipids is altered and arachidonic acid released by phospholipases, is metabolized into a number of biologically active intermediates and products. Within a few minutes, the leukocyte changes its shape that is oriented along the direction of chemotactic gradient. Reorganization of cytoskeletal contractile elements, particularly actin microfilaments and microtubular structures, contributes to the change in shape.

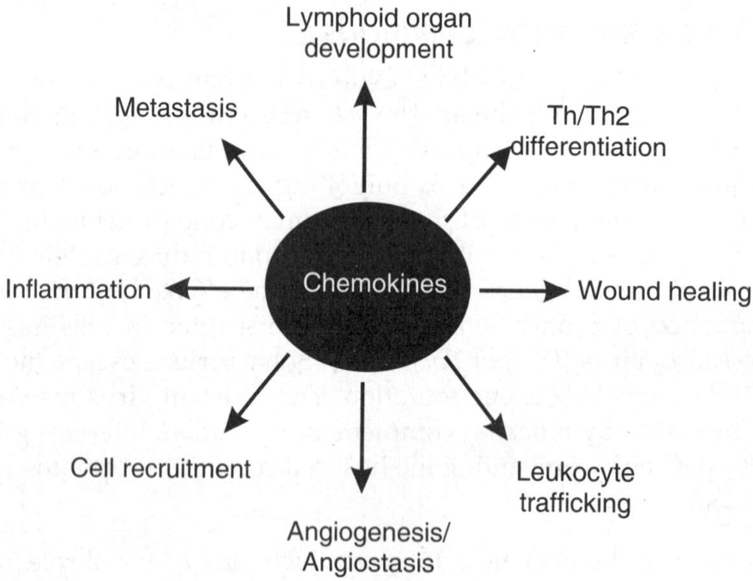

Fig. 10.2

The amino acids such as cysteines that are important for creating three dimentional tertiary structures are conserved in all chemokines. All the chemokine molecules share 20-50% structural similarities, including four conserved cysteine residues which form disulphide bonds in the tertiary structure of the proteins. The first two cysteines are situated near the N-terminal end of the mature protein, the third cysteine resides in the centre of the molecule and the fourth is in C-terminal end.

Approximately 50 human chemokines that are known segregate into four families on the basis of differences in structure (especialy on the spacing of their first two cysteine residues) and function. They are as follows:

(1) CC chemokines: The largest family of chemokines is named as "CC chemokines" due to the presence of first two of the four cysteine residues in adjacent position to each other. About 27 distinct members of this subgroup have been reported in mammals. A small number of CC chemokines possess six cysteine amino acids instead of four. CC chemokines attract mononuclear cells to the site of chronic inflammation. The most thoroughly characterized CC chemokine is monocyte chemoattractant protein 1 (MCP-1), termed as "chemokine ligand or CCL2" in the systematic nomenclature. It is a potent agonist for monocytes, dendritic cells, memory T cells, and basophils. Other CC chemokines include macrophage inflammatory protein-1 alpha (MIP-1α) (CCL3), MIP-1-beta (CCL4) and RANTES (CCL5).

(2) CXC chemokines: The second family CXC chemokines consists of a single amino acid residue between the first two canonical cysteines. The letter "X"represent the amino acid present between the two cysteines. 17 different CXC chemokines have been described in mammals and are subdivided into two categories based on the presence of specific amino acid sequence "glutamic acid-leucine-arginine" or ELR for short before the first cysteine. ELR-positive CXC chemokines eg. interleukin-8 (CXCL8) specifically induce neutrophils to leave the bloodstream and enter into the surrounding tissue. Other CXC chemokines that lack the ELR e.g. interleukin-13 (CXCL13) tend to be chemoattractant for lymphocytes. The prototype CXCL8 also activates monocytes and may direct the recruitment of these cells to vascular lesions.

(3) C chemokines: The third group of chemokines is known as the C chemokines (or chemokines). Unlike all other chemokines the C (gamma) subfamily lacks the first and third cysteine residues. Lymphotactin (also known as SCM-1 alpha) and SCM-1 beta are currently the only two family members. Both have chemotactic activity for lymphocytes and NK cells.

(4) CX3C chemokines: The fourth group of chemokines have three amino acids between the two cysteines hence it is termed as 'CX3C chemokine" or "d-chemokines". The only CX3C chemokine discovered to date is fractalkine or CX3CL1. It is both secreted and tethered to the surface of the cell that expresses it, thereby serving as both a chemoattractant and as an adhesion molecule.

Within the fascinating world of chemokines, C and CX3C chemokines have long been regarded as two minor components, even though they present unique features and show less redundancy than the other chemokine families. Nevertheless, the body of data on their expression and role in various inflammatory disorders has grown in the past few years.

RANTES: A cytokine that is a member of the interleukin-8 superfamily of cytokines. RANTES is a protein. It is a selective attractant for memory T lymphocytes and monocytes. It binds to CCR5, a coreceptor of HIV. RANTES is an acronym for Regulated on Activation, Normal T Expressed and Secreted. It is also known as CCL5.

Fractalkine (FKN), the sole member of the CX3C chemokine family, is named for its fractal geometry. The CX3C motif, with three amino acids between the two terminal cysteines, makes fractalkine distinct from other chemokines.The structure of fractalkine, a membrane-bound glycoprotein with the chemokines domain atop an extended mucin-like stalk, is unique. Membrane-bound FKN can be markedly brought on primary endothelial cells by inflammatory cytokines; this form promotes the robust adhesion of monocytes and T lymphocytes.

Soluble FKN can be released by proteolysis at an efficient chemotactic activity level for monocytes and T cells. Thus, FKN is a versatile molecule regulating regulating both cell-cell interactions in its membrane-bound form and directed-cell migration in its soluble form. The receptor of FKN, CXC3R1, is a G protein-couple protein, which expresses T lymphocytes, monocytes, natural killer (NK) cells, microglia, and neurons.Sulfation of tyrosine enhances the function of CX3CR1 in cell capture and firm adhesion. Fractalkine is expressed constitutively in the kidney, heart, lung, and brain. Fractalkine has demonstrated an important role in CNS inflammation, cardiac allograft rejection, arteriogenesis, renal disease, psoriasis, and during pregnancy. Silverman et.al. demonstrated the presence of FKN in normal cultured microvascular endothelial and stromal cells of iris and retina in vitro. Upon inflammatory cytokine stimulation, EC also express FKN and its receptors with FKN secretion in an autocrine manner. In addition to EC chemotaxis and tube formation, FKN is an angiogenic mediator in rheumatoid arthritis.

11

HISTOCOMPATIBILITY COMPLEX

HISTOCOMPATIBILITY MOLECULES

The specific glycoprotein molecules expressed on the surface of almost all vertebrate cells are referred as "histocompatibility molecules". Histocompatibility molecules are unique in nature. Except in identical (Monozygotic) twins, no two individuals show the same type of molecules. The histocompatibility molecules of one individual act as antigens, when they are introduced into another individual. Hence they are often referred as histocompatibility antigens or transplantation antigens. With reference to their role in graft rejection histocompatibility molecules are classified in to two types. One is major histocompatibility molecules (MHC) that have major influence on transplant (graft) and the other type is minor histocompatibility molecules that have negligible impact on graft rejection.

Histo compatibility Molecules

Minor Histo compatibility Molecules   Major Histo compatibility Molecules

Major histocompatibility molecules (MHC): Discovery of the MHC was one of those numerous 'fortuitous' things in science. During 1970s, immunologists recognized the role of certain genes in acceptance or rejection of a graft. Genetic mapping revealed that these genes were all clustered in the same genetic context with three general regions. Since the protein molecules that they encode determine the compatibility of tissues of different individuals, they play a major role in graft rejection, hence they are collectively referred as "Major histocompatibility complex" (MHC). MHC loci are some of the most genetically variable coding loci in mammals.

The MHC molecules displayed on the surface of the cells help immune system in distinguishing "self" from "non-self" molecules, to get rid of the foreign agents entered into the body, before they generate any problem. Hence rapid and severe graft rejection occurs when there is mismatch of donor and recipient tissue major histocompatibility molecules. For this reason the function of the MHC can be described as pleiotropic (multiple and unrelated). Even though MHC is best known for its role in histocompatibility and in immune regulation, many other functions are not much appreciated yet.

As in most species, each class of MHC genes in man and mouse are represented by more than one locus (polygeny), in man the MHC gene cluster is referred as HLA system (Human Leucocyte Antigen system) and in mice it is referred as H2 system. The physical map of the MHC of man and mouse has been determined by cloning, mapping and sequencing techniques. Since MHC genes are codominant genes, proteins encoded by both the sets inherited from father and mothers are expressed on the surface of cells. In about 97% of cases the entire linked MHC complex is inherited intact, i.e. without recombination. The set of linked MHC alleles found on the same chromosome is called as "haplotype".

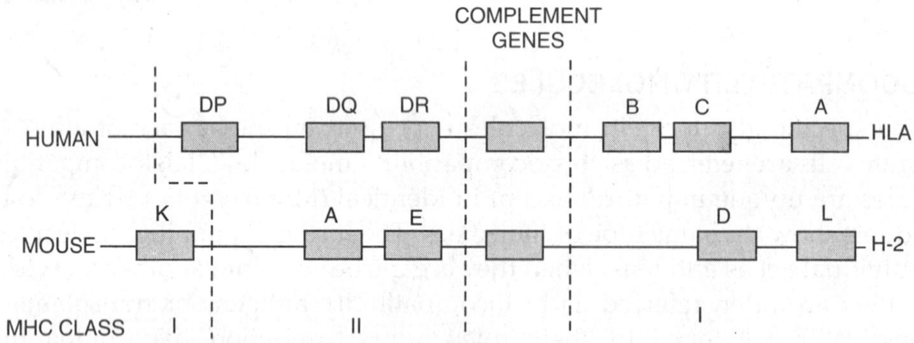

Fig. 11.1

The products of the MHC play a fundamental role in regulating immune responses. T cells recognize antigens as a complex with MHC molecules only. Since each allelic product has a unique set of peptides, with which it can bind with high affinity (though rarely certain peptides may bind to more than one MHC allele), the allelic variation of MHC molecules is functionally reflected in the selection of peptides to which it can bind. In a normal cell majority of MHC molecules are complexed with self peptides; empty MHC molecules are less stable.

PRINCIPLES OF MHC

The MHC loci are polymorphic, Many alternative forms of the gene, or alleles, exist at each locus. The diversity of the MHC within a species stems from its polymorphism. It is one of the most polymorphic genetic complexes known in higher vertebrates. For instance, HLA-A has 240 alleles, HLA-B 470 alleles, HLA-C 110 alleles

The theoretical class I diversity possible for the human is 240x470x110.

The MHC loci are closely linked. The large segment (from HLA-B to HLA-DQB) is almost always inherited as a whole.

Most individuals inherit two sets of MHC genes one from each parent. Each set of MHC genes are referred as a haplotype. A haplotypical association is usually stronger and more meaningful than an allelic association.

INHERITANCE:

MHC genes are inherited as a group (haplotype), one from each parent. Thus, a heterozygous human inherits one paternal and one maternal haplotype, each containing three class-I (B, C and A) and three class II (DP, DQ and DR) loci. A heterozygous individual will inherit a maximum of six class I specificities. Similarly, the individual also inherits DP and DQ genes and express both parental antigens. Since each chromosome is found twice (in diploid condition) in an individual, a normal tissue type involves 12 loci in HLA antigens production. Ever since each chain, and DR □- and □-chains can associate in cis (both from the same parent) or trans (one from each parent) combination. An individual can have additional DR specificities. Also, there are more than one class II MHC molecules comprising two chains (□ and □), with some antigenic determinants (specificities) on functional DR □-chain genes. Hence, many DR specificities can be found in any one individual. Haplotypes, normally, are inherited in intact condition. Hence antigens encoded by different loci are inherited together. However, on occasions, there is crossing over between two parental chromosomes, thereby resulting in new recombinant haplotypes. There is no somatic DNA recombination that occurs for antibodies and for the TCR, so the MHC genes lack recombinational mechanisms for generating diversity. Many alleles of each locus permit thousands of possible assortments. There are at least 1000 officially recognized HLA alleles.

NOMENCLATURE:

HLA specificities are identified by a letter for locus and a number (A1, B5, etc.), and the haplotypes are identified by individual specificities (e.g., A1, B7, Cw4, DP5, DQ10 DR8). Specificities which are defined by genomic analysis (through PCR), are named with a letter for the locus and a four digit number (e.g. A0101, B0701, C0401, etc.)

Specificities of Mouse MHC (H-2) are identified by a number. Since laboratory mice are inbred, each strain is homozygous and has a unique haplotype. The MHC haplotype in these strains is designated by a small letter (a, b, d, k, q, s, etc.). For example, the MHC haplotype of Balb/c, an inbred strain of mouse is H2d.

HLA

HLA stands for human leukocyte antigen; because in humans MHC antigen molecules were first studied on leukocytes. In humans the MHC complex is located on chromosome 6 and it covers a region of about 3.6 million base pairs (depending on the haplotype) and consists of more than 70 genes. There are multiple alleles, or forms, of each HLA gene. This diversity is important in maintaining an effective system of specific immunity. Jan Klein in 1977 proposed three regions in human HLA complex and they are class I, II, and III regions.The telomeric region of the classical HLA complex is now referred as class Ib region; and there has also been a suggestion for a class IV region located at the telomeric end of the class III region.

MHC class I: All class I genes are between 3 and 6 kb, the classical HLA antigens encoded in this region are HLA - A, B, and C. Class I HLA genes are highly polymorphic (multiple forms). There are at least 57 HLA-A alleles, 111

HLA-B alleles, and 34 HLA-C alleles. HLA antigens are expressed on the surface of almost all cells and form functional receptors. They are important for displaying antigens of viruses or parasites to killer T-cells in cellular immunity. The peptides that they present are produced from digested proteins that are broken down in the proteasomes inside the cell. Generally the peptides are small polymers of about 9 amino acids in length. Class I MHC is also particularly important in organ and tissue rejection following transplantation. In addition to the portion of class I MHC, that was coded by the genes on chromosome 6, each class I MHC protein contains a small, non-variable protein component called beta 2-microglobulin also. It is coded by a gene on chromosome 15. The 1998 Nomenclature Committee recognized more HLA genes, in class I and Ib regions: they are HLA-E, -F, -G, -H, -J, -K and -L. Among those, only HLA-E, -F and -G are expressed antigens and are considered as minor histocompatible molecules.

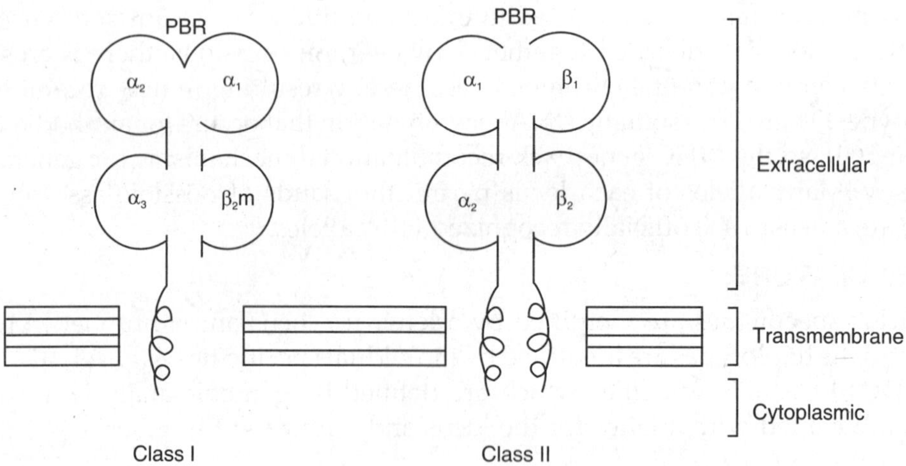

Fig. 11.2

CLASS I MOLECULES

Almost all the cells of an animal's body have thousands of class I molecules present on the plasma membrane. Class I molecules are composed of two polypeptide chains; one is heavy alpha (□) chain encoded by the BCA region and another is a light chain- beta-2-globulin (ß2-microglobulin) that is encoded elsewhere. The MHC-encoded alpha chain is about 350 amino acids long and glycosylated, giving a total molecular weight of about 45 kDa. Alpha chain can be divided into three extra cellular domins, alpha1, alpha 2 and alpha 3, in addition to a trans membrane domain, where the polypeptide chain passes through the plasma membrane of the cell; and a cytoplasmic domain (with the C terminal) within the cytoplasm of the cell. The alpha 3 domain is highly conserved, as is beta-2-microglobulin. Both alpha 3 domain and beta-2-microglobulin are homologous to the CH3 domain of human immunoglobulins. Except the alpha 3 domain, the remaining domains are stabilized by disulfide (S-S) bridges.

ß2-microglobulin is a 12 kDa polypeptide that is non-covalently associated with the alpha-3 domain. The □1 and □ 2 domains fold to make up a groove for peptides to bind. MHC class I molecule binds peptides that are 8-10 amino acid in length and present to a T-cell. Without the beta-2 microglobulin, the class I antigen cannot be expressed on the cell surface. Individuals with a defective beta-2 microglobulin gene does not express any class I antigen and hence have a deficiency of cytotoxic T cell function.

MHC Class II

MHC Class II genes include HLA-DP, HLA-DQ, and HLA-DR. The antigens encoded by these genes are found only on a few specialized cell types, including macrophages, dendritic cells and B cells, all of which are professional antigen-presenting cells (APCs). Hence unlike class I molecules, only certain specialized cells can present antigens with class II molecules. They are particularly important in humoral immunity.

CLASS II MOLECULES

Class II molecules are heterodimeric glycoproteins, with 34kD alpha chain (about 230 amino acids) and 29kD beta chain (about 240 amino acids), both anchored in the membrane. Unlike class I molecules both alpha and beta chains of class II molecules are encoded by the MHC. Each of these two chains has 2 extracellular domains, togethere with the trans membranous and cytoplasmic domains. The membrane-proximal alpha 2 and beta 2 domains are homologous to immunoglobulin CH domain (Refer chapter 6 for immunoglobulins). The two chains interact to form a groove at their outer end which, like class I molecules, always contains a fragment of antigen. But the fragments bound to class II molecules are derived from foreign antigens that the cell has taken in from its surroundings. They present the foreign antigen to helper T-cells, which stimulate B-cells to elicit an antibody response. Unlike class I molecules, the foreign antigen (peptide) presented by class II molecules are derived from extracellular proteins and it is longer (about15 to24 amino acid residues) than the peptide presented by the class I molecules. Like Class I MHC, there are hundreds of alleles that make up the class II HLA gene pool. Class II molecules interact exclusively with CD_4^+ (helper) T cells. Within the DQ molecule both the alpha chain and the beta chain contain the polymorphisms specifying the peptide binding specificities, resulting in up to 4 different molecules.

MHC Class III and Class III molecules:

MHC Class III region has the highest gene density but some of the genes are not involved in the immune system. Since class III genes encode several components of the complement system (i.e. C2, C4a, C4b, Bf), they are responsible for the levels of components of compliment system. In addition to components of the complement system MHC III genes code inflammatory cytokines, tumor necrosis factor α and β (TNF α and β), two heat shock proteins (HSP) etc. They are not membrane proteins and have no role in Ag presentation. MHC Class III molecules are not structurally related to class I and class II molecules but are important in immune response. Complement proteins help to activate and maintain the inflammatory process of an immune response. The heat shock proteins are highly conserved proteins produced by cells at the time of shock including heat shock.

The MHC of humans is now completely sequenced. A consortium of laboratories reports in the 28 October 1999 issue of Nature says that they have determined the sequence of 3,673,800 nucleotides on chromosome 6 that encode the genes of the MHC as well as many other genes involved in immune function.

HLA TYPING

HLA typing is a testing process that is used to match patient's and donor's Leukocyte antigens. HLA Typing helps to assess the chance of survival of transplant. Since some HLA antigens are recognized on almost all of the tissues of the body (with few exceptions), the identification of HLA antigens is also described as "Tissue Typing". HLA matching between donor and recipient is desirable for allogenic transplantation. For a successful transplant, at least 4 of the 6 HLA markers must match. In some cases even a 3/6 match has been successful. However, it is best to have 4 or more markers that match, as it reduces the risk of graft versus host disease. Ever since HLA antigens are inherited, the best chances of finding matches are between siblings. As every one inherits half of their HLA antigens from their mother and half from their father, a sibling has a 25% chance of matching with another. During transplantation, the patient's parents and/or children are also tested to confirm the HLA typing and to make sure no possible donors are overlooked.

In general HLA typing is accomplished by serologic methods which are complement-dependent cytotoxicity assays, detecting gene products from the HLA complex. The class I loci gene products are readily detected by this method of testing, but practice indicated that certain gene products present are not being detected. In view of the fact that all gene products are not easily detected by serology, a cellular testing method has been developed. The detection and subsequent characterization of class II loci ensued, using known cell lines and cell-culture methods. Continued practice of HLA typing and development of new reagents demonstrated that even the alleles detected could be divided into subtypes or splits within an allele. An example would be HLA-B12, the original allele detected, being further split to HLA-B44 and B45. Both HLA-B44 and -B45 are reactive with the broad-reacting HLA-B12 antisera, but they are suitably differentiated by more specific antisera.

Class I typing methods include tests such as microcytoxicity (for typing A, B, C loci) and cellular techniques such as Cell mediated lympholysis or CML (for HLA-DPw typing). Class II typing involves cellular techniques such as Mixed Leukocyte Reaction or MLR/ Mixed Leukocyte Culture or MLC (for DR typing) and molecular techniques such as polymerase chain reaction or PCR and direct sequencing (for DR, DQ typing).

SEROLOGIC METHODS FOR HLA TYPING:

The following are some of the serological methods used for HLA Typing:

Microcytotoxicity assay: This is done by exposing the unknown lymphocyte to a battery of antisera of known HLA specificities. Lymphocytes isolated from the peripheral blood or from lymph node or spleen of cadaver is separated from other cells by buoyant density gradient centrifugation. For HLA I antigens test T lymphocytes are chosen and for HLA II antigens B lymphocytes are chosen. An array of anti-HLA sera covering full range of HLA types is used in the test. Individual serum with approximately 2000 lymphocytes per well is dispensed into the microtitre wells and incubated by adding compliment to it. The duration of incubation is different for T and B lymphocytes. If the antibodies bind to lymphocytes, complement gets activated and results in lysis of that lymphocyte. The damaged cells are not completely lysed but suffer sufficient membrane damage to allow uptake of vital stains such as eosin Y, Trypan Blue or fluorescent stains such as Ethidium Bromide. Live cells do not stain but the dead cells take up the stain.

Antibody screening: This is used to detect the presence of HLA antibodies in the potential transplant recipients. A highly sensitive solid phase ELISA is used to detect antibodies in recipient's serum. Purified preparations of HLA antigens are adsorbed on the solid phase of plastic plates. Recipient's serum is then added to different HLA antigen coated wells. After the removal of unbound antibodies by washing, the wells are treated with enzyme-labeled anti-gamma globulin. The wells are then washed and treated with colour generating substrate. If the recipient is positive for the HLA antigens of the donor (that means recipient has antibodies directed against donor's antigens), survival of transplant is not possible in the recipient's body.

CELLULAR ASSAYS:

Lymphocytes of one donor, when cultured with lymphocytes of an unrelated donor, they get stimulated to proliferate or become cytotoxic. This proliferation is due to a disparity in the class II MHC (DR) antigens. This character has been used in different cellular assays.

Mixed Leukocyte Reaction (MLR) or Mixed Leukocyte Culture (MLC):

When lymphocytes from individuals of different class II haplotypes are cultured together, blast cell transformation and mitosis takes place in the culture. When irradiated or mitomycin-C treated lymphocytes/stimulator cells of recipient (usually containing B cells, macrophages, dendritic cells) are mixed with CD4 cells of donor, donor cells respond to different class II antigens on stimulator cells and undergo transformation (DNA synthesis and enlargement) and proliferation (mitogenesis). These changes can be recorded by the addition of radioactive thymidine into the culture. Monitoring radioactive thymidine incorporation into DNA helps to understand the compatibility levels of recipient and donor cells.

Cell mediated lympholysis (CML):

The responder cell not only undergoes blast transformation and proliferation on contact with different MHC II molecules, they also give rise to cytotoxic cells. These cytotoxic cells in turn identify the HLA I antigen on the stimulator cells and kill them. Lysis of stimulator cells indicates incompatibility of donor and recipient cells.

MOLECULAR TECHNIQUES:

These methods involve detection of the genes coding for the antigens rather than detecting the antigen itself. Methods currently in use for HLA typing, through available commercial kits are sequence-specific oligonucleotide probe (both dot blot and the reverse blot dot), sequence-specific primer amplification, restriction fragment length polymorphism of amplified products, double-stranded sequence conformation polymorphism (with and without reference strand), sequence-based typing, and microarray technologies.

SIGNIFICANCE OF HLA TYPING:

Applications of Histocompatibility Testing

Anthropology: HLA-typing has proved to be an invaluable tool in the study of the evolutionary origins of human populations. The fact that HLA types vary very widely among different ethnic populations has allowed anthropologists to establish or confirm relationship among populations and migration pattern. This information, in turn, contributes to an understanding of cultural and linguistic relationships and practices among and within various ethnic groups.

Paternity Testing: If a man and child share a HLA haplotype, there is a possibility to consider the man as father for the child but it's not a proven. However, if they don't match or share a haplotype then it is agreed that he is not the father.

Transplantation: Since HLA plays such a dominant role in transplant immunity, pre-transplant histocompatibility testing is very important for organ transplantation.

Transfusion: During transfusion of whole blood or blood components, HLA typing helps to prevent transfusion reactions.

Forensic science: HLA-typing can provide valuable DNA-based evidence contributing to the determination of identity in criminal cases. This technology has been used in domestic criminal trials. Additionally, it is a technology that has been applied internationally in the human-rights arena.

Disease Correlation: A number of diseases have been found to occur at a higher frequency in individuals with certain MHC haplotypes. Tissue typing helps to detect the cause of disease. Most prominent among these are ankylosing spondylitis (B27), celiac disease (DR3), and Reiter's syndrome (B27).

Ankylosing spondylitis (B27), Reiter's disease (B27), Acute anterior Uvietis (B27), Psoriasis vulgaris (Cw6) are associated with Class I HLA genes.

Hashimoto's disease (DR5), Primary myxedema (DR3), Graves thyrotoxicosis (DR3), Insulin-dependent diabetes (DQ2/8), Addison's disease (adrenal) (DR3), Goodpasture's syndrome (DR2), Rheumatoid arthritis (DR4), Juvenile rheumatoid arthritis (DR8), Sjogren's syndrome (DR3), Chronic active hepatitis (DR3), Multiple sclerosis (DR2, DR6), Celiac disease (DR3) and Dermatitis herpetiformis (DR3) are Disease associated with Class II HLA.

Even though no definite reason is known for this disease association with

HLA genes, several hypotheses have been proposed to explain the reason. Antigenic similarity between pathogens and MHC, antigenic hypo- and hyper-responsiveness controlled by the class II genes are some of the hypothesises proposed to explain the relationship of the disease with HLA genes.

In addition to autoimmune diseases, HLA genes less commonly play a role in susceptibility to other diseases, including cancer, certain infectious diseases and metabolic diseases. Conversely, some HLA-types confer a protective advantage for certain types of infectious disease. In addition, there are rare immune deficiency diseases that result from inherited mutations of the genes of components of the major histocompatibility complex.

Ankylosing Spondylitis: *Ankylosing spondylitis* (AS) is one of the many types of arthritis. "Ankylosing" means joining together or stiffening; "spondylitis" means inflammation of the vertebral bones of the spine. Inflammation of the bones in Ankylosing Spondylitis can lead to degeneration, pain, and loss of joint motion. AS typically affects the spine but can be seen in other areas, especially the hips also. Ankylosing spondylitis can range from a mild to more severe disease in patients and it is approximately three times more common in males than females. It is usually diagnosed in young adults, with a peak onset between 20 and 30 years of age. Children may also be affected by a form of AS termed "*juvenile ankylosing spondylitis*", seen in children younger than 16 years of age. There is evidence suggesting a strong genetic component in the development of the disease. Those with a family history of AS involving a first degree relative (i.e. mother, father, siblings) will be 5 to 16 times more likely to develop AS.

Celiac disease: Celiac disease is a digestive disease that damages the small intestine and interferes with absorption of nutrients from food. People who have celiac disease cannot tolerate gluten, a protein in wheat, rye, and barley. Gluten is found mainly in foods but may also be found in everyday products such as medicines, vitamins, and lip balms. Symptoms of celiac disease vary from person to person. Symptoms may occur in the digestive system or in other parts of the body. Digestive symptoms are more common in infants and young children and may include abdominal bloating and pain, chronic diarrhea, vomiting, constipation, pale or foul smelling or fatty stool and weight loss. The only treatment for celiac disease is a gluten-free diet.

Reiter's disease: Reiter's disease is an autoimmune disorder that usually occurs following infection of the genitals or gastric mucosa (stomach lining). Reiter's disease usually causes an acute arthritic syndrome that spontaneously resolves within 2-12 months, although symptoms may reoccur and lead to chronic disease. Reiter's disease is named after the physician Hans Reiter, who first reported the condition in 1918 in a young Prussian soldier. Reiter's disease primarily affects young men, and affected individuals often have the HLA B27 marker seen in the autoimmune condition ankylosing spondylitis. This suggests that patients with Reiter's disease are genetically predisposed to its development after exposure to certain infectious organisms, including those causing urogenital (affecting the urinary or genital tract) and enteric (involving the stomach or gastrointestinal tract) infections, such as *Chlamydia trachomatis, Shigella flexneri, Yersinia enterocolitica, Ureoplasma, Campylobacter* species, *Salmonella* and possibly *Neisseria gonorrhoeae,* which causes gonorrhea. Chlamydia infection is seen in about 50 percent of patients, and their Chlamydia antibody titers (evidence of current or past infection) are much higher than those seen in patients with Chlamydia who do not develop Reiter's disease.

Psoriasis vulgaris: Psoriasis vulgaris is the medical name for the most common form of psoriasis ("vulgaris" means common). It is also called plaque psoriasis because of the characteristic plaques, the well-defined patches of red raised skin that can appear on any area of skin, although knees, elbows, scalp, trunk and nails are the most common locations. The flaky silvery white buildup on top of the plaques is called scale; it is composed of dead skin cells. This scale comes loose and sheds constantly from the plaques. Skin affected with psoriasis is generally very dry, and other possible symptoms include skin pain, itching and cracking.

Uveitis: Uveitis specifically refers to inflammation of the middle layer of the eye, termed the "uvea" but in common usage it may refer to any inflammatory process involving the interior of the eye, with inflammation specifically of the uvea termed iridocyclitis.

H-2 SYSTEM

The major histocompatibility complex in mouse is referred as H-2 system or complex. Since an antigen (antigen-2) in the blood cells of mice is recognized by an antibody, co-segregates with the MHC, the mouse MHC locus is called an H-2 locus. H-2 is a complex of genetic loci on chromosome 17 that define the major histocompatibility complex of the mouse. It is homologous to HLA in man, and is responsible for the production of antigens located on the surface of nucleated cells and components of compliment system. The H-2 complex consists of several major genes whose products are important in tissue acceptance and rejection. Haplotypes of the H-2 complex are determined by the combination of alleles of the class I (K, D, L, Qa, and Tla) and class II (Aβ, Aε, Eβ, Eα) genes.

THE MOUSE MHC COMPLEX

MHC Class I

It consists of two major loci, K and D. Unlike the human MHC, the mouse class I gene complex loci are not together but they are separated by class II and class III genes as shown in the figur.

MHC Class II:

The class II gene complex contains two loci A and E, each loci code for one α- and one ß- chain polypeptide, to produce one class II molecule. The mouse class II gene complex is also known as the I-region. Since they determine the magnitude of immune responsiveness of different mouse strains to certain antigens, the genes in this complex are referred as Immune response genes or Ir genes. Products of each loci A and E are termed as IA and IE antigens and collectively they are known as

Ia antigens.

MHC Class III:

The class III gene complex code components of the complement system.

MINOR HISTOCOMPATIBILITY (mHC)

Genetic loci responsible for encoding histocompatibility antigens other than those encoded by the MHC molecules are referred as minor histocompatibility genes. The proteins produced by them are "Minor histocompatibility (mHC) antigens". Minor histocompatibility antigens are normal proteins and polymorphic in a given population. Minor histocompatibility antigens or mHAgs are targets of graft-versus-host disease and graft-versus-leukemia responses after allogeneic HLA identical hematopoietic stem cell transplantation. Hence human minor histocompatibility antigens (mHags) have been recognized as barriers to successful hematopoietic cell transplantation (HCT) from normal donors.

Only a few human minor H antigens have been molecularly characterized and in all cases, amino acid differences between homologous donor and recipient proteins due to nucleotide polymorphisms in the respective genes were responsible for immunogenicity. Ideal minor histocompatibility antigens would be derived from proteins that are not only selectively expressed on hematopoietic cells, including leukaemia cells, but are also necessary for cell function. The problems created by the minor histocompatible molecules are less frequent than those of the major histocompatibility complex (MHC).

Several human minor histocompatibility antigens, such as HA-1, HA-2, HB-1 and BCL2A1, are expressed by hematopoietic cells only. They are investigated as potential targets for a graft-versus-leukemia (GVL) effect. The minor histocompatibility antigen (mHag) HA-1 is the only known mHag for which mismatching is correlated with the development of severe graft versus host disease (GvHD) after human leukocyte antigen-identical bone marrow transplantation. The location of some of mHC loci on the X and Y chromosomes explains why grafts from males to females may be rejected while grafts from females to males are accepted.

In the mouse roughly 30 minor histocompatibility loci have been recognised, comprising more than 500 genes.Some investigators suggests that there may be nearly 1,000 genes scattered through out the mouse genome.

12

IMMUNE RESPONSE

If a foreign agent enters in to the body, immune system responds in different ways to get rid of it from the body. Response of immune system is not same for all foreign agents. The response depends on the type of antigen or foreign substances which entered the body. Responses of immune system to any foreign agent are broadly classified in to two main types one is "Humoral immune response" and the other one is "Cell mediated immune response". Even though the aim of both is removal of the foreign agent, the way they work is different and the cells as well as cell components involved in the reaction are different. Immunoglobulins secreted by activated B cells play a major role in humoral immunity. Binding of antibodies to the pathogen is not sufficient to remove the foreign agent from the body. However it makes the foreign agent susceptible for further actions of immune system. In cell mediated immunity, cells chiefly T cells and other accessory cells involve directly in immune reactions. Binding of the immune cell to the target confirms its destruction and removal from body. Cell that is binding to the foreign agent becomes cytotoxic in cell mediated immunity. Irrespective to the difference in function both humoral and cell mediated immune responses exhibit complex interrelationship to fine-tune immune reactions to almost any antigen, or molecule that stimulates the immune response.

HUMORAL IMMUNITY OR HUMORAL IMMUNE RESPONSE:

Immunity provided by humus (body fluid), through antibodies is known as "humoral immunity". It is also referred as "antibody-mediated immunity" because of the major role played by antibodies in this immune response. In humoral immunity, binding of antibodies to microorganism (foreign agents) results in the formation of immune complex (Ag-Ab complex). Immune complex initiates activation of complement system and other factors such as attraction of other immune cells near to it, inhibition of their migration from the site of Ag-Ab complex etc., to complete the reaction (removal of foreign agent from the body). Binding of Antibodies to soluble toxins neutralizes the toxic nature of the toxin. Antibody binding to viral particles stops subsequent binding of virus to host cells. Immune system executes humoral response in three steps.

1. ACTIVATION OF B CELLS: Activation of B cells is the first step in humoral response to produce antibodies necessary for the humoral immune response. Activation of B cells may be direct or indirect. In direct B cell activation, B cells interact with the T cell independent antigens and start multiplying to produce plasma cells and memory cells (Refer Chapter 5 for related information). In indirect activation, B cells get stimulation from T helper cells. T helper cells induce B cells differentiation and colony formation after interacting with the antigen, processed and presented by the antigen presenting cell.

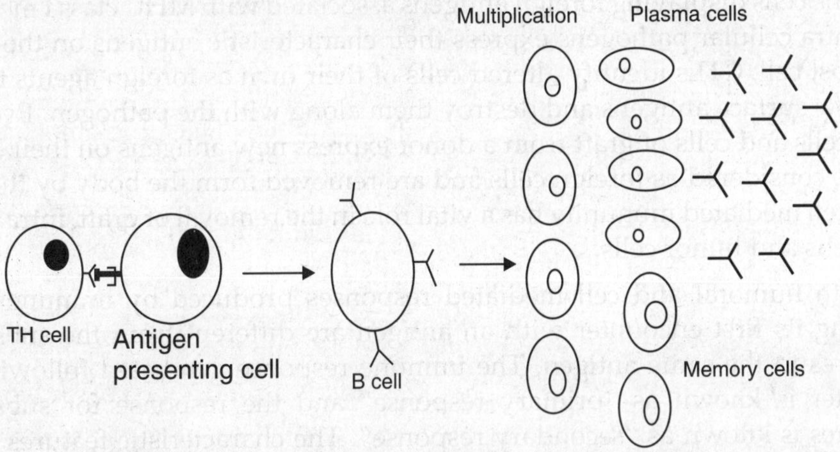

Fig. 12.1

2. EFFECTOR PHASE: Communication between helper-T cells and B-cells through lymphokines released by activated T cells initiate differentiation and multiplication of B cells to produce a colony. Some cells from the colony become plasma cells to secrete antibodies that can react with the antigens responsible for their production. The remaining cells become memory cells to retain "memory" of the foreign invader (antigen) and remain in the body in G_0 phase till they are used in future. If the immune system encounters with the same antigen for the second time, memory cells react very quickly and remove the pathogen very efficiently. Life span of memory cells is much longer than life of plasma cells and it depends upon the strength and nature of antigen that has induced its production. Memory of certain antigens such as polio virus, small pox virus etc. remains for the whole life to give life long protection.

3. ANTIBODY BINDING WITH ANTIGENS: Antibodies secreted by plasma cells interact with their respective antigens resulting in the formation of Ag-Ab complex. The Ag-Ab complex initiates subsequent immune reactions for its removal from the body. Characteristic features of Ag-Ab complex and the subsequent reactions depend upon the type of antigen (Refer Chapter 8 for information on antigen antibody interaction).

CELL MEDIATED IMMUNITY:

Unlike humoral immunity, cell-mediated immunity is mediated by the cells, especially T cells of immune system. When a pathogen enters the body, the antigen presenting cells phagocytise the pathogen and processes the antigenic molecules to present the same to T cells through MHC class II complex. As soon as TH cell interacts with antigen and MHC class II molecule complex of antigen presenting cell, it gets activated and starts secreting cytokines. Cytokines released from T cells activates B cells, TC cells and various other phagocytic cells. Activated phagocytic cells are capable of killing microorganisms such as bacteria, protozoa etc. more efficiently. Activated T cells differentiate into cytotoxic T lymphocytes (CTLs) and proliferate under the influence of cytokines produced by activated TH cells. CTLs kill all the cells displaying foreign antigens associated with MHC class I molecules. Since intra cellular pathogens express their characteristic antigens on the surface of its host cell, CTLs identify altered cells of their own as foreign agents through their new surface antigens and destroy them along with the pathogen. Ever since tumor cells and cells of graft from a donor express new antigens on their surface, they are considered as foreign cells and are removed form the body by the CTLs. Hence cell mediated immunity has a vital role in the removal of graft, intra cellular pathogens and tumor cells.

Both humoral and cell mediated responses produced by immune system following its first encounter with an antigen are different from the subsequent exposures to the same antigen. The immune response generated following first encounter is known as "primary response" and the response for subsequent exposures is known as "secondary response". The characteristic features of both primary and secondary immune responses are different. Generally the secondary response is faster than the primary response due to the presence of memory cells.

(1) PRIMARY IMMUNE RESPONSES:

Immune response to new antigens is known as primary response. When a new pathogen enters in to the body, immune system takes little time to mount response. During this period immune system learns about the pathogen and gets ready to eliminate it from the body. The preparation period that is the period between entry of pathogen and expression of immune response is known as "latent period". Latent period in humoral immunity indicates activation and proliferation of naive B cells to produce plasma cells and memory cells. Plasma cells secrete antibodies and memory cells store information of the pathogen. Generally IgM type antibodies with a half life of 5 days are produced in primary response.

Concentration of secreted antibodies is different at different stages of latent period. In the initial, stage antibodies against the new antigens are almost absent, and this period is known as "Lag phase". Antibodies gradually rise from zero stage to a maximum and this raising period is referred as "Log phase". After attaining maximum, antibody levels remain constant for some time and the period with constant antibody levels is referred as "plateau phase". Maintenances of Abs at constant level in plateau phase indicate production of Abs proportionate to the loss. Plateau phase is accompanied by a decline phase, indicating reduction of Abs.

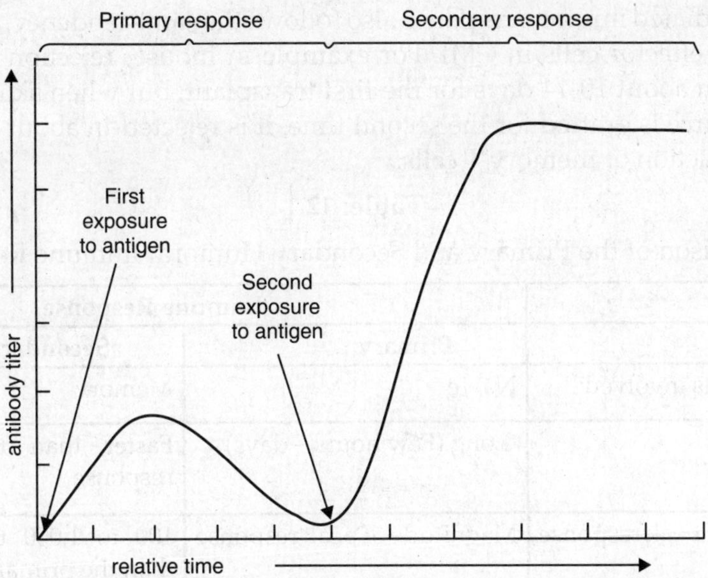

Fig. 12.2

Presence of antigen is necessary for the production of plasma cells. Since the antigens are removed by the action of antibodies, B cells fail to get stimulation from antigens and stops producing plasma cells. The number of plasma cells producing Abs gradually decreases due to their short life. Death of plasma cells producing antibodies and drop in the formation of plasma cells leads to a reduced Abs level in the decline phase. If a graph is plotted for the Abs titer against time in an immune response, it gives a typical sigmoid curve with an extended decline phase as shown in the figure. Duration of latent period in primary immune response varies from several hours to days. It depends on many factors such as type of antigen, amount of antigen entered, rout of entry, health status of the individual etc. For instance latent period is few hours for **pneumococcal** antigen but 2- 3 weeks for **diphtheria**.

(2) SECONDARY IMMUNE RESPONSE:

When an individual encounters the same antigen for second time, immune system responds very quickly due to the presence of memory cells. Secondary immune response is different from the primary response, both qualitatively and quantitatively. The log phase in secondary response is very short or negligible. Since the population of memory B cells specific for the antigen is present, the antibody levels peak with in a short time. Hence lag face is absent in secondary response. Raise of antibody concentration is about 100 to 1,000 fold higher than the primary response resulting a short log phase. Like the sharp raise in Abs, the plateau phase is also much extended in secondary response. The decline in the Abs level is much gradual than the decrease in primary response. Generally the Abs produced in secondary response is IgG type.

Since IgG type Abs have longer life span (about 25 days), their concentration declines very steadily even in the absence of new plasma cells production. This results much extended plateau phase and gradual drop in the decline phase.

Cell mediated immune response also follows the same tendency, but cytotoxic cells are the effector cells in CMI. For example in mouse, rejection of skin graft takes place in about 10-14 days for the first transplant, but when skin tissue from the same source is grafted for the second time, it is rejected-in about 7-9 days due to the faster action of memory T cells.

Table: 12.1

Comparison of the Primary and Secondary Humoral Immune Responses

Feature	Immune Response	
	Primary	**Secondary**
Type of B cells involved	Naive	Memory
Duration	Long (Few hours – days)	Faster than the primary response
Magnitude of peak response	Magnitude of peak response	100 to 1,000 times higher than the primary response
Predominant antibody type produced	IgM	IgG
Antigens	Both thymus-dependent and thymus-independent	Thymus-dependent
Affinity of antibodies	Lower	Higher

13

INFLAMMATION

Humans or animals must defend themselves against multitude of different pathogens including viruses, bacteria, fungi, protozoan and metazoan parasites as well as tumors and a number of various harmful agents that are capable of deranging their homeostasis, resulting in infection and injury. Inflammation is a complex defense mechanism that evolved in higher organisms to protect them from infection and injury. The term inflammation is derived from the Latin word "**inflamatio**"means "to set on fire" to signify heat associated with inflammation. The complex stereotypical reaction of the body is a protective attempt to remove the injurious stimuli, damaged tissue components and also to initiate healing process of the damaged cells and vascularized tissues. In vascular tissues such as cornea of eye, the true inflammation does not occur. The inflammatory reaction is the oldest defense mechanism both phylogenetically and ontogenetically. In the absence of inflammation, wounds and infections would never heal and progressive destruction of the tissue would compromise the survival of the organism. Since the cells of the immune system are widely distributed throughout the body, inflammation concentrates them and their products at the site of damage, to remove damaged tissue components and to initiate healing process.

The five basic symptoms of inflammation - redness (rubor), swelling (tumour), heat (calor), pain (dolor) and deranged function (functio laesa) have been known since long time. The first four classical signs were described by Celsus (ca 30 BC–38 AD), while loss of function was added later by Virchow in the year 1870. Early investigators considered inflammation a primary host defense system. But inappropriate activation of inflammatory responses is the underlying cause of many common diseases such as arthritis and gout. Some times it can lead to death also, as in anaphylactic shock.

Inflammation

Inflammatory reactions involve a wide variety of interconnected cellular and humoral (soluble) mechanisms. The major events occur during this response are:

(1) Vasodilation, i.e. widening of the blood vessels to increase the blood flow to the infected area.

(2) Increased vascular permeability, which allows diffusible components to

enter the site. Increased blood flow to the area of damage may result in redness and warmth.

(3) Cellular infiltration by chemotaxis, or the directed movement of inflammatory cells through the walls of blood vessels into the site of injury.

(4) Changes in biosynthetic, metabolic, and catabolic profiles of many organs.

(5) Activation of cells of the immune system as well as of complex enzymatic systems of blood plasma.

(6) Elevation of body temperature followed by the synthesis of acute phase proteins in the liver.

Of course, the degree to which these occur is normally proportional to the severity of the injury and the extent of infection. Influx of antigen non-specific but highly destructive cells (neutrophils) is one of the earliest stages of the inflammatory response. The inflammatory process may stimulate nerves and cause pain. Inflammation in different tissues is referred by suffixing "-it is" to the tissue name for eg. "pancreatitis" - inflammation of pancreas, "myocarditis" - inflammation of the heart, "colitis" - inflammation of the large intestine, "nephritis" - inflammation of the kidneys etc.

According to different criteria, inflammatory responses can be divided into several categories. The criteria include:

(1) Time -- acute and chronic inflammation.

(2) The main inflammatory manifestation - alteration, exudation, proliferation;

(3) The degree of tissue damage - superficial, profound.

(4) Characteristic picture - nonspecific, specific;

(5) Immunopathological mechanisms such as allergic (reaginic) inflammation, delayed-type hypersensitivity reactions etc.

Inflammation classified with reference to time (acute and chronic) is most appropriate to study the reactions in detail.

ACUTE INFLAMMATION: It occurs over seconds, minutes, hours, and days, of the tissue injury and end when the injurious stimulus has been removed. The initial response is essentially the same regardless the nature of the stimuli. During acute local inflammation, the response remains specific to a particular region of the body (for example, tennis elbow or a mosquito bite). It is the initial response of the body to harmful stimuli resulting the basic symptoms (redness/**rubor**), heat / **calor**, swelling /tumor, and pain /**dolor** and deranged function /**functio laesa**) of inflammation in the affected area. Redness is caused by the dilation of small blood vessels in the area of injury. Heat results from increased blood flow through the area (experienced only in peripheral parts of the body such as the skin). Fever is brought about by chemical mediators of inflammation and contributes to the rise in temperature at the injury. Swelling, called edema is caused primarily by the accumulation of fluid outside the blood vessels. Certain chemical mediators of inflammation, such as bradykinin, serotonin, and the prostaglandins, distortion of tissues due to edema and compression of nerves by swollen tissue, generate pain. Loss of function may result from pain that inhibits mobility or from severe swelling that prevents movement in the area.

All these five symptoms of inflammation can be seen if the inflammation occurs on the body's surface. If the inflammation occurs in internal organs all these five signals may not appear. Since in most cases it remains localized to a specific area of the body it is relatively easy to treat with medicines and proper care. Although acute inflammation is usually beneficial, it often causes unpleasant sensations, (usually temporary) such as the pain of a sore throat or the itching of an insect bite. Occasionally, an acute inflammatory reaction is severe and becomes systemic eg. major trauma, a severe and overwhelming infection that spreads outside of a local area, a very strong allergic reaction etc. In each of these cases, there is a major acute response that is mediated by the immune system.

MECHANISM OF ACUTE INFLAMMATION: The body has the capacity to respond to both minor injuries such as bruising, scratching, cuts, and abrasions, as well as to major injuries such as severe burns and amputation of limbs through inflammation. Inflammation initiates a series of catabolic and anabolic processes that occur in a defined order to re establish homeostasis. The body responds to injury by healing and repairing the damaged tissue, as well as by eliminating the infectious agents and their toxins that might have entered the wound.

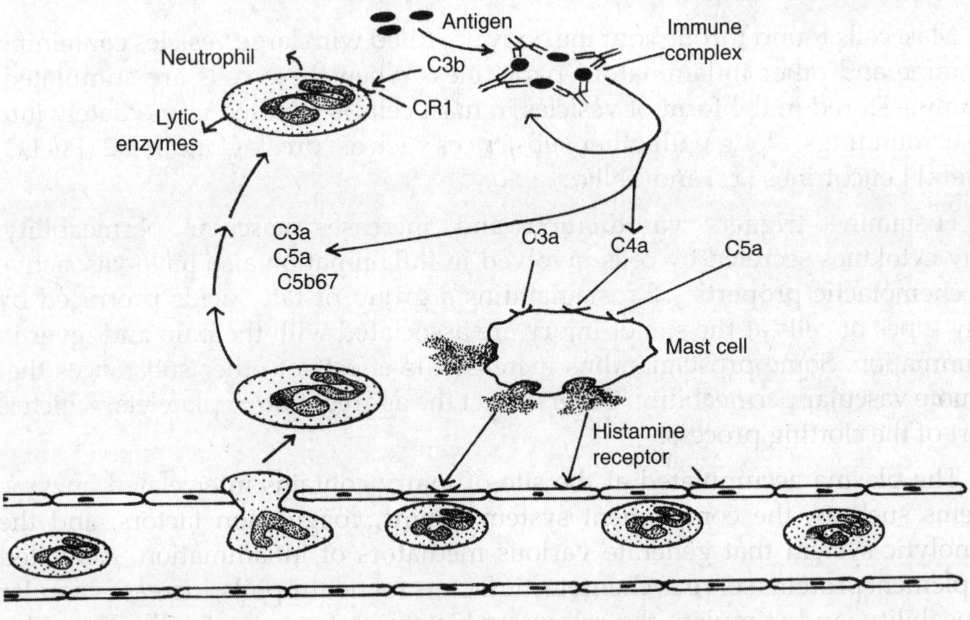

Fig. 13.1 Mechanism of Inflammation

When there is any damage to living tissues, inflammatory response begins in a cascade fasion. The factors that can stimulate inflammation includes microorganisms, physical agents, chemicals, tissue death, and inappropriate immunological responses also. The events that occur in inflammation are (1) the activation of resident cells (mast cells, resident macrophages and dendritic cells) and rapid entry of granulocytes in response to injury, (2) further recruitment of macrophages, (3) infiltration of effector immune cells (lymphocytes) to enable specific immune responses, (4) recruitment and activation of mesenchymal cells such as endothelial cells and fibroblasts to form new blood vessels and a collagenous matrix; and (5) tissue remodelling. In its initial stages, inflammation is an aggressive state that can destroy both exogenous pathogens and host tissues. This is followed by a switch to a state that promotes cell survival and tissue regeneration.

Factors associated with tissue damage trigger inflammation, the sequence of changes are as follows:

1. Release of chemical mediators: Although injury starts the inflammatory response, chemical factors released upon this stimulation bring about the vascular and cellular changes, necessary for inflammation. Most of the mediators involved in inflammation originate from blood plasma, white blood cells (basophils, neutrophils, monocytes, and macrophages), platelets, mast cells, endothelial cells lining the blood vessels, and damaged tissue cells. Histamine is one of the best-known chemical mediators released from cells during inflammation. In the presence of the foreign substance or injury phagocytes of surrounding area especially mast cells liberate cytokines, lipid messengers, and various other mediators of inflammation.

Mast cells found throughout the body are filled with large vesicles containing histamine and other inflammatory paracrines. When these cells are stimulated, histamine stored in the form of vesicles in mast cells is released immediately into the surroundings, along with other substances such as, prostaglandin D2 (PG D2) , several Leucotrines (Ts) and TNFα.

Histamine triggers vasodilation and increases vascular permeability. Many cytokines secreted by cells involved in inflammation also have vasoactive and chemotactic properties. Prostaglandins a group of fatty acids produced by many types of cells at the site of injury are associated with the pain and fever in inflammation. Some prostaglandins increase the effects of other substances that promote vascular permeability. Others affect the aggregation of platelets, which is a part of the clotting process.

The plasma accumulated at the site of injury contains interrelated enzyme systems such as, the complement system, kinins, coagulation factors, and the fibrinolytic system that generate various mediators of inflammation. Activated complement proteins serve as chemotactic factors for neutrophils, increase vascular permeability, and stimulate the release of histamine from mast cells. They also adhere to the surface of bacteria, making them easier targets for phagocytes. The kinin system, which is activated by coagulation factor XII, produces substances that increase vascular permeability. Bradykinin, the most important of the kinins, is responsible for much of the pain and itching experienced with inflammation. The coagulation factors convert the plasma protein fibrinogen into fibrin, a major component of the fluid exudates. The fibrinolytic system contributes to inflammation primarily through the formation of plasmin, which breaks down fibrin into products that affect vascular permeability.

2. Vascular changes: The first vascular change is vasoconstriction. When a tissue is injured, the small blood vessels in the damaged area constrict momentarily. Following this transient event, the blood vessels dilate (vasodilation), under the influence of regulatory molicules on endothelial cells of blood vessels. When blood vessels dilate the walls of the blood vessels become more permeable and allow protein-rich fluid (exudates) along with water and salts into the tissues of damaged area. Substances in the exudate include clotting factors that help in preventing the spread of infectious agents throughout the body. Other proteins include antibodies that help in destroying invading microorganisms. As fluid and other substances leak out of the blood vessels, blood flow becomes more sluggish and white blood cells begin to fall out of the axial stream in the centre of the vessel to flow nearer the vessel wall. Vasodilation may last from 15 minutes to several hours.

3. Cellular changes: Accumulation of white blood cells (phagocytic cells) at the site of injury is the most important feature of inflammation. The main phagocytes involved in acute inflammation are the neutrophils. Within an hour after injury or infection large number of neutrophils reach the site of injury. When tissue damage is minor, an adequate supply of neutrophils can be obtained from those already circulating in the blood. But, when damage is extensive, neutrophils from reservoirs move to perform their tasks. If the demand is high, even immature forms of neutrophils directly from the bone marrow also reach the site. The movement of neutrophils from the blood vessel (diapedisis) towards the area of tissue damage is made possible by chemical substances that diffuse from the area of tissue damage and create a concentration gradient followed by the neutrophils.

In many cases subsequent to 24 to 28 hours of the inflammation another group of white blood cells, the monocytes, reach the site and mature into cell-eating macrophages. Hence macrophages usually become more prevalent at the site of injury only after days or weeks of injury and are a cellular hallmark of chronic inflammation. If the inflammation is caused by parasitic worms, against which neutrophils have little success, eosinophils rather than neutrophils predominate in acute inflammation. Eosinophils release several proteins that are often effective against parasites. Generally eosinophils are linked to certain types of allergies.

ROLE OF CELL ADHESION MOLECULES AND CHEMOTAXIS: In the migration of neutrophils from blood vessels into the tissues, the first step is binding of the neutrophils to the endothelium of the blood vessels (marginalization). Marginalization is due to certain molecules, called cell adhesion molecules (CAMs), found on the surfaces of neutrophils and on endothelial cells. The binding of adhesion molecules occurs in two steps. In the first step, adhesion molecules called selectins lightly tether the neutrophil to the endothelium, so that it begins rolling along the surface, in a second step, a much tighter binding occurs through the interaction of CAMs on the endothelial cells with integrins on the neutrophils. Once outside the blood vessel, a neutrophil is guided towards an infection by various diffusing chemotactic factors. Examples include the chemokines and the complement peptide C5a that is released when the complement system is activated either via specific immunity or innate immunity.

CHRONIC INFLAMMATION:

Inflammation that has a slow onset and persists for weeks or more is referred as chronic inflammation. The symptoms are not as severe as with acute inflammation, but the condition is insidious and persistent. Chronic inflammation may follow on acute inflammation or exist by itself. An acute inflammation becomes chronic, if the immune system fails to clear the offending foreign agents from the body eg. Asbestosis. Acute inflammation due to persistent infections such as tuberculosis, auto antigens responsible for certain autoimmune diseases such as rheumatoid arthritis also induce chronic inflammation in some people.

Appearance of a mononuclear cell infiltrate composed of macrophages and lymphocytes, presence of granulation tissue are the characteristic features of chronic inflammation. Macrophages are involved in microbial killing, in clearing up cellular and tissue debris, and they also seem to be very important in remodelling the tissues. The activities of Macrophages and Lymphocytes are interdependent. Activation of one stimulates the actions of the other. In cases of chronic inflammation due to the presence of foreign agent macrophages can fuse together to form multinucleated/giant cells. For example **Tuberculosis** cause macrophage cells to unite in this manner.

Collagen production is a key feature of chronic inflammation. If too much collagen is formed, this can lead to the condition known as fibrosis. Connective tissue cells known as fibroblasts enter the area of tissue injury and produce collagen which is necessary to replace the tissue lost during long term inflammation. The over production of collagen can lead to scarring that can cause permanent distortion of the tissue, interfering with its function. Chronic inflammation can be continually stimulated by substances with low antigenic properties or by auto-immunity.

Asbestosis or interstitial fibrosis: Asbestos particles are long, extremely thin, microscopic fibers. When asbestos is in the air, these particles are inhaled by those in close proximity. The fibers are so thin and light that they cannot be properly filtered by the lungs. The asbestos can become embedded in various parts of the lungs, including the interstitium (the area surrounding the alveoli).

Once embedded, the asbestos particles are attacked by the body's immune system. Since asbestos is a hard, fibrous mineral, the macrophages are unable to eliminate them from the lungs. As the macrophages attempt to wipe out the asbestos, they create scar tissue in the area where the asbestos is embedded. As macrophages are unable to remove the asbestos, the body's immune system sends more and more macrophages, creating more scar tissue. This creates a chain reaction that cannot be stopped. When scar tissue in the interstitium becomes advanced and there is large-scale injury to tissue of the lung, this is called as "fibrosis"; or, more specifically, "interstitial fibrosis or asbestosis".

Mycobacterium tuberculosis: Mycobacterium tuberculosis is one of the most ubiquitous pathogen infecting about one-third of the world's population. Immune responses to tuberculosis rarely result in complete eradication of the infection. Instead, TB-infected immune cells promote the generation of chronic inflammation and the formation of granulomas, which are areas where the bacteria are contained but not destroyed.

On the basis of histological alterations chronic inflammation can be divided in to four forms. They are as follows:

1. Chronic fibrous inflammation: This Indicates severe inflammatory condition and is characterized by exudation rich in fibrin that does not clear easily. The fibrous tissue producing fibrin in the region of inflammation differentiates in to myofibroblasts. Contraction of these myofibroblasts like smooth muscles results in mechanical defects. Stiffened joints, stenosis (narrowing) of ducts are the best examples for mechanical defects developed by fibrous inflammation.

2. Chronic serous inflammation: Serous inflammation is the mildest form of reaction characterized by accumulation of clear fluid (without any cells) due to minimal increase in vascular permeability. Although it occurs in very mild inflammation, it may have grave consequences. Serous inflammation is marked by the outpouring of a thin fluid that is derived from either the plasma or the secretions of mesothelial cells lining the peritoneal, pleural, and pericardial cavities depending on the size of injury. For example, the skin blister resulting from a burn or viral infection represents a large accumulation of serous fluid, either within or immediately beneath the epidermis of the skin. Serous pericarditis, pleuritis, peritonitis; rheumatoid arthritis (serous fluid in joints) etc. are some more examples for serous inflammation.

3. Chronic suppurative inflammation: It is a type of acute inflammation characterized by infiltration of neutrophils at the microscopic level and formation of puss at the gross level. Abscess is a special type of suppurative inflammation marked by collection of dead neutrophils (pus formation) in the cavity formed by the tissue on the basis of an infectious process and encapsulated from the rest of the body by inflammatory cells and decaying tissues. The encapsulation is an attempt to keep the puss from infecting neighboring structures. Some abscesses are easily diagnosed clinically, as they are painful and may "come to a head" such that puss becomes visible, but deep and chronic abscesses may just look like a tumor clinically and require biopsy to distinguish them from neoplasm.

The infecting organisms responsible for the formation of abscesses vary. Staphylococcus bacteria are prevalent in skin abscesses, but a multitude of other organisms, including viruses, bacteria, fungi, amoebas and worms, can be involved as well, depending on the site of the abscess. In some cases, the cause for abscess formation is unknown. If not treated properly an abscess, may progress to a life-threatening infection and death also, especially in people susceptible to infection, such as diabetics or people on steroid medication. When an abscess enlarges it may develop in to "sinus" (abnormal passage leading from a suppurating cavity to the body surface) or fistula (an abnormal tunnel connecting two body cavities).

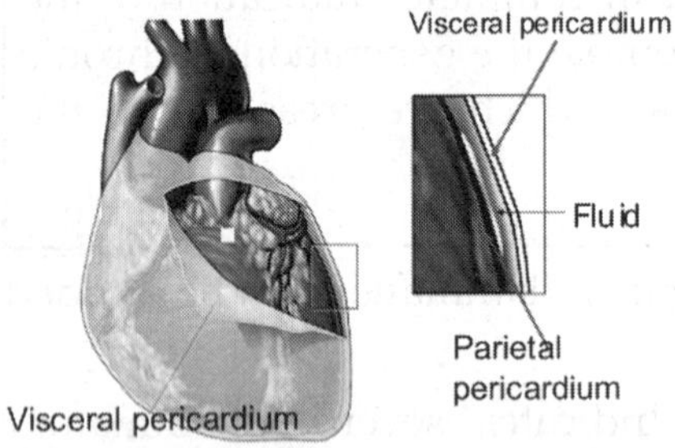

A. Serous pericarditis

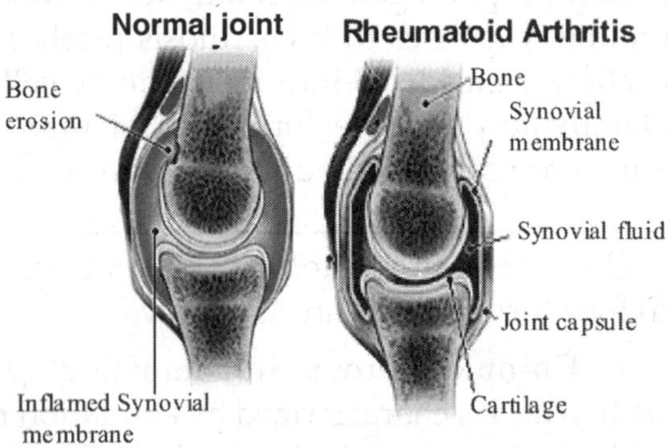

B. Rheumatoid arthritis

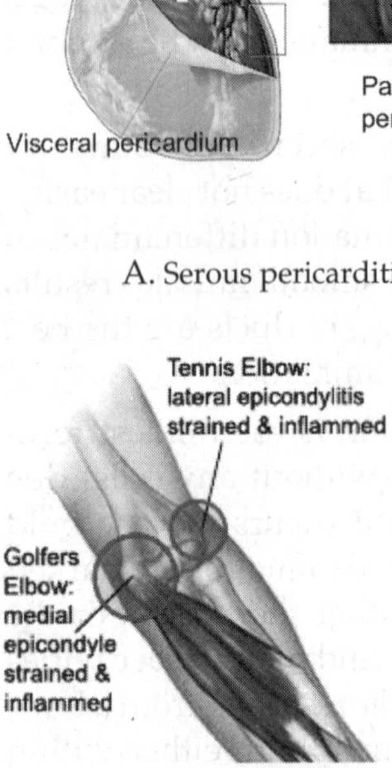

C. Stiffened joints

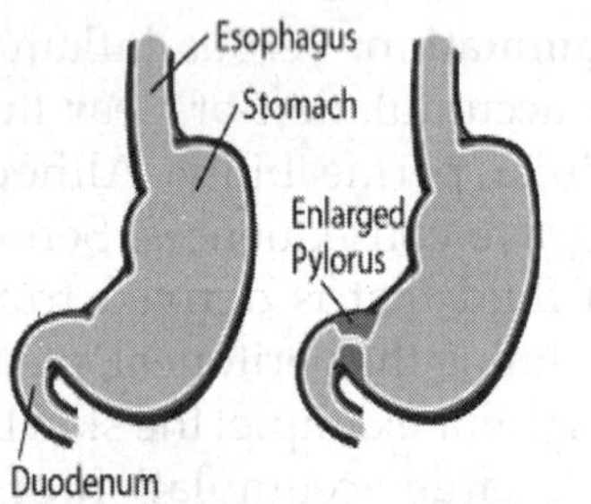

D. Normal Pyloric stenosis

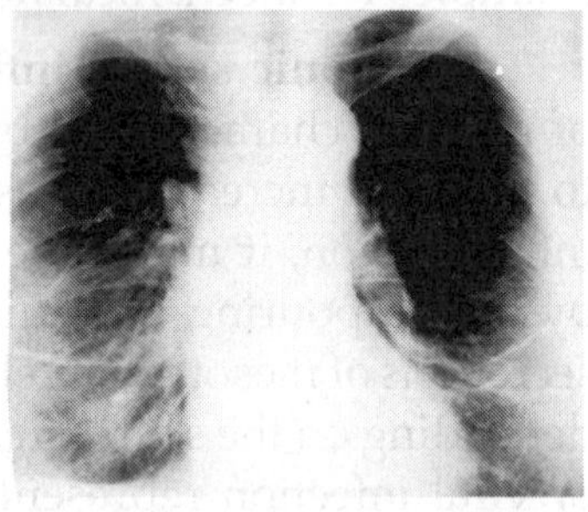

E. Asbestosis Lung Xray

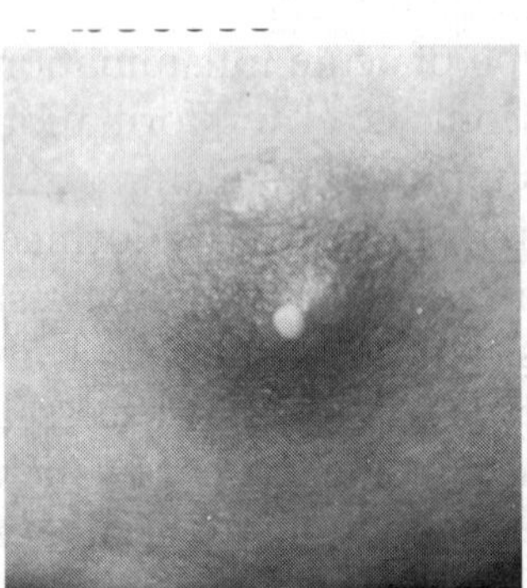

F. Abscess

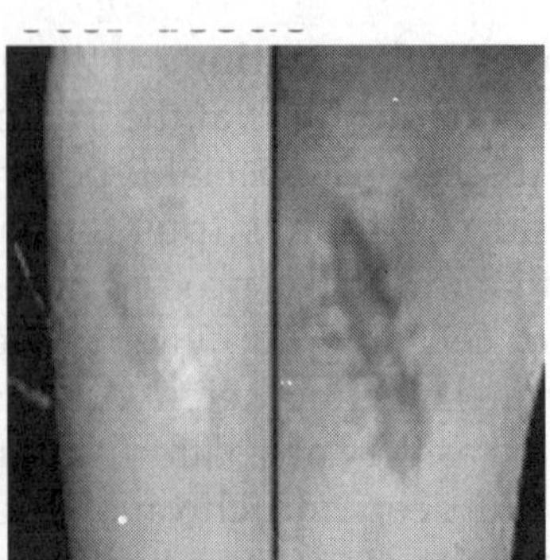

G. Scar tissue

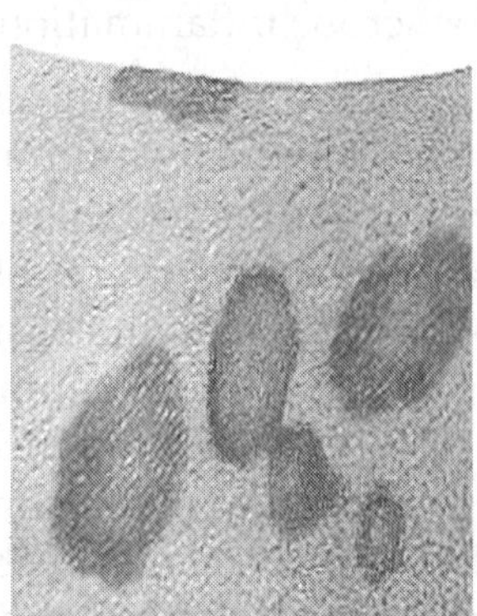

H. Inflammation

Fig. 13.2

4. Chronic granulomatous inflammation: With somewhat more vascular permeability, high molecular weight solutes also pass from the intravascular to the extravascular space. There are many different plasma proteins in the high molecular weight category, but the most conspicuous of these is fibrinogen. Contact of coagulation factor XII (Hageman factor) with collagen activates the coagulation system and ultimately leads to proteolytic cleavage of soluble fibrinogen to form insoluble fibrin, which precipitates on every available surface, grossly the serosal surfaces become shaggy and rough. The inflamed pericardium and pleurae emit friction rubs due to this. Microscopical study of inflamed pericardium suggests the presence of a shaggy coat of preciptated fibrin on the serosal surfaces.

MECHANISM OF CHRONIC INFLAMMATION

Chronic inflammation is a product of the Type 4 hypersensitivity mechanisms (Refer Chapter 14 for Hypersensitivity).

TISSUE REPAIR AND WOUND HEALING:

While removing the agent responsible for inflammation, the defense mechanism of body causes some damage to the tissue in and around the region of inflammation. To get back the normal status, healing and repair of the damaged tissue is necessary. Hence healing and repair of damaged tissue is the end phase of inflammation. Restoring cellular structures and tissue layers is a complex and dynamic process. It takes place in two steps one is regeneration of tissue and the other is fibroplasia and fibrosis or replacement. Depending upon the injury, tissue involved in injury, the wound may be healed by regeneration alone or by a combination of both regeneration and replacement. Balance between these two processes determines the out come of the final response of inflammation.

Tissue regeneration: If basement membranes and the underlying extra cellular matrix of damaged tissue are intact, regeneration occurs through active division of the remaining cells. Mitogenic factors released from the cells of inflammation or availability of increased nutrients indirectly produced by the reduced tissue mass may trigger proliferation of healthy cells that remain at the site of injury. If the damage is repaired by regeneration the regenerated tissue is indistinguishable from the original tissue.

Tissue replacement: Since non-dividing or quiescent cells such as nerve cells, skeletal muscle cells and cardiac muscle cells etc. are not capable of undergoing division's, granulation tissue take up the job of filling the damaged region. Granulation tissue is combination of abundant new blood vessels and immature collagen admixed with plump fibroblasts. Eventually, many of the blood vessels regress and all that is left is collagen. The excess collagen is recognized as a "scar" or "scar tissue". The human body has a limited capability for regeneration and the amount of excess collagen depends on the extent of tissue damage, the regenerative capacity of the injured tissue, as well as an individual's tendency, to produce excess collagen.

SYSTEMIC INFLAMMATION: Chronic inflammation that lasts for days, months, or longer, can cause damage to many body tissues. For example, Crohn's disease - a disorder involving severe abdominal pain and intestinal problems. Like Crohn's, other diseases such as multiple sclerosis, autoimmune disease, arthritis, and even some forms of cancer, are the consequence of unchecked, ongoing inflammation.

INFLAMMATION GONE AWRY:

The intention of inflammation is certainly beneficent; however, the consequences of inflammation are not always predictable or desirable. When neutrophils and macrophages are digesting bacteria some of the free radicals and hydrolytic/proteolytic enzymes may leak from the phagosome causing local destruction of tissue and cells eg. pulmonary emphysema, osteoarthritis. Recruitment of inflammatory cells, secretion of growth factors may cause over-exuberant granulation tissue with subsequent scarring. The inflammatory system may also be an unwitting accessory in processes such as fistula formation (eg. inflammatory bowel disease), atherosclerotic plaques, autoimmune diseases, immune hypersensitivity responses (eg. anaphylaxis, allergies), etc. Since chronic inflammation can cause considerable damage to the tissues of the body, it can lead to a variety of problems. In many cases, inflammation can spread across the body. Hence chronic inflammation is a growing concern among health care professionals. Some of the diseases associated with inflammation are arthritis, type 1 diabetes, asthma, crohn's disease, colitis etc. Many of them are life threatening.

> Crohn's disease: Crohn's disease is an ongoing disorder that causes inflammation of the gastrointestinal (GI) tract. It is also called as "ileitis or enteritis". Crohn's disease can affect any area of the GI tract, from the mouth to the anus, but most commonly affects the ileum. The swelling extends deep into the lining of the affected organ. The swelling can cause pain and make the intestines empty frequently, resulting in diarrhea. In Crohn's disease, all layers of the intestine may be involved, and normal healthy bowel can be found between sections of diseased bowel.

SOME EXAMPLES OF INFLAMMATION ASSOCIATED DISEASES:

Heart Disease: Inflammation (triggered by environmental factors or genetic influences) plays a role in certain heart diseases, because LDL cholesterol (bad cholesterol) gets embedded inside artery walls as well, where the immune system sees it as an invader to be attacked. The ongoing inflammation in arteries, essentially a revved up immune response, can eventually damage arteries and cause vulnerable plaque to burst, resulting in damage to the vessel walls. In trying to heal this damage, inflammatory cells come into the vessel walls and induce a sequence of inflammatory actions in the coronary artery, such as plaque rupture, thrombus formation and embolization into the blood vessels within the heart etc., placing one at increased risk for heart attack. Since inflammation prompts the liver to produce a protein in the blood known as C-reactive protein (CRP), a test for

CRP can help in predicting the risk of heart attack and stroke as well.

Arthritis: "Arthr" refers to joints between bones "itis" indicates inflammation. The complete word "Arthritis" means inflamed joint or joints" In many types of arthritis, the body's inflammatory response is misdirected. In arthritis, the secretions of inflammatory cells called cytokines lead to the production of enzymes that break down cartilage in joints. The pain, redness, heat, swelling and other harmful effects of inflammation can be treated with medication, diet and exercise.

Diabetes: It's long been known that type 1 diabetes is an autoimmune disease, because the body's immune system attacks the cells that make insulin, resulting in type I diabetes. In recent years, the immune system has also been implicated in type II diabetes. Type II diabetes often begins with insulin resistance, in which cells stop responding properly to insulin. TNF (tumor necrosis factor) released in chronic inflammation makes cells more resistant to insulin.

Alzheimer's disease (AD): It is an irreversible, progressive and degenerative disorder that destroys the higher structures of the brain. There is mounting evidence that chronic inflammatory processes play a fundamental role in the progression of neuro pathological changes of Alzheimer's disease. Whenever the brain is injured or infected, cells in the brain called glia pump out cytokines. Normally, this response shuts down when the injury or infection is over. But in chronic neurodegenerative diseases like Alzheimer's, these glial cells are activated too high or too long or both, making them pump out even more cytokines to try to repair this damage and creating chronic inflammation, which in turn results degenerative disorder.

Inflammatory bowel disease (IBD): It is an inflammatory condition of the colon and small intestine. Crohn's disease and ulcerative colitis are the major types of IBD. The main difference between Crohn's disease and ulcerative colitis is the location and nature of the inflammatory changes. In Crohn's disease inflammation can affect any part of the gastrointestinal tract, from mouth to anus (skip lesions), although a majority of the cases start in the terminal ileum. Ulcerative colitis, in contrast, is restricted to the colon and the rectum. Microscopically, ulcerative colitis is restricted to the mucosa (epithelial lining of the gut), while Crohn's disease affects the whole bowel wall.

Tumour: Recent data have expanded the concept that, inflammation is a critical component of tumour progression. Many cancers arise from sites of infection, chronic irritation and inflammation. Inflammation aids in the proliferation and survival of malignant cells, promotes angiogenesis and metastasis, subverts adaptive immune responses, and alters responses to hormones and chemotherapeutic agents. In addition, tumour cells have co-opted some of the signaling molecules of the innate immune system, such as selectins, chemokines and their receptors for invasion, migration and metastasis. In certain types of cancer, an oncogenic change induces an inflammatory microenvironment that promotes the development of tumors. Recent data suggest that an additional mechanism involved in cancer related inflammation (CRI) is induction of genetic instability by inflammatory mediators, leading to accumulation of random genetic alterations in cancer cells. These insights are fostering new anti-inflammatory therapeutic approaches to cancer development.

INFECTION:

Infection can be defined as the injurious colonization of a host organism, by a foreign species. In such a case, the foreign species, which can also be called the infecting organism, starts utilization of the resources of the host. The result is that the normal functioning of the host is adversely affected. In human beings, the negative effects might manifest themselves in the form of chronic wounds, loss of an infected limb, gangrene and in some cases even death. The foreign species usually comprise of microscopic organisms like bacteria, viruses, parasites, fungi, prions, viroids, and so on.

The term "infection" has some exceptions. For example, the normal growth of the usual bacterial flora in the intestinal tract is not usually considered as an infection. The same consideration applies to the bacteria that normally inhabit the mouth.

General infections can be divided into two categories, namely systemic infection and local infection.

SYSTEMIC INFECTION

The cause of a systemic infection comprises of bacteria or virus. The main characteristic of such an infection is that it affects the bloodstream of an individual, with the result that the symptoms spread to the whole of the body. In this case, the pathogen is distributed throughout the body, rather than being concentrated in one area. Bacterial toxin is the major reason that leads to systemic infection. The most common examples of a systemic infection are cold, flu, mononucleosis, strep throat etc.

Signs and Symptoms of Systemic Infection

Aches: When a person is suffering from systemic infection, he/she experiences ache in areas such as the forehead and back. In extreme cases, the person experiences body ache too.

Chills: Systemic infection triggers chills, which make a person shiver even after wearing layers of woolen clothes.

Fever: Fever is a telltale sign of systemic infection. Depending upon the severity of the infection, the person might suffer from low to high fever.

Nausea: Systemic infection triggers a feeling of nausea. The person reacts to certain smells by vomiting.

Vomiting: Vomiting is one of the major symptoms of systemic infection. The person would have the tendency of puking, even after consuming regular food.

Weakness: Overall weakness in the body is another symptom of systemic infection.

LOCAL INFECTION

A local infection can be explained as that infection, which does not affect the whole body of an individual. Rather, it is limited to a specific portion of the body. It does not attack the bloodstream and is limited to the outer surface of the body. Some of the most common examples of a local infection include an infected wound, an infected cut, etc.

Signs and Symptoms of Local Infection

Fever: Fever is the only systemic symptom that can be caused by a local infection.

Foul Odor Discharge: A foul odor discharge from the affected area is a telltale sign that the person has incurred a problem of local infection.

Heat at the Site: In some cases, local infection might cause swelling in the affected area, which would in turn cause heat at the site.

Pain: Pain in the area, which has been infected, is a very visible sign of local infection.

Pus: One can figure out whether a wound is infected or not, by observing the amount of pus released from there.

Redness and Swelling: Local infection might cause redness and swelling in the affected area.

14

HYPER SENSITIVITY

Immune system is meant for giving protection against the problem causing foreign agents, but some times, over enthusiasm of immune system results in damage to its own body organs and tissue. The violent and destructive action of immune system is referred as "hypersensitivity reaction" or "allergic reaction". Here the term hypersensitivity is used in a negative sense to explain the destructive action of immune system. The factors or antigens causing hypersensitivity or allergic reactions are known as allergens. An allergen may be a protein or a complex chemical substance with low molecular weight that generally may not cause any immunological response in non allergic people. The allergens responsible for hypersensitive reactions may be food products or pollutants or drugs. Usually, first encounter with an allergen will not generate any hypersensitive reactions, but the immune system produces memory cells for that particular allergen. Production of memory cells for exposed allergen is known as "sensitization". The person with memory cells for an allergen is considered as sensitized, and shows clinical symptoms of allergy, when he encounters with the same allergen for the second time. The hyper sensitivity reactions can be classified into two types based upon the time taken for pathogenicity.

(1) Immediate Hyper sensitivity(2) Delayed Hyper sensitivity

1. Immediate Hyper sensitivity: If the sensitized person shows allergic reactions in less than 24 hours after exposure to an allergen, the reactions are considered as immediate hyper sensitivity reactions. A hyper sensitivity reaction to drugs like penicillin belongs to this category. Interaction of antibodies with antigen results in immediate hypersensitivity and the reactions are handled by B lymphocytes. Humoral immunity or antibody-mediated action is responsible for immediate hypersensitivity reactions. Therefore they are transferable from one individual to the other through serum or antibody (Ab) transfer.

2. Delayed Hyper sensitivity reactions: If a sensitized person shows Hyper sensitivity reactions after 24 hours of antigenic exposure, the reactions are considered as Delayed Hyper sensitivity reactions. Delayed hyper sensitivity reactions are cell mediated and T lymphocytes are responsible for this type of reactions. The inflammatory response can not be transferred through antibodies, but can be transferred through sensitized T cells to a non allergic person. The clinical symptoms of delayed hyper sensitivity are **Erythema** (redness of skin), and **Induration** (hardening of tissue).

In 1963 Coombs and Gell classified hyper sensitivity reactions into 4 types, based on the mechanism of pathogenesis. They are (1)Type I or Anophylactic hyper sensitivity (2)Type II or Antibody dependent cytotoxic hyper sensitivity (3)Type III or Immune complex mediated hyper sensitivity (4) Type IV or Cell mediated hyper sensitivity. Apart from these 4 types, Type V or Stimulatory hyper sensitivity has been included later to Coombs and Gell nomenclature.

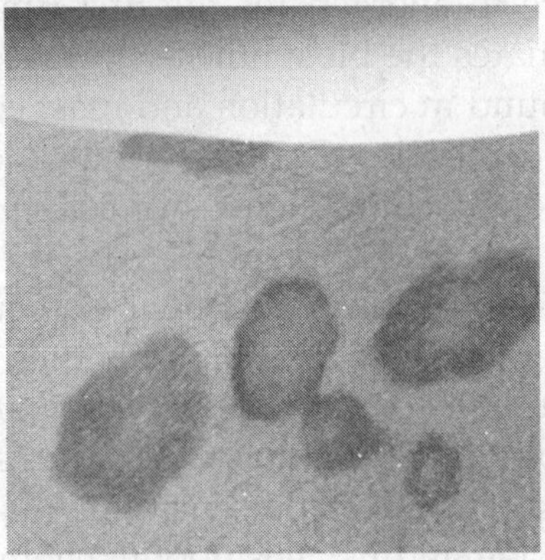

Erythema

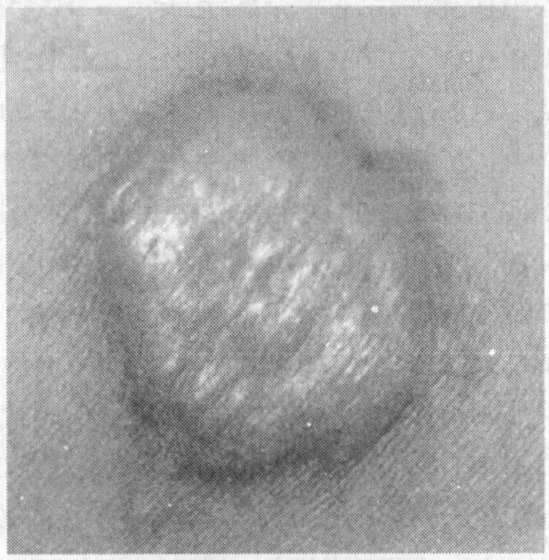

Induration

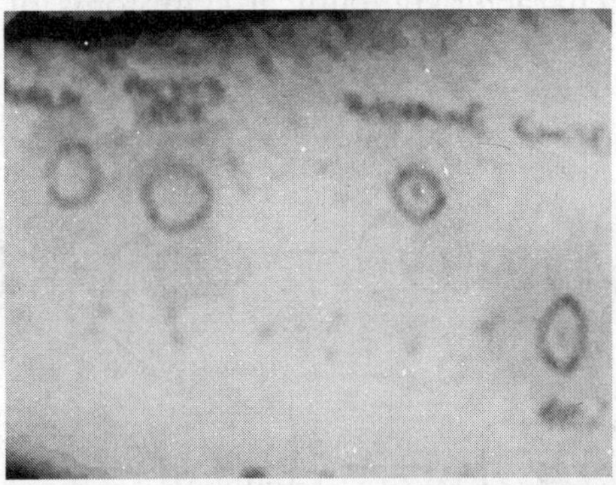

Wheal and Flare test

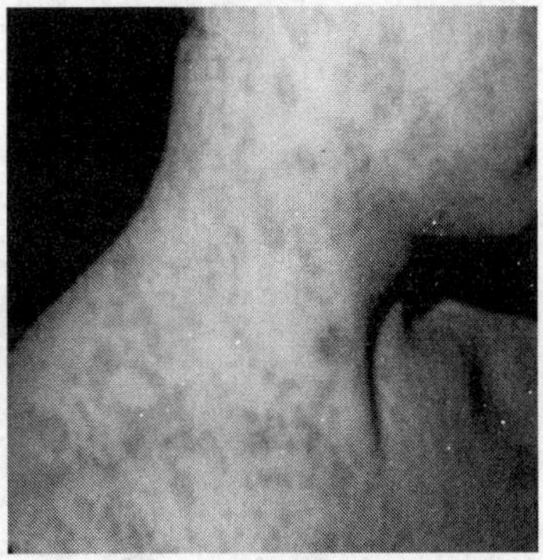

Anaphylaxis

Fig. 14.1

Type I Hypersensitivity or Anaphylaxis: This is an immediate type of hypersensitivity; a pre sensitized host produces immediate pathological changes after subsequent exposure to the same allergen. The pathological changes are due to de granulation of mast cells or basophils, following an antigen binding to their surface bound IgE antibodies. IgE Abs production is very low in normal people, usually at an average of 0.0004mg/ml of serum. Individuals prone to allergy produce more number of IgE antibodies than the normal people. The exact reason for the production of IgE antibodies instead of IgG antibodies in allergic persons is not yet known. Antigens such as pollen grains helminth antigens are potent stimulators of IgE Abs in all individuals. Clinical symptoms developed in sensitized persons after exposure to allergen are referred as anaphylactic reactions. (Ana-without, phylaxis - protection) and high level IgE antibodies producing tendency is referred as atopic condition. The factors that are influencing the production of IgE antibodies are mostly genetic and the analysis of conditions suggests that the interaction of IgE regulatory gene and one or more genes of HLA region are responsible for generating atopic conditions.

MECHANISM OF IgE MEDIATED HYPER SENSITIVITY (ANAPHYLAXIS): The first step in the development of Anaphylactic or Type I hypersensitivity is sensitization. Exposure to allergen for the first time does not generate any clinical symptoms, but initiates the biosynthesis and release of humoral IgE Abs. Generally basophils are found in circulation and mast cells are distributed in connective tissues, including capillaries. Both basophils and mast cells contain different pharmacologically potent components in vesicles. Since mast cells and basophils are having receptors for FC region of IgE Abs, they bind to the membranes of both mast cells and basophils. In subsequent exposures to the same allergen, the allergen molecule interacts with the IgE antibodies bound to the mast cells and basophils. The antigen antibody complex then triggers the release of pharmacological substances from basophils and mast cells. The released pharmacological substances responsible for Type I hypersensitivity reactions are histamines, certonins, leucotrines, prostaglandins, eosinophil chemotactic factor of anaphylaxis, (ECFA), platelet activating factor, heparin, kinin, etc. The released biological products induce characteristic clinical symptoms of Type I hypersensitivity in atopic persons.

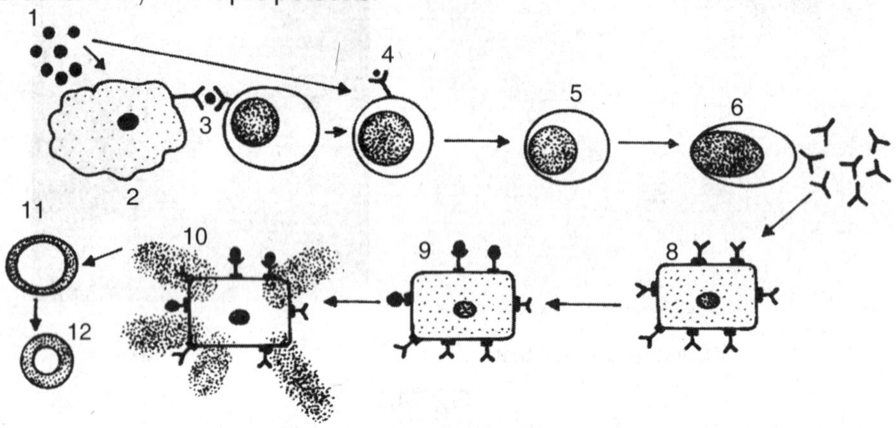

1. Antigen 2. Antigen presenting cell 3. Antigen presentation 4. B cell
5. Activated B cell 6. Plasmacell 7. Antibodies 8. Mast cell with bound antibodies
9. Antigens bound to mast cells 10. Release of pharmacological substances
11. Normal bronchiole 12. Asthmatic bronchiole

Fig. 14.2 Mechanism of IgE mediated hyper sensitivity.

HISTAMINE: Histamine is the abundant and fast acting substance of all pharmacological substances. It induces smooth muscle contractions, release of mucus, vasodilation and increased capillary permeability. The target areas for the action of histamines are respiratory tract, uterus etc. Action of histamine on respiratory tract results in suffocation, leading to anoxic conditions. Under the influence of histamine, uterus shows inappropriate contractions and these contractions may cause abortion in pregnant women. Histamines release also causes less toxic conditions for instance edema (excess fluid accumulation) in the tissue due to increased capillary permeability. Extensive loss of fluid in the tissue due to vasodilatation may cause circulatory shock through reduced supply of oxygen and nutrients.

SEROTONIN (5-Hydroxytryptamine): In addition to histamine, serotonin is another substance that acts as a chemoeffector of smooth muscles and it also increases the respiratory rate, heart rate and causes vasoconstriction leading to a raise in blood pressure. It appears to have little effect on vascular permeability but stimulates further release of histamine.

LEUCOTRINES: These are slow reacting substances of anaphylaxis and are very potent muscle spasmogens .They act as chemotactic substances for neutrophils, and eosinophils to attract them towards the site of reaction. Other actions of leucotrines are similar to the actions of histamine and serotonin but at a slower level.

PROSTAGLANDINS (PGS): They are a family of complex lipids with a wide range of activities. They act as vasodilators, brancho constrictors and regulators of blood coagulation.

PLATELET ACTIVATING FACTORS (PAFS): It provokes aggregation of platelets and release of their contents, especially serotonin.

EOSINOPHIL CHEMOTACTIC FACTOR (ECF): ECF attracts eosinophils and neutrophils to the site of mast cell degranulation, to prevent their movement from the site of inflammation and to desensitize them. This reaction overturns some of the deleterious effects of anaphylaxis.

OTHER BIOLOGICALLY ACTIVE FACTORS: As the mast cell granules are modified lysosomes they contain some hydrolytic enzymes. Heparin is one of the substance released from the mast cells and basophils during allergic reactions. Since it is anticoagulant in character, coagulation of blood in anaphylactic condition may be stopped or delayed. Kenin is another substance released in small quantities. It is a small peptide and it enhances capillary permeability, mucous secretions and leucocyte migration from blood vessels in to the tissues. The collective action of all the substances released from mast cells and basophils are responsible for the cause of anaphylactic reactions.

CONSEQUENCES OF TYPE-I HYPER SENSITIVITY REACTIONS:-

The consequences of Type I Hyper sensitivity reactions may be local or systemic. Since mast cells are located in diverse areas of the body such as respiratory tract, gastro intestinal tract, reproductive tract and skin, exposure to allergen may lead to development of local responses like eczema, fever etc., or systemic response like asthma. Generally the clinical symptoms of Type I hyper sensitivity reactions depend on the release of pharmacological products from mast cells and basophils. The severity and area of the reactions depends on the number of mast cells stimulated, the amount of antigen administered, the route of administration etc. If small quantities of mild antigens are administered through intradermal injection, mild and localized reactions develop due to body's response for harmonizing the changes developed under the influence of mast cell derived factors. If a strong antigen in little large quantity is injected intravenously the reaction may be systemic and faster. Systemic anaphylaxis is a shock like condition and occurs in a very short time. A wide range of antigens such as venom of bees, penicillin drugs, antitoxins, sea food, etc have been shown to trigger Type - I hyper sensitivity reactions in humans. Allergic rhinitis, hay fever, allergic bronchitis, vomiting, diarrhea, utricaria, atopic dermatitis etc. are some of the examples of Type I hyper sensitivity reactions. Since Type I hypersensivity reactions are developed by humoral immunity, it can be transferred from an allergic person to other non allergic persons through serum transfer.

Since all the clinical signs of Type I hypersensitivity are related to the release of vasoactive substances from mast cells and basophils, the severity and site of the reactions depends on the number of mast cells stimulated, amount of antigens, and route of administration. If the antigens are administered slowly in small quantities clinical signs would be very less. Because the individual gets an opportunity to balance the vascular changes provoked by the factors derived from mast cells.

CLINICAL TESTS FOR ALLERGY:

If a person is suspected to be allergic to any particular substance/allergen, it can be confirmed by simple wheal and flare test. In this clinical procedure a small dose of allergen is injected under the skin and the injected area is marked and studied in less than 30 minutes. If the person is allergic to the injected allergen, a wheal and flare response at the site of infection is developed. PK test or Prausnitz-Kustner procedure is one of the skin testing techniques for allergy, to detect reactive antibodies for specific antigens. This test is based on repetition of intra dermal injection of serum from an allergic individual to non allergic person once in 24 hours, to observe inflammatory response. If the individual is positive (allergic) to that specific allergen, inflammatory response develops within 1 or 2 minutes. This test can be carried to test certain life threatening allergens such as bee venom, scorpion venom etc.

THERAPY: The first step in therapy is identifying and stay away from contact with the allergens. Otherwise desensitization or immuno therapy with repeated injections of antigens in increasing doses (hyposensitization) can be done to reduce the strength of reactions in allergic people. In this procedure repeated encounter with antigens may cause a shift in antibody production from IgE to IgG and the IgG antibodies may block or minimize binding of antigen with the mast cell bound IgE antibodies. Use of anti histamines, to block histamine binding with the target cells through their receptors would work in the prevention of development of clinical symptoms.

Stabilization of mast cells can be done with the help of certain drugs like isoprenaline, sodium cromoglycate etc. The drugs stabilize mast cells and prevent release of pharmacological products that are totally responsible for pathogenesis.

TYPE II OR ANTIBODY DEPENDENT CYTOTOXIC REACTION:- Type II hypersensitivity reactions are mediated by IgG antibodies, raised against the allergen and activated complement enzymes. Lysis due to complement fixation is the cause for pathogenesis in this reaction.

MECHANISM OF TYPE II HYPER SENSITIVITY REACTIONS: Antibodies present in the sensitized person bind to the antigen of the foreign cell and the antigen antibody complex triggers the cascade of complement system. The activated components of the complement system binds to the membrane of the foreign cell as membrane associated complex, leading to the development of pore, that causes leakage of the cell contents resulting in its death. In addition to this the released components of the complement system C3a,C5a express chemotactic action and induce accumulation of Tc cells, macrophages, phagocytes and other immunological cells near the area of reaction. Since macrophages show affinity to FC region of IgG antibodies the cells bound with IgG are susceptible for phagocytosis. The remaining Killer cells of immune system also kill the foreign cells through surface bound antibody. Since antibody binding with antigen makes the foreign cell cytotoxic, Type II Hyper sensitivity is also referred as antibody mediated cytotoxic reaction. The antigen inducing these reactions may be an isoantigen or an auto antigen (self antigen). With reference to the type of antigen responsible for Type II Hyper sensitivity the reactions can be subdivided into (1) Isoimmune hyper sensitivity reactions and (2) auto immune hyper sensitivity reactions.

ISOIMMUNE HYPER SENSITIVITY REACTIONS: If Hyper sensitivity reactions are induced by antigens derived from individuals of same species, the reactions are referred as isoimmune Hyper sensitivity reactions. Blood transfusion reactions, graft rejection reactions, Rh incompatibility reactions are some of the examples for this hypersensitivity.

BLOOD TRANSFUSION REACTIONS: In blood transfusion procedures hemolytic reactions may develop due to mismatch of blood groups, between donor and recipient. In these reactions the serum factors of the recipient may agglutinate the RBCs of the donor, or serum of the donor may agglutinate RBCs of the recipient. The agglutination of the red blood cells and their lysis in circulation leads to various pathological changes such as jaundice, fever, kidney failure etc. Some times hemolytic reactions may lead to death of the recipient due to systemic shock brought about by massive erythrocyte destruction and kidney failure due to excessive function for the removal of debris of red blood cells. Minor hemolytic reactions like anemia occur when the lysis of RBCs is slow.

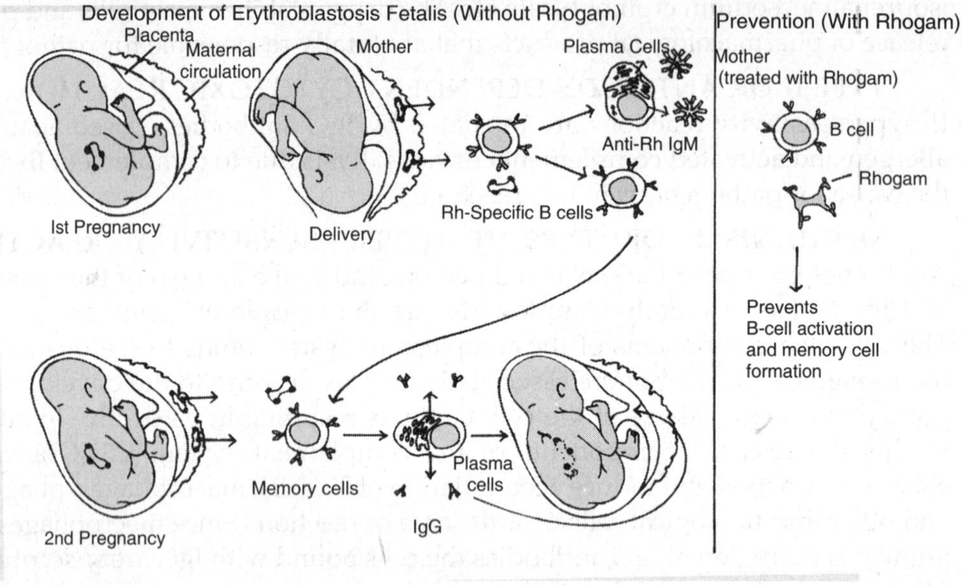

Fig. 14.3 Erythroblastosis fetalis

Rh INCOMPATIBILITY / ERYTHROBLSTOSIS FETALIS: If Rh⁻ women bear Rh⁺ fetus in her womb, Rh⁻ mother may get sensitized to Rh+ antigens produced by fetus and synthesize antibodies against to fetal Rh⁺ antigens. Normally maternal circulation does not mix with fetal circulation during gestation period. Hence the first baby rarely gets affected, but at the time of parturition (delivery) rupture of blood vessels and excessive bleeding during placental separation ensures entry of fetal Rh+ antigens into mothers circulation, triggering production of antibodies against Rh+ antigens. Once antibodies for Rh⁺ antigens are produced by mother subsequent pregnancy become risky. Since maternal antibodies produced are IgG type, they can enter fetal circulation crossing the placental barrier and bound to fetal RBCs inducing Type II hypersensitive reactions. As a consequence the baby may born with a disease called "Erythroblastosis fetalis" or "hemolytic disease" (Refer Chapter 20 for further information). The clinical symptoms include severe jaundice, enlargement of the infant spleen and liver. The treatment of this disease depends upon the severity of symptoms. In extreme cases total blood transfusion might be performed in order to save the baby from death due to shock.

This disease is not common with the first pregnancy as there is no inter mixing of maternal and fetal blood before delivery. But rarely hemorrahage can occur during the last trimester when the fetus is relatively large. However hemorrhage is usually slight and the concentration of fetal Rh+ factor is too low to induce Ab production in the mother.

GRAFT REJECTION: Since HLA antigens present on all nucleated cells are diverse in different individuals, immune system recognizes them on the graft tissue and triggers cytotoxic response against the graft (Refer Chapter 16 for transplantation).

AUTO IMMUNE REACTIONS: Immune system can distinguish self MHC antigens of their own cells from those of foreign cells and develop tolerance to self antigens. Yet some physiological autoimmune reactions against self antigens can occur and serve as physiological regulators of the immune system and are carefully controlled. But some times this carefully controlled activity goes away and large quantities of auto antibodies are produced leading to auto immune reactions.

MECHANISM OF ANTIBODY DEPENDENT CYTOTOXIC HYPER-SENSITIVITY: Type II or cytotoxic hypersensitivity reactions develop when interaction of serum IgG Abs & IgM Abs with foreign antigens on the cell membrane. The Ag & Ab complex initiates activation and fixation of complement system enzymes on the surface of foreign cell. The fixed complement enzymes such as C4b, C5b, C6, 7, 8, 9 produce membrane attack complex on foreign cell surface and develop a pore, leading to death of the cell due to leakage of cytoplasm. In addition to activated complement enzymes activity, some of the fragments of activated complement enzymes such as C3a, C5b, etc. are released in to the surroundings. Since these fragments are chemotactic for phagocytic cells, a phagocytic response is generated against the target cell. In addition to the complement dependent cytotoxic reactions, Ab dependent cytotoxic reactions are also induced due to the affinity of NK Cells to Fc region of IgG and IgM antibodies. If the foreign antigen happens to be a haptane and is adsorbed on to any of the cell, the cell with absorbed haptane also be removed by antibody dependent cytotoxic hypersensitivity reactions. Drug induced immune hemolytic anemia is a familiar example for this kind of reactions. Since penicillin like drug molecules show characters of heptane and bind to the surface of RBC and initiate Type II hyper sensitivity reactions leading to severe anemia. Individuals with this kind of problem show clinical symptoms like fever, weakness, jaundice etc.

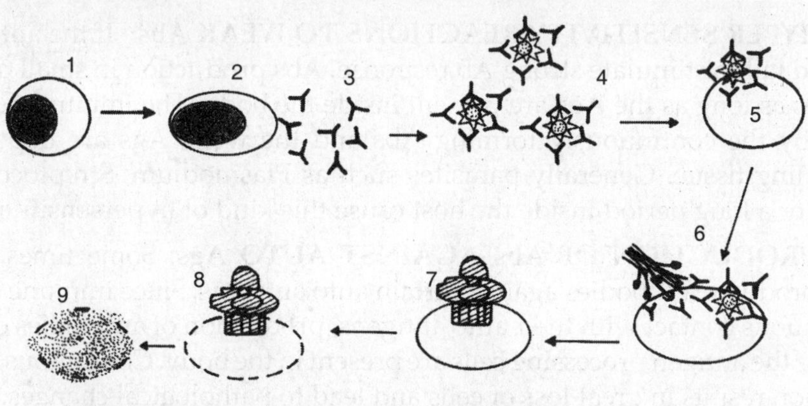

1. Activated B cell 2. Plasmacell 3. Antibodies
4. Ag-Ab complex 5. RBC with bound Ag-Ab complex
6. Activation of complement 7. MAC formation
8. Lysis of RBC 9. Broken RBC

Fig. 14.4. Mechanism of Type II Hypersensitivity

THERAPY: Treatment for blood transfusion reactions involves prompt termination of transfusion and maintenance of urine flow with diuretic drugs to minimize stress on kidneys. Treatment for hemolytic disease depends on the severity of the reactions. In severe cases the fetus can be given an intra uterine blood transfusion for every 10-21 days to replace fetal Rh+ red blood cells with Rh- cells until delivery. In less severe conditions blood transfusion is not necessary, but after birth the infant has to be exposed to low levels of UV light to remove the bilurubin and to avoid cerebral damage by bilurubin (Exposing infants to UVradiation helps to reduce high bilirubin levels). In certain cases mothers blood has to be screened for Rh+ antibodies by separating RBC and Plasma. If Rh+ antibodies are present, the plasma has to be replaced with fresh plasma solution without Rh+ antibodies. The consequences of A, B, O and AB blood group incompatibility are very minor, in case bilurubin is produced due to their incompatibility; exposure to UV light is enough to break down the bilurubin. Hemolytic disease can be prevented successfully through injection of Rh+ antibodies within 72 hours after delivery. Because the injected Rh+ Abs bind to Rh+ antigens of fetus, even before the activation of mother's immune system. When mother is not sensitized to Rh+ antigens, production of Rh+ Abs and memory cells does not take place to cause hemolytic disease.

TYPE III OR IMMUNE COMPLEX MEDIATED HYPERSENSITIVITY: This type of hypersensitivity develops when the immune system encounters large number of free antigens. Interaction of antibodies with free antigens results in the formation of precipitating antigen antibody complexes Normally monocytes or macrophages (MΦ) remove these precipitates very efficiently, but their efficiency is minimized, if the precipitate is formed in antigen excess resulting Type III hypersensitivity reactions. The diseases brought about by Type III or immune complex mediated reactions is broadly classified into 3 categories

1. HYPER SENSITIVITY REACTIONS TO WEAK Abs: If the antigens are weak and fail to stimulate strong Ab response, Abs production in small quantities continues as long as the Ags are present inside the body. The immune complexes formed by the continuously forming Abs and the weak Ags are deposited on surrounding tissue. Generally parasites such as Plasmodium, Streptococcus etc. staying for a long period inside the host cause this kind of hypersensitivity.

2. PRODUCTION OF Abs AGAINST AUTO Ags: Some times immune system produces antibodies against certain auto antigens. Since immune system is in continuous contact with their auto antigens, production of antibodies continues as long as the antigen processing cells are present in the body. Continuous antibody production results in great loss of cells and lead to pathological changes.

3. EXCESSIVE Ag - Ab COMPLEX FORMATION: When the scavenger systems such as phagocytes, complement system etc. get over loaded, certain Ag-Ab complexes are left in the body. The left out Ag- Ab complexes then settle on several surrounding tissues causing diseases like Systemic Lupus Erythematosus (SLE).

MECHANISM OF TYPE III HYPER SENSITIVITY: When Ag-Ab complexes are not properly removed from the system, they get deposited on the surrounding tissue, and trigger a variety of inflammation processes. The activation of complement system is one of them. The C3a and C5a fragments of activated components of the complement system are anaphylactic in nature and initiate release of vasoactive amines such as histamine serotonin etc. from mast cells and basophils ensuing inflammation. Usually activity of complement system helps in the removal of foreign bodies through lysis or phagocytosis, but in Type III Hyper sensitive reactions, the cells that are removed by this process are normal cells to which left out Ag- Ab complexes are attached resulting in necrosis (destruction of cells).

Through chemotactic action of C5a, Polymorphonuclear cells (PMNs) also reach the site of inflammation and attempt to ingest Ab - Ag complexes. Since the complexes are trapped in the tissue they fail to ingest them. Therefore they release their lytic enzymes in the vicinity of the reaction, ensuing lysis of host cells around the reaction site. In normal conditions lysosomal secretions released in to the blood or tissue are rapidly neutralized by certain inhibitor enzymes. But in Type III Hyper sensitivity reaction, the phagocytes gather close to the tissue trapped immune complexes through Fc binding, hence serum inhibitors are excluded and destruction of tissues is continued by the activity of lytic enzymes.

In addition to complement system platelets also interact with the left out immune complexes through their receptors for Fc region of Abs, release their secretions ensuing microthrombus formation, followed by an increase in vascular permeability. Since the platelets are a rich source for growth factors, their release may result in abnormal proliferation of immune cells also in the site of reaction. The increased vascular permeability allows immune complexes deposition on tissues. The turbulence in blood flow and high blood pressure will also induce deposition of immune complexes leading to pathological conditions like arthus reaction, glomerulonephritis etc. The intensity of reactions generally depends upon the concentration of antigen to that of Ab and the reactions may be local or systemic like other hyper sensitivity reactions.

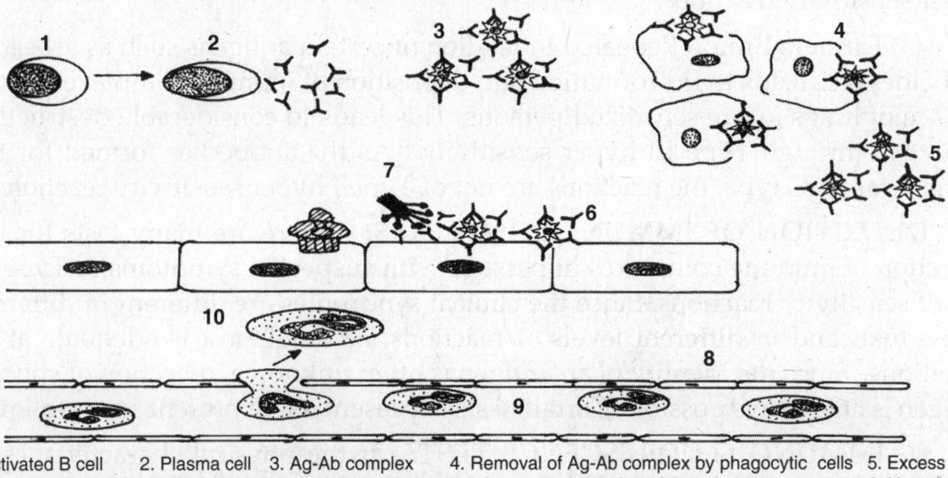

1. Activated B cell 2. Plasma cell 3. Ag-Ab complex 4. Removal of Ag-Ab complex by phagocytic cells 5. Excess Ag-Ab complex 6. Deposition of AgAb complex on surrounding tissue 7. Activation of complement enzymes 8. Vascular changes 9. Marginalization 10. Migration of neutrophils

Fig. 14.5. Mechanism of type III hyper sensitivity

EXAMPLES FOR TYPE III HYPER SENSITIVITY:

(1) Arthus Reaction (A Local Type III Hyper Sensitivity):- It was named after the scientist who first observed it in rabbits. It is a local reaction that has been formed on the skin after intra dermal injection of antigen. Binding of an antigen with circulating antibodies results in this kind of reaction. Symptoms of the reaction may appear in 2 to 8 hours after the injection of antigens and persists for about 12 to 24 hours. The reaction starts as an erythematosus edema due to local hemorrhage and thrombosis in average limits. The reactions begin with marginalization (attachment of the cells to the wall of blood vessel) and migration of neutrophils through the walls of blood capillaries. Infiltration of the neutrophils continue till the reaction has reached to maximal intensity (for about 6-8hours). As the reaction progresses, destruction of walls of blood vessels take place, resulting in edema and hemorrhage. This vascular destruction is associated with platelet aggregation and thrombosis

The antigen injected into the body diffuses away from the site of injection through tissue spaces and crosses the walls of small blood vessels, enters into the circulation and encounters the Abs. As a result, immune complex is generated and deposited in between and beneath the epithelial cells leading to the initiation of Type III Hyper sensitivity reactions.

(2) Serum Sickness (Systemic Hyper sensitivity reaction): - It is a systemic hyper sensitive reaction. When antigens are administered intravenously to animals with a high level of circulating Abs, development of immune complexes takes place in circulation. The larger complexes are removed by phagocytosis, but small complexes formed in antigen excess escape phagocytosis. These escaped small complexes induce complement fixation, platelet aggregation and release of vasoactive amines and thus alter the properties of vascular endothelium. When the escaped immune complexes adhere to the cells of certain vital parts such as glomeruli, choroid plexus, vascular filters etc., they get damaged by systemic hyper sensitivity reaction.

(3) Farmers lung: - Repeated inhalation of certain antigens such as asbestos, pesticides etc., leads to the formation and deposition of immune complexes on the surface of lungs in pre sensitized persons. This leads to considerable destruction of alveoli through Type III hyper sensitivity. As the antibodies formed for the antigens are IgG type, the reactions are not of Type I hyper sensitivity reactions.

DETECTION OF IMMUNE COMPLEXES: - There are many tests for the detection of immune complexes in persons with suspected symptoms of Type III hyper sensitivity reactions. Since the clinical syndromes are different in different individuals and in different levels of reactions, no single test is adequate at all situations. Since the identity of an antigen is often unknown, detection of specific antigen is not always possible. Certain tests in present use at present are as follows.

(1) IMMUNO FLUORESCENCE TEST: - If the physical characteristics of antigen are known, tissue samples can be studied by immunoflurescence for the presence of antigen and Ab complex by laser nephelometry. Since polyethylene glycol (PEG) has the capacity to precipitate high molecular weight immune complexes, serum samples can be added to buffer, containing PEG, to precipitate Ag -Ab complex that can be monitored by laser nephelometry.

(2) PLATELET AGGREGATION TEST: If we know the adhering tendency of antigen to cell membrane, Ag -Ab complexes can be detected via the platelet aggregation test. Since Ag-Ab complexes interact with membrane surface of blood platelets and cause aggregation the presence of platelets in test sample can be studied either visually with a microscope, or electrically by means of changes in turbidity measurements. The platelet aggregation test measures the rate and degree to which dispersed platelets in a sample of plasma (the liquid portion of blood) form clumps after the addition of a material that normally stimulates aggregation. These materials may include adenosine diphosphate (ADP), epinephrine, arachidonic acid, collagen, or ristocetin. Clumping of platelets causes the sample to be more clear (less turbid). A machine measures the changes in turbidity (cloudiness) and prints a graphic recording of the results.

TEST WITH RADIO LABELED ANTI-IgG Abs: - In this assay the property of Ag-Ab complex interaction with certain components of the complement system is exploited. The serum samples are exposed to Clq component of complement system bound to the sides of the test tube. If immune complexes are present, they bind to the Clq. Following incubation, sample is removed and again incubated with radio labelled Anti-IgG Abs. The amount of radioactivity correlates with the concentration of immune complexes in the serum sample. This character has provided a basis for a novel therapeutic procedure called Plasmaphoresis. Individuals with certain immune complex disorders can be treated by Plasmaphoresis, to remove immune complxes from their serum. The therapy is performed with an automatic continuous flow of blood through cell separator machine that removes the large immune complexes and returns the cleared plasma to the individual.

SOME COMMON IMMUNE COMPLEX DISORDERS:-

(1) Acute post streptococal glomerulonephritis: If the simple and common problem sore throat developed by simple *streptococcal* infection is neglected, it can lead to kidney failure. When immune complexes formed by streptococcal bacteria and antibodies get deposited on the glomerular basal lamina of kidney, they induce Type III hyper sensitivity. Tissue damage through Type III hyper sensitivity reactions leads to chronic renal failure.

(2) Lepromatous Leprosy: Systemic invasion of *Mycobacterium leprae* (leprosy causing bacteria) produce a high titer of antigenic fragments. The immune complex formed with this antigen induces hundreds of sore, red skin lesions all over the body due to the deposition of immune complexes in capillary beds beneath the skin. Another complication of lepromatous leprosy is deposition of immune complexes in the joints and kidneys leading to arthritis and kidney malfunctions.

(3) Seconday Syphilis: This sexually transmitted disease is caused by *Treponema pallidum*. If the disease is not treated in the initial stages with antibiotics, it progresses to secondary stage due to the formation of immune complexes developed in the body with the released antigens of *Treponema pallidum*, resulting in Type III hyper sensitivity related pathological conditions.

(4) Malaria: The *Plasmodium* parasites invade blood and hepatic cells and induce hyper sensitivity reactions resulting in pathogenesis. Raise of body temperature, with chills at regular intervals is due to hyper sensitivity reactions induced by the toxins released by the parasites. Rheumatoid arthritis, Goodpastures syndrome etc. (Refer Chapter15 for further information) are examples for type III hyper sensitivity.

TYPE IV OR TD CELL MEDIATED HYPER SENSITIVITY: Symptoms of certain hyper sensitivity reactions appear after 24 to 72hours of exposure to allergen and such reactions are referred as delayed type hyper sensitivity reactions. The term delayed hyper sensitivity was first coined by Koch in late nineteenth century, while studying immunity to tuberculosis. When certain antigens are injected into the skin of sensitized animals an inflammatory response develops after many hours of injection. Several evidences suggest that, type IV reaction is important in host defense against parasites. Unlike other forms of hyper sensitivity reactions Type IV hyper sensitivity cannot be transferred from one animal to another thorough serum, but can be transferred by T cells. Three types of delayed hyper sensitivity reactions have been recognized (1) Contact hyper sensitivity (2) Tuberculin-Type hyper sensitivity (3) Granulomatus hyper sensitivity.

(1) Contact Hyper sensitivity: This kind of hyper sensitivity reaction produces eczematous response at the site of contact with the allergen which is generally a haptane like chemical. The small antigenic molecules (haptanes) penetrate epidermis and bind to the proteins inside and act as sensitizers. The protein bound haptens are first internalized by epidermal langerhans cells and later carried to paracortical areas of lymphnodes by circulation and finally they are presented to T Cells. Release of lymphokines from the stimulated cells results in manifestation of clinical symptoms after 12 to 15hours of contact.

(2) Tuberculin Type hyper sensitivity (Mantoux Reactions): When a small dose of tuberculin (antigen derived from the tubercle bacillus) is injected intradermally into a sensitized individual, hardening and swelling develops at the site of injection. Soluble antigens from a number of organisms including *Mycobacterium tuberculosis, M leprae* and *Leishmania tropica* induce similar type of reactions in sensitive people. Granulomatous reaction due to persistence of antigens in the tissues may be responsible for the development of lesions.

(3) Granulomatous hyper sensitivity: It is the most important from of delayed hyper sensitivity reactions rooting many of the pathological effects. If macrophages fail to destroy the engulfed microbes or their Ag particles, the persistent immune complex induces **epithelioid cell granuloma** formation. In the same way **granuloma** formation occurs with a variety of foreign bodies or particulate agents, when macrophages fail to digest the inorganic matter of foreign agents or particulate matter. Epithelioid granuloma cells are large flattened cells with increased endoplasmic reticulum. The region affected by Type IV hyper sensitivity reactions typically show a core of epithelioid cells and macrophages, with or without giant cells and the core is surrounded by a cuff of lymphocytes and a considerable fibrosis. Increased proliferation of fibroblasts and collagen synthesis ensue fibrosis in reaction areas. Delayed hyper sensitivity reaction manifests many chronic diseases in man. Some of the important diseases developed by delayed hyper sensitivity reactions are Tuberculosis, Leprosy, Leishmaniasis, Deep fungal infections and Helminth infections.

MECHANISM OF CELL MEDIATED HYPER SENSITIVITY REACTIONS: Mechanism of delayed hyper sensitivity reactions involve activation of T cells by Ags that are bound to the cell. The activated T cell proliferates to produce clones of T_D and T_C lymphocytes. Interaction of Ags with primed T cells induces release of lymphokines from T cells. Since the lymphokines contain macrophage stimulating factor, macrophage migration inhibiting factor etc., the macrophages are accumulated to phagocytize and destroy foreign cells at the site of infection. The degradative lytic enzymes released from activated macrophages produce localized inflammatory response, resulting in necrosis and fibrosis in the host tissue along with destruction of foreign agents.

MEASUREMENT OF DELAYED HYPERSENSIVITY: There are different tests to measure delayed hyper sensitivity. They are grouped in to four categories. (1) Skin tests (2) Lymphocyte activation tests (3) T Lymphocyte assays and (4) T cell function tests.

Skin test: This test is used to establish previous exposure to particular antigen. The antigen to be tested is injected into the skin and studied for positive delayed inflammation reaction at the site of injection.

Lymphocyte activation test: This test is commonly used to Judge' cellular immunity in individuals with immune deficiency, autoimmunity, infections, diseases and cancer. The test depends on culture of purified lymphocytes of patients in media containing mitogens. (Mitogene is a plant or bacteria derived product that have the ability to stimulate lymphocytes division). Since DNA synthesis is very active during cell division, a radio active precursor of DNA has to be added to the media, before leaving it for incubation. The radioactivity levels are measured after incubation to estimate the rate of division. High quantity of radioactive substance indicates high rate of cell division in the subject tested.

E Rosette test : The test helps to estimate the number of stimulated T cells in an individual to identify immune disorders. As human cell bind with sheep erythrocytes, they form flower like rosettes with centrally located sheep erythrocyte. The role of this test is being superseded by the use of the fluorescence activated cell sorter.

Macrophage migration inhibition test:-This test helps to judge the functioning capacity of lymphocytes through liberated lymphokines. It is a test which measures the presence of migration-inhibitory factor. Usually peritoneal macrophages are placed in a capillary tube in the presence or absence of supernatants from activated T-cells. If migration inhibition factor is present, the migration of monocyte/macrophages is reduced.

TYPE V OR STIMULATORY HYPER SENSITIVITY : This hyper sensitivity is some what similar to Type II hyper sensitivity but here the hyper sensitivity reaction stimulates an inappropriate and enhanced function of the target cells. Thyrotoxicosis or graves disease is a very good example for the stimulatory hyper sensitivity.

Thyrotoxicosis:- It is a disease condition due to over activity and secretion of thyroid (Refer Chapter 15 for autoimmune diseases). The reaction causing agent is an IgG antibody, which mimics the thyroid stimulating hormone molecules released from pituitary gland.

15

AUTOIMMUNITY

The healthy person's body is equipped with a powerful set of tools in the form of "immune system" to resist the attack of invading microorganisms such as viruses, bacteria, and parasites. Immune system responds in a regulated fashion towards microbes and eliminates them, but it does not respond to self-antigens. Several regulatory mechanisms terminate immune response to foreign antigens to return the immune system in to the normal condition following clearance of the antigens. Regulatory mechanisms also maintain immune unresponsiveness, or tolerance, to self-antigens. Unfortunately, in spite of these regulatory mechanisms, immune system sometimes goes awry and attacks its own body. Failure of immune systems tolerance to self antigens ensues in pathological state. The misdirected immune response results in debilitating illness and sometimes death is referred as "autoimmunity". This can be demonstrated by the presence of auto antibodies or T lymphocytes reactive with self antigens. Generally immune system tolerates their own potentially antigenic substances, and failure of self tolerance is the fundamental cause for autoimmunity.

To some extent autoimmune response (sometimes termed as natural autoimmunity) is an integral part of vertebrate immune systems. Auto antibodies are believed to be a product of natural selection and have been suggested to play an important role in "housekeeping" functions. They serve as physiological regulators of the immune system and act as components of body's homeostasis. Indeed, natural autoimmunity performs several functions that include the scavenging of metabolic waste and senescent cells, a first line of protection against viral and bacterial infection.

The role of Natural autoantibodies (NAb) in health and Disease

- Antikeratin antibodies enhance the elimination of keratin after keratinocyte death.
- IgG NAb anti-band 3 proteins participate in the elimination of senescent red blood cells.
- IgM NAb increase resistance to tumors.
- NAb may be cytotoxic.

- NAb may inhibit interferon action by binding to the cell surface.
- NAb may inhibit NK cell activity.
- IgM NAb anti-IgG inhibits the binding of IgG to self-antigens.
- NAb anti-idiotype antibodies to pathogenic autoantibodies may have therapeutic potential.
- Some NAb posess proteolytic activity on the vasoactive intestinal peptide.
- IgM (but not IgG) NAb enhance phagocytosis of parasites.
- Natural anti-trinitrophenyl autoantibodies protect against viral infection.

Yet the appearance of normal auto antibodies is a carefully controlled event. Autoimmune disorders might simply arise as a consequence of the dysregulation of natural physiological autoimmunity. The mechanisms involved in the shift fom physiological to pathological autoimmunity are unknown.

Several theories have been proposed since the mid-twentieth century to explain origin of self tolerance but the exact mechanism of induction and maintenance of tolerance is not fully understood. Different possible ways for origin of self tolerance are as follows.

CLONAL DELETION THEORY : Burnet has proposed clonal deletion theory to explain origin of self tolerance. According to his theory destruction of self-reactive lymphoid cells takes place during the development of the immune system. T and B lymphocytes undergo positive and negative selection during their development and maturation within the primary lymphoid organs. During this process, cells that can react with self antigens undergo clonal deletion. Thus clonal deletion plays a key role in ensuring tolerance to self antigen. If any T and B cells fail to undergo deletion, the immune system has devised several additional check points to maintain tolerance. For example T cells upon activation not only produce cytokines or carryout their effector functions but also die through programmed cell death or apoptosis.

CLONAL ANERGY: According to Nossal, self-reactive T- or B-cells become inactivated in the normal individual and cannot amplify the immune response. T cells when exposed to auto-reactive antigenic peptides on antigen presenting cells (APC) that do not possess the co-stimulatory molecules become anergic (nonresponsive) to the antigen. B cells when exposed to large amounts of soluble antigen down-regulate their surface IgM and become anergic.

CLONAL IGNORANCE : Host immune responses are directed to ignore self-antigens. T cells reactive to self-antigen, not represented in the thymus may mature and migrate to the periphery but they may never encounter the appropriate antigen because it is sequestered in inaccessible tissues (tissue not drained directly by the lymphocytes) such as central nervous tissue, testicular tissue etc. Hence cells reactive to self-antigen may die for lack of stimulus. Auto-reactive B cells that escape deletion may not find the antigen or the specific T-cells help and thus not get activated and die out.

ANTI-IDIOTYPE ANTIBODY: According to this theory a network of antibodies capable of neutralizing self-reactive antibodies exists naturally within the body. Anti-idiotypic antibodies are produced during the process of tolerization and have been demonstrated in tolerant animals. These antibodies may prevent the B cell receptor from interacting with the antigen

SUPPRESSOR POPULATION OR REGULATORY T CELLS: Regulatory T-lymphocytes (commonly CD_4^+ $FoxP_3^+$ cells, among others) prevent, down regulate, or limit autoaggressive immune responses. The precise mechanism/s through which regulatory T cells suppresses the function of other T cell is not yet clear. One of the mechanisms is production of immunosuppressive cytokines such as, TGF-β and IL-10. Genetic mutations in Foxp3 in human beings leads to development of a severe and rapidly fatal autoimmune disorder known as Immune dysregulation, Polyendocrinopathy, Enteropathy, X-linked (IPEX) syndrome. This disease provides the most striking evidence that regulatory T cells play a critical role in preventing autoimmune diseases.

In spite of this regulation and mechanisms for clonal deletion of many self-reactive T and B cells, immune system occasionally attack auto antigens and produce autoimmunity. Autoimmunity can be the cause of a broad spectrum of human illnesses, known as autoimmune diseases. The concept of autoimmunity is first predicted by the Nobel Laureate Paul Ehrlich in the beginning of the twentieth century, and he described it as "horror autotoxicus".

Clonal deletion and anergy of self-specific lymphocytes greatly reduces but does not eliminate the possibility of low affinity self-specific responses. Transient autoimmune responses are common but usually cause no lasting damage. The random generation of many diverse T cell receptors (TCR) and B cell receptors (BCR) makes autoimmunity possible. Since self antigens are continually present in the body, prolonged autoimmune responses cause tissue damage, which may be life-threatening. Autoimmune diseases caused by auto antibodies or T cells, may be systemic or organ-specific. Autoimmune diseases are initiated by activation of antigen-specific TH cells. TH cells in turn activate B cells, to produce auto antibodies, which damage tissues by activating complement system directly or initiating prolonged inflammation. Cytotoxic T lymphocytes and macrophages activated by TH cells are directly cytotoxic and also promote inflammation. The events that initiate specific autoimmune diseases are not clearly understood. Various factors that cause break down of self tolerance may result in autoimmune reactions.

MECHANISM OF BREAK DOWN OF SELF TOLERANCE:

EXPOSURE OF SEQUESTERED ANTIGEN: Some times the hidden or sequestered antigens get exposed to the circulating lymphocytes due to their release from inaccessible tissues such as central nervous tissue, testicular tissue, eye lens etc., either by accidental traumatic injury or surgery. Exposure of sequestered antigens results in the stimulation of auto immune response leading to an autoimmune disease. For example, inflammation of the testis known as "orchitis" occurs in males followed by mumps. Since mumps virus damage the basement membrane of seminiferous tubules, leading to the release of sperms in to the circulation. As the production of spermatozoa begins in puberty (at the age of 13 to 15), sperm antigens are not exposed to the developing immune system, hence immune system fails to develop tolerance to them. Production of antibodies against sperm antigens takes place when sperm antigens enter in to the blood. The circulating antibodies enter the testis and initiates immune response.

Inflammatory eye diseases also develop in the same manner. Antibodies produced against the lens proteins are responsible for the pathogenesis. The development of lens takes place around tenth week of gestation and thereafter they are isolated from fetal circulation. Since the lens proteins are encapsulated prior to the development of immune system, they can not induce tolerance. Therefore if lens proteins escape into the circulation due to surgery or any other injury they induce production of antibodies against them resulting different inflammatory eye diseases and damage of lens.

The exact etiology of autoimmune diseases is not yet known. However, various theories have been offered. These include sequestered antigens, escape of auto-reactive clones, loss of suppressor cells, cross reactive antigens including exogenous antigens (pathogens) and altered self antigens (chemical and viral infections).

ESCAPE OF AUTO-REACTIVE CLONES : The negative selection in the thymus may not be fully functional to eliminate self reactive cells. Not all self antigens may be represented in the thymus or certain antigens may not be properly processed and presented. Hence, to some extent autoimmunity is present in everyone and facilitates autoimmune pathology in some individuals, but in others they are components of protective mechanism. The escape of auto reactive cones allows immune system to mount an effective and specific immune response against self determinants.

DEVELOPMENT OF NEW ANTIGENIC DETERMINANTS : The development of new antigenic determinants on normal proteins may provoke formation of auto antibodies, ensuing autoimmune disease. Formation of rheumatoid factors and immunoconglutinins are the best examples for auto antibodies generated in this fashion. Rheumatoid factors are antibodies produced by the immune system against newly exposed antigenic determinants of other immunoglobulins. In affected people, when antigens bind to certain IgG antibodies, new antigenic determinants are exposed in the Fc region of the molecule, and these new determinants stimulate the formation of rheumatoid factors. Most strikingly, arthritis can be transferred with serum or with purified antibody of the systemic auto antigen.

HORMONES : Hormones affect function of immune cells and consequently immune system activities. For example, estrogen influences the production of regulatory factors produced by immune cells and tissues. As immune cell functions are dependent on these regulatory factors, estrogen levels alter the functioning of immune system to a certain extent. Onset of some autoimmune diseases may coincide with pregnancy or menopause. For example, autoimmune thyroiditis (Hashimoto's and Grave's) and rheumatoid arthritis generally improve during pregnancy (pregnancy is associated primarily with elevated progesterone and to a lesser extent estrogen), but tend to return post partum. In addition, the typical age of onset varies among autoimmune diseases. For example, SLE (systemic lupus erythmatosis) onset commonly occurs after puberty and during the reproductive years, while rheumatoid arthritis onset tends to occur later with a peak around the age of menopause and declining estrogen levels.

INFECTIONS : There are intimate links between infectious agents (viruses, bacteria, etc) and autoimmunity. Microbial attack may be one of the key environmental factors that trigger autoimmune disease. Although the microorganisms present are too low to be detected even by the most sensitive clinical tests, they are detected by the immune system. Even the most virulent microbes fail to cause disease in such low quantity, but the immune system attempts to flush out and destroy them, which could cause extensive damage to apparently normal tissues.

Exposure of auto-antigens on the surface of microbial cells is another possibility for induction of autoimmune reactions. Molecular mimicry (resemblance of auto antigens) is another possibility for induction of autoimmune reactions. Some times antigens present on the foreign agents show resemblances with the host's auto antigens hence antibodies produced against the foreign agents' cross-react with auto cell antigens leading to damage their own cells. Inflammation of valvular endocardium in acute rheumatic fever, hemolytic anemia in syphilis are very good examples for this kind of auto immunity. Cross reaction of antibodies produced against *Streptococus* bacteria in rheumatic fever, with cells of cardiac valves leads to their dysfunction resulting in dilation and congestive heart failure. Cross reaction of antibodies produced against *Treponema palidum* antigens with certain erythrocyte blood group antigens results in the destruction of RBC's leading to hemolytic anemia.

Adjuvants (usually bacterial) when administered with self-antigens activate the innate immune response similar to pathogen-specific manner; this process results in organ-specific autoimmune disease in animal models. Microorganisms are likely to provide not only the adjuvant effect to stimulate the immune response but also the damage necessary to make self-antigens available to the immune system, resulting in autoimmune disease. Viruses also induce autoimmune diseases through polyclonal activation of lymphocytes.

DEVELOPMENT OF PREVIOUSLY SUPPRESSED IMMUNE CELLS: It is not uncommon to find autoimmune disease associated with lymphoid tumors. For example, myasthenia gravis may be associated with the presence of thymoma (tumor originating from the thymus). In humans there is a four fold increase in the incidence of rheumatoid disease in patients with malignant lymphoid tumor, and there is evidence for a similar association in other animals. Since development of tumor is an indication of failure in immunological control mechanism, a simultaneous failure in self tolerance may also occur. Alternatively, some tumors may represent the development of a "forbidden clone" of cells producing auto antibodies.

BINDING OF CERTAIN DRUGS/CHEMICALS: Some drugs or chemicals fasten to the surface of certain cells. Immune response raised by the antibodies attachment to this foreign substance destroys the cell also along with the removal of foreign substance. Hemolytic anemia following exposure to antibiotic drug penicillin is a very good example for this kind of auto immunity.

DEFECTS IN IMMUNE SYSTEM: Defects in lymphoid organs, mutations in lymphocytes or defective function of lymphocytes could result in autoimmune reactions. Thymus atrophy is often encountered with systemic lupus erythmatosis (SLE). If elimination of self reacting lymphocytes is not properly done during their development in primary lymphoid organs and released in to the circulation, they may induce autoimmune problems. Since proper antigen presentation is essential for proper action of immune cells, defects in antigen presenting cells could result in auto immune reactions. Cytokine imbalances or defective immune regulatory circuits may also contribute to the emergence of autoimmunity. For example, decreased apoptosis, diminished production of tumor necrosis factor (TNF) and interleukin- 10 (IL-10) has been reported to be associated with the development of autoimmunity.

Intense stimulation of T lymphocytes can produce nonspecific signals that bypass the need for antigen-specific helper T cells and lead to polyclonal B cell activation with the formation of multiple auto antibodies. For example, antinuclear, anti erythrocyte and anti lymphocyte antibodies are produced during the chronic graft-versus-host reaction.

ANTI-IDIOTYPE ANTIBODIES: One of the mechanisms that regulate normal humoral immune responses is production of *anti-idiotype antibodies*. These are immunoglobulin molecules directed against antigen-binding determinants of the specific antibodies originally elicited by the immunogen. Even the initial immunogen is T cell independent, production of anti-idiotype antibodies may depend on TH cells activity. Therefore, it is possible that abnormalities in the synthesis of appropriate anti-idiotype antibodies, either at the B or T cell level are responsible for the development of autoimmunity in certain circumstances.

GENETIC FACTORS: Since genes influence overall reactivity of the immune system, they may predispose an individual to autoimmunity. Three main sets of genes are suspected in many autoimmune diseases they are genes for immunoglobulins, T-cell receptors and the major histocompatibility complexes (MHC). The first two are concerned in the recognition of antigens and are inherently variable and susceptible to recombination. These variations enable the immune system to respond to a very wide variety of invaders, but some times the variation may result in the production of self reactive lymphocytes. Some of the MHC class II allotypes are strongly correlated with specific autoimmune diseases. Other allotypes may affect the ability of the target tissue to resist or modify immune attack.

LACK OF REGULATORY T CELLS: Regulatory T-cells are important for the maintenance of peripheral tolerance. Fundamentally regulatory T cells have a suppressive effect on the neighboring immune cells, thus contributing to the local modulation and control of immune response. There are fewer regulatory T-cells in many autoimmune diseases, In the IPEX syndrome (immunodysregulation, poly endocrinopathy and enteropathy, X-linked), which is caused by mutation in Foxp3 gene. The Foxp3 gene influences the development and function of regulatory T cells. Mutations in the gene results in severe autoimmune reactions that may produce the following auto immune problems;

Autoimmune endocrine disorders eg. Type 1 diabetes, thyroiditis etc.,

- Respiratory and nutritive allergies.
- Eczema and severe infections.
- Different types of allergies eg. allergy for pollen grains, dust mites, nutritive allergens.
- Autoimmune diseases eg. rheumatoid arthritis, multiple sclerosis type 1 diabetes
- Lower number or decreased functional capability of regulatory T cells.

It is clear that no single mechanism can explain all the varied manifestations of autoimmunity. Indeed, it appears clearly in systemic autoimmune diseases, where a number of abnormalities converge to induce the complete syndrome. Moreover, one abnormality may cause a second, which, in concert with the first facilitates the expression of autoimmunity.

COMMON FEATURES IN AUTOIMMUNE REACTIONS:

1. An elevated level of immunoglobulins.
2. Demonstrable levels of auto antibodies.
3. Deposition of immunoglobulins or their derivatives at the site of trouble such as renal glomeruli.
4. Accumulation of lymphocytes and plasma cells at the site of lesions.
5. Temporary or lasting benefit from immunosuppressive therapy.
6. Occurrence of more than one type of autoimmune lesion in an individual.
7. Genetic predisposition towards autoimmunity.

PATHOGENIC MECHANISMS IN AUTOIMMUNITY

Pathogenic mechanisms in autoimmunity are not similar in all cases; different mechanisms are involved in different diseases. Damage may be caused by complement fixing antibodies raised against auto antigens, or binding of auto antibodies to cells surface receptors to initiate destructive inflammatory response or by activated cytotoxic cells against auto antigens.

Pathogenesis may be due to destruction of a particular type of cell or tissue, or stimulation of an organ into excessive growth, or interference in the function of certain organs. Organs and tissues frequently affected by autoimmune processes include the endocrine glands such as the thyroid, pancreas, adrenal glands, components of the blood and the connective tissues, skin, muscle, and joints.

CLASSIFICATION OF AUTOIMMUNE DISEASES

Autoimmune diseases can be broadly divided into a) Autoimmune anemias (b) localized or organ specific diseases (c) systemic or non organ specific diseases and (d) transitory diseases depending on the principal clinico-pathologic features of each disease.

(A) AUTOIMMUNE ANEMIAS: Autoimmune anemias results in destruction of the components of blood due to auto antibodies formed against one's own RBCs eg. Hemolytic anaemia, pernicious anemia, dug induced anemia etc.

Autoimmune hemolytic anemia: Production of auto antibodies against RBC antigens leads to anemic condition in some people. Hemolysis is usually extra vascular. There are two groups of antibodies responsible for hemolytic anemia they are, warm and cold antibodies. Generally the cold auto antibodies are complete agglutinating antibodies and belong to the IgM class. They agglutinate erythrocytes at < 37°C but not at > 37° C. Cold agglutinins are seen in paroxysmal cold hemoglobulinuria, trypanosomiasis, black water fever and primary atypical pneumonia.

Warm antibody hemolytic anemia is the most common form of autoimmune hemolytic anemia (AIHA); it is more common among women. Warm antibodies are frequently seen in patients taking drugs like sulphonamides, antibiotics, and alpha methyl dopa. Auto antibodies in warm antibody hemolytic anemia generally react at temperatures > 37° C. They may arise spontaneously or in association with certain diseases such as SLE, lymphoma, chronic lymphatic leukemia etc. The warm auto antibodies generally, incomplete non agglutinating antibodies, usually belong to the IgG class.

It can be seen coating the erythrocytes in the direct Coombs test. The direct antiglobulin (Coombs') test establishes the diagnosis and may suggest the cause. If symptoms are mild or if destruction of red blood cells seems to be slowing on its own, no treatment is needed. If red blood cell destruction is increasing, a corticosteroid such as prednisone is usually the first choice for treatment. When people do not respond to corticosteroids or when the corticosteroid causes intolerable side effects, surgery to remove the spleen (splenectomy) is often the next treatment. The spleen is removed because it is one of the places where antibody-coated red blood cells are destroyed. When destruction of red blood cells persists after removal of the spleen or when surgery cannot be done, immunosuppressive drugs, such as **cyclophosphamide or azathioprine** are used. When red blood cell destruction is severe, blood transfusions are sometimes needed, but they do not treat the cause of the anemia and provide only temporary relief.

Pernicious anemia: Pernicious anemia or Megaloblastic anemia is a disease where large, immature, nucleated cells (megaloblasts, which are forerunners of red blood cells) circulate in the blood, and do not function as blood cells. Megaloblasts are produced in the bone marrow when vitamin B-12 or folic acid levels are low. It is due to an inability to absorb vitamin B-12 (also known as cobalamin or Cbl) from the gastrointestinal tract. Vitamin B12 substitute is a nutrient found in animal products; both meat and dairy products. Normally, vitamin B-12 binds to intrinsic factor in the stomach, and this facilitates its absorption by the small intestine. Auto antibodies against intrinsic factor (IF), attacks the IF protein and lowers IF levels in stomach secretions resulting in the failure of absorption of vitamin B-12. Pernicious anemia is sometimes associated with other autoimmune diseases such as Graves' disease, Hashimoto's thyroiditis and vitiligo (depigmentation or blanching of skin areas). Megaloblastic anemia can also be caused by other disease of the bone marrow and can be a side effect of some cancer chemotherapy drugs. In addition to weakness and other anemia associated problems, severe or long-lasting pernicious anemia can damage the heart, brain, and other organs in the body. Pernicious anemia also can cause other complications, such as nerve damage, neurological problems (such as memory loss), and digestive tract problems. People who have pernicious anemia also may be at higher risk for stomach cancer. Pernicious anemia usually is easy to treat with vitamin B12 pills or shots. With ongoing care and proper treatment, most people who have pernicious anemia can recover, feel well, and live normal lives.

Drug-induced immune hemolytic anemia: Drug-induced immune hemolytic anemia is a blood disorder that occurs when a medicine triggers the body's immune system to attack its own red blood cells. About 16 to 18 per cent of cases of acquired immune haemolytic anaemia are caused by drug administration. In some cases, a drug can cause the immune system to mistakenly think its own red blood cells are dangerous, foreign substances. Antibodies then develop against the red blood cells. The antibodies attach to red blood cells and cause them to break down too early. Drugs that can start an immune reaction against red blood cells are Penicillin and its derivatives, Cephalosporins, Levodopa, Methyldopa, Quinidine and Some anti-inflammatory drugs.

Autoimmune thrombocytopenia: Autoimmune disorder causes lack of blood platelets. It is one of the most common autoimmune disorders. It occurs in 2 distinct clinical types, one is acute self-limiting form observed almost exclusively in children (5 cases per 100,000 persons), and another is chronic form, observed mostly in adults (3-5 cases per 100,000 persons) and rarely in children. It may be acute or chronic or idiopathic autoimmune disorder. For reasons unknown, platelets can be mistaken by the immune system as invaders. When this happens, antibodies coat the platelets and the spleen's phagocytes remove them in numbers up to 10 times greater than the normal platelet removal rate. The megakaryocytes in the bone marrow respond by getting larger and growing in numbers so that they may increase their production of platelets. The platelets produced under these circumstances tend to be larger and more effective than normal platelets and are called "stress platelets." The bone marrow attempts to overcome the accelerated platelet destruction rate but during immune-mediated destruction activity, human platelet can expect to survive only one day in the circulation instead of its normal 6-8 days. If antibody levels are very high, a platelet may survive only minutes or hours after its release from the bone marrow and, making matters worse. Antibody coated platelets still circulating does not function normally.

Autoimmune thrombocytopenia is a relatively common disorder. This is primarily a disease of younger women. 70 percent of autoimmune thrombocytopenia patients are women, and 72 percent of these women are under age 40. Also, it is seen in association with other diseases, such as the autoimmune disorders of systemic lupus erythematosus or rheumatoid arthritis. The acute form of this disease is a childhood disorder. Onset is abrupt. It usually follows an infectious illness, and it spontaneously remits in six months. The chronic form of autoimmune thrombocytopenia has a duration of greater than six months, and is an organ-specific autoimmune disease. Antibodies actually are directed to important platelet glycoprotein receptors, which not only leads to a decrease in platelet count but also to functional abnormalities.

Thrombocytopenia usually improves by treating the underlying cause. Sometimes, medications or surgery can help to treat chronic thrombocytopenia. If bleeding is severe, blood or platelet transfusion can save the life.

Autoimmune leucopenia: Leukopenia is generally defined as reduction in the total white blood cell count to less than 4,000 cells per decilitre. The terms "autoimmune leukopenia," "autoimmune granulocytopenia," and "autoimmune Neutropenia" are often used synonymously to describe conditions in which auto antibodies to mature neutrophils, or their precursors, lead to cell destruction and a reduced blood neutrophil count.

(B) LOCALISED (ORGAN SPECIFIC) AUTOIMMUNE DISEASES

In localized auto immune diseases a particular organ is affected due to auto antibodies. The antibodies produced are specific for the antigens present on cells of a specific organ. Some of the organ specific autoimmune diseases are as follows.

AUTOIMMUNE DISEASES OF THYROID GLAND:

(a) Hashimoto's Disease (Lymph Adenoid Goitre): Chronic thyroiditis or Hashimoto's disease is a common thyroid gland disorder that can occur at any age, but it is most often seen in middle aged women. It is an autoimmune disorder, characterized by the production of antibodies (IgG, IgM type) in response to thyroid antigens (antibody producing) and the replacement of normal thyroid structures with lymphocytes and lymphoid germinal centres. The thyroid, typically enlarged, pale yellow, and lumpy on the surface shows dense lymphocyte infiltration, and the remaining thyroid tissue frequently contains small empty follicles. Hashimoto's disease is also known as chronic lymphocytic thyroiditis.It is a T cell associated autoimmune disease. The disease leads to an under activity of thyroid gland (hypothyroidism).

Hashimoto's disease does not have unique signs and symptoms. The first indication of this problem may be a goiter (a gradual painless enlargement of the thyroid gland). The disease typically progresses slowly over a number of years and causes chronic thyroid damage, leading to a drop in thyroid hormone levels. The signs and symptoms of hypothyroidism vary widely depending on the severity of hormone deficiency. Fatigue and sluggishness, increased sensitivity to cold, constipation, pale dry skin, puffy face, hoarse voice, elevated blood cholesterol level, unexplained weight gain, muscle aches, tenderness and stiffness, etc. are some of the symptoms to indicate the problem.

Essentially, the diagnosis of Hashimoto's disease is based on presence of thyroid antibodies in the blood. The level of these antibodies often increases as the disease progresses. In the late stages when the whole of the thyroid gland has been destroyed, the level of the auto-antibodies may fall to low or undetectable levels

Since the problem is associated with auto immune reactions the basic cause of Hashimoto's thyroiditis cannot be not treated. In general, the treatment is the management of the consequences of thyroid failure, although a goiter is sometimes prevented from becoming larger or is reduced in size by giving thyroxine.

(b) Thyrotoxicosis (Grave's disease): Graves' disease, Hashimoto's thyroiditis, and idiopathic thyroid failure are closely associated and in fact overlapping syndromes. The common features of the autoimmune thyroid diseases include the immune reactivity to specific thyroid antigens. Patients can move from one or the other category, depending upon the stage of their illness. For example, an individual might first be observed with thyroid enlargement and positive antibodies tests for anti-thyroglobulin or anti-TPO antibodies, and thus qualify as having Hashimoto's thyroiditis. Later on the person might become hyperthyroid and fit in the category of Graves' disease or, the patient might have progressive destruction of the thyroid, or develop blocking antibodies, and become hypothyroidic or ultimately develop myxedema. The immunological basis of thyrotoxicosis is supported by the identification of the 'long acting thyroid stimulator' (LATS) which is an IgG antibody to the thyroid membrane antigen.

(c) Addison's disease: Addison's disease is an endocrine or hormonal disorder that occurs in all age groups and afflicts men and women equally. Since Addison's disease arises when the adrenal glands do not produce enough of the hormone cortisol or hormone aldosterone, the disease is thought to be caused by their hypo secretions. Addison's disease can cause irritability and depression. Because of salt loss, a craving for salty foods is also common. Hypoglycemia, or low blood glucose, is more severe in children than in adults. In women, menstrual periods may become irregular or stop. The disease is also called adrenal insufficiency, or hypocortisolism.

Since the symptoms progress slowly, they are usually ignored until a stressful event like an illness or an accident makes the conditions worse. This situation is called as an addisonian crisis, or acute adrenal insufficiency. In most cases, symptoms are severe enough that patients seek medical treatment before a crisis occurs. However, in about 25 percent of patients, symptoms first appear during an addisonian crisis. Symptoms of an addisonian crisis include sudden penetrating pain in the lower back, abdomen, or legs, severe vomiting and diarrhea, dehydration, low blood pressure, loss of consciousness etc. In its early stages, adrenal insufficiency can be difficult to diagnose. A diagnosis of Addison's disease is made by laboratory tests. X-ray exams of the adrenal and pituitary glands are also useful to establish the cause.

Treatment of Addison's disease involves replacing, or substituting the hormones that the adrenal glands are not making. Cortisol is replaced orally with hydrocortisone tablets, (a synthetic glucocorticoid) taken once or twice a day. If aldosterone is also deficient, it is replaced with oral doses of a mineralocorticoid called fludrocortisone acetate (Florinef).

Autoimmune orchitis: It is inflammation of the testis caused by autoimmune disease after viral infections like mumps. It can manifest as enlargement of the testis. It is most common in boys past puberty and rare before the age of 10. Approximately 30% of patients who have mumps develop orchitis during the course of the illness. Lymphocytic infiltration in to testis and circulating antibodies to the sperms and the germinal cells leads to this disease. It usually develops 4 to 6 days after the attack. In one-third of orchitis cases it is induced by mumps. It leads to testicular atrophy (shrinking of the testicles). Chronic orchitis may cause mild testicular pain or swelling and may look like a tumor. Hence distinguishing autoimmune orchitis from a tumor is the main challenge. This is determined by biopsy and deoxyspergualin (an immunosuppressant) might be useful in prevention or treatment of human immuno inflammatory orchitis.

Myasthenia gravis: Myasthenia gravis is a chronic autoimmune neuromuscular disease characterized by an abnormal fatigability of muscles due to malfunctioning of the myoneural junction. The name myasthenia gravis is derived from Latin and Greek words that literally means "grave muscle weakness." It is caused by a defect in the transmission of nerve impulses to muscles. It occurs when normal communication between the nerve and muscle is interrupted at the neuromuscular junction. Auto antibodies produced against acetyl choline receptors block, alter, or destroy the acetylcholine receptors of striated muscles at the neuromuscular junction. In the absence of acetyl choline receptors nerve impulses fails to reach the muscle ensuing failure of muscle contraction followed by weakness and rapid fatigue in the affected muscles. It occurs in all ethnic groups and both genders. Most commonly it affects young adult women (under 40) and older men (over 60), but it can occur at any age.

Certain muscles such as those that control eye and eyelid movement, facial expression, chewing, talking, and swallowing are often, but not always, involved in the disorder. The muscles that control breathing, movements of neck and limb may also be affected. In neonatal myasthenia the auto antibody is passively acquired from the mother.

A special blood test can detect the presence of immune molecules or acetylcholine receptor antibodies. Most patients with myasthenia gravis have abnormally elevated levels of these antibodies. Another test is called the edrophonium test. This approach requires the intravenous administration of edrophonium chloride or Tensilon(r), a drug that blocks the degradation (breakdown) of acetylcholine and temporarily increases the levels of acetylcholine at the neuromuscular junction. In people with myasthenia gravis involving the eye muscles, edrophonium chloride will briefly relieve weakness.

A different test called single fiber electromyography (EMG), in which single muscle fibers are stimulated by electrical impulses, can also detect impaired nerve-to-muscle transmission. EMG measures the electrical potential of muscle cells. Muscle fibers in myasthenia gravis, as well as other neuromuscular disorders, do not respond as well to repeated electrical stimulation compared to muscles from normal individuals.

There are several therapies available to help, reduce and improve muscle weakness. Medications used to treat the disorder include anticholinesterase agents such as neostigmine and pyridostigmine, which help improve neuromuscular transmission and increase muscle strength. Immunosuppressive drugs such as prednisone, cyclosporine, and azathioprine may also be used. These medications improve muscle strength by suppressing the production of abnormal antibodies. Thymectomy, the surgical removal of the thymus gland (which often is abnormal in myasthenia gravis patients), reduces symptoms in more than 70 percent of patients without thymoma and may cure some individuals, possibly by re-balancing the immune system. Other therapies used to treat myasthenia gravis include plasmapheresis, a procedure in which abnormal antibodies are removed from the blood, and high-dose intravenous immune globulin, which temporarily modifies the immune system and provides the body with normal antibodies from donated blood. These therapies may be used to help individuals during especially difficult periods of weakness.

Autoimmune disease of the eye: Two types of autoimmune eye diseases are seen

(a) Cataract surgery sometimes leads to intra ocular inflammation caused by the autoimmune response to the lens protein; this is known as "phacoanaphylaxis".

(b) Perforation injury of the eye, particularly those involving the iris and ciliary body are often followed by sympathetic ophthalmia (a kind of inflammation) of the opposite eye.

Autoimmune diseases of nervous system: This is a group of diseases where the body's immune system attacks its own nervous system. Examples include opsoclonus myoclonus syndrome, Guillain-Barre syndrome and multiple sclerosis. Numbness, Paralysis, Vision impairment, Neurological symptoms, Incoordination, Movement problems, Weakness, Impaired sensation etc. are the symptoms of the disease.

Autoimmune diseases of skin: Autoimmune skin diseases sometimes pose a serious health threat and may cause symptoms such as skin blisters or rashes.

Psoriasis is a common skin disorder characterized by patches of raised, inflamed lesions. Phemphigus vulgaris is another skin disease caused by auto immunity. Pemphigus complex" is a group of four autoimmune skin disorders characterized by "vesicles" and "bullae" (blisters), erosions, and ulcers. In "pemphigus vulgaris", the lesions are usually found in the mouth and at mucocutaneous junctions, those borders of haired skin and mucosal tissues. Such areas include the eyelids, lips, nostrils, anus, and prepuce or vulva. There may also be skin lesions in the groin or axillae (armpits). The blisters are thin, fragile, and rupture easily. The skin lesions are described as red, weeping, ulcerated placques. Phemphigus vulgaris may be caused by an antibody to the intercellular cement substance. In bullous phemphigoid, antibodies are directed against the dermal epithelial junction.

(C) SYSTEMIC OR NON-ORGAN-SPECIFIC DISORDERS:

In non-organ-specific disorders, autoimmune activity is widely spread throughout the body. These conditions tend to be associated with auto antibodies to antigens which are not tissue specific. Rheumatoid Arthritis, Scleroderma dermatomyositis, Systemic lupus erythematosus (SLE), Sjögren's syndrome, etc. are examples for systemic or non-organ-specific disorders. This group includes conditions characterized by immune response against a variety of self-antigens and damage to several organs and tissues systems.

Systemic lupus erythematosus (SLE): Lupus is an autoimmune disease characterized by acute and chronic inflammation of various tissues of the body. Lupus has the potential to affect a variety of areas. Sometimes lupus can cause disease of the skin, heart, lungs, kidneys, joints, and/or nervous system. When internal organs are involved, the condition is referred to as systemic lupus erythematosus (SLE).

The precise reason for the abnormal autoimmunity that causes lupus is not known. Inherited genes, viruses, ultraviolet light, and certain medications may all play some role. Patients have a variety of antibodies which are directed against cell nuclei, intra cytoplasmic cell constituents, immunoglobulins, thyroid and other organ specific antigens. The first immunological feature is lupus erythematosus (LE) cell phenomenon; here LE cell is a neutrophil containing a large pale homogenous body (LE body). LE body is the immunologically damaged nucleus of a leucocyte.

Anti nuclear antibody test are sensitive but not specific for SLE. High titre of anti-ds(double strand) DNA antibody is relatively specific for SLE. Another SLE specific antibody is anti-sm (smooth muscle) antibody. Common complaints and symptoms include fatigue, low-grade fever, loss of appetite, muscle aches, arthritis, ulcers of the mouth and nose, facial rash ("butterfly rash"), unusual sensitivity to sunlight (photosensitivity), inflammation of the lining that surrounds the lungs (pleuritis) and the heart (pericarditis), and poor circulation to the fingers and toes with cold exposure (Raynaud's phenomenon). There is no permanent cure for SLE. The goal of treatment is to relieve symptoms and protect organs by decreasing inflammation and/or the level of autoimmune activity in the body.

Rheumatoid disease: Rheumatoid arthritis (RA) is an autoimmune disease that causes chronic inflammation of the joints. Rheumatoid arthritis can also cause inflammation of the tissue around the joints, as well as in other organs in the body. There is a genetic predisposition, although the cause remains unknown. Women are more affected. The symptoms of rheumatoid arthritis come and go, depending on the degree of tissue inflammation. In rheumatoid arthritis, multiple joints are usually inflamed in a symmetrical pattern (both sides of the body affected). When the disease is active, symptoms can include fatigue, lack of appetite, low-grade fever, muscle and joint aches, and stiffness. Muscle and joint stiffness are usually most notable in the morning and after periods of inactivity. Since rheumatoid arthritis is a systemic disease, its inflammation can affect organs and areas of the body other than the joints.

The diagnosis is based on the pattern of symptoms, the distribution of the inflamed joints, and the blood and x-ray findings. A blood antibody called "rheumatoid factor" is found in 80% of patients. Citrulline antibody (also referred to as anti-citrulline antibody, anti-cyclic citrullinated peptide antibody, and anti-CCP) is present in most patients with rheumatoid arthritis. There is no known cure for rheumatoid arthritis. To date, the goal of treatment in rheumatoid arthritis is to reduce joint inflammation and pain, maximize joint function, and prevent joint destruction and deformity.

Sjogren's syndrome: Sjogren's syndrome is an autoimmune disease characterized by the abnormal production of extra antibodies in the blood that are directed against various tissues of the body. This particular autoimmune illness features inflammation in certain glands of the body. Inflammation of the glands that produce tears (lacrimal glands) leads to decreased water production for tears and eye dryness. Inflammation of the glands that produce the saliva in the mouth (salivary glands, including the parotid glands) leads to dry mouth and dry lips. The diagnosis of Sjogren's syndrome involves detecting the features of dryness of the eyes and mouth. There is no cure for Sjogren's syndrome. The treatment of patients with Sjogren's syndrome is directed toward the particular areas of the body that are involved and complications, such as infection.

Scleroderma dermatomyositis: Scleroderma is a group of rare, progressive diseases that involve the hardening and tightening of the skin and connective tissues. The main abnormality is excess formation of fibrous tissue, particularly collagen that leads to rigidity of the affected part. Localized scleroderma affects only the skin. Systemic scleroderma also harms internal organs, such as the heart, lungs, kidneys and digestive tract. Symptoms of scleroderma vary, depending on which organ systems are involved. The most prevalent signs and symptoms of scleroderma include; an exaggerated response to cold temperatures or emotional distress, Gastroesophageal reflux, Skin changes etc. Blood tests and biopsy are some tests for diagnosis of Scleroderma. There is no known cure and no drug will stop the overproduction of collagen. But medications can help control the symptoms of scleroderma or help prevent complications.

16

TRANSPLANTATION IMMUNOLOGY

The term "transplantation" means removing something from one location and introducing it in another location, hence in immunology the term transplantation is used to refer the procedure involved in the replacement of a nonfunctional or damaged organ or tissue with a good, and functional organ or tissue to safe guard the life of an individual. The implanted tissue or organ is known as "graft". Organs that can be transplanted are heart, kidneys, liver, lungs, pancreas, penis, eyes and intestine. Tissues include bones, tendons, cornea, heart valves, veins and skin. The advancement in surgical techniques introduced the idea of transplantation of required organs or tissues. It is now possible to transfer a variety of tissues and organs from a healthy donor to an ailing recipient or from one site to another in the same individual (eg. skin grafting in burn cases) through sugery. Even though development in surgical techniques allowed clinicians to perform transplantation of organs or tissues, certain barriers such as availability of donors, expenditure for the clinical procedure and implant rejection reactions etc. made it a difficult and cumbersome procedure.

Since the immune system has been evolved to protect its own self from the attack of foreign bodies, it holds the power of identifying its own cells from foreign cells. Cells express a set of membrane bound antigens called auto antigens. The auto antigens act as identification marks for the immune system to identify its own cells from foreign cells. Immune system identifies the graft through the antigens present on their cells and reacts in a similar way as it reacts to a pathogen. Hence the unique power of immune system is responsible for graft rejection. But immunological rejection is exempted for genetically identical or allograft (Own tissue taken from some other region), because the antigens present on the graft tissue are identical with its own antigens and immune system fails to identify them as foreign cells to mount any action.

First systematic study of transplantation was reported in 1908 by Alexis Carrel. In 1935 a Russian surgeon attempted the first human kidney transplant, but mismatch of blood group between donor and recipient induced a rejection reaction. The first successful human kidney transplant between identical twins was succeeded in 1954. Many failures in transplantation procedure insist the importance of knowledge in immunobilogy. Discovery of human blood groups was one of key event that helped to understand the cause for transplant rejection. Now it is understood, that matching of donor and recipients blood groups is essential for the survival of tissue grafts, because the vascular endothelium express blood group antigens. Matching of blood group antigens other than A, B, AB, O is not critical for transplantation, because they are expressed only on red Blood cells.

Study of Mouse skin graft rejection further improved the knowledge of transplantation immunology, and it helped a lot in understanding major histo compatibility antigens. As recognition of foreign cells by recipient T cells is associated with MHC antigens of foreign cells, knowledge about MHC is essential to understand transplantation reactions. Success of transplantation between identical twins proposes that the success rate depends on the amount of sharing of histo compatibility genes. Histocompatibility genes are responsible for the production of antigens on cell surface. With reference to the surface antigens, the grafts or transplants are differentiated in to four types. They are as follows:

1. Auto graft or Autogenic graft, 2. Isograft or Syngraft or Syngenetic graft, 3. allografts or Homografts, 4. Xenograft.

1. Auto graft or Autogenic graft: When tissue is transplanted from one site to another in the same individual, the transplant is referred as "auto graft" or "autogenic graft" (From Greek Auto=Self). Immune system of recipient accepts the auto graft very easily, because antigens of recipient cells, and the transplanted tissue are alike.

2. Isograft or Syngraft or Syngentic graft: The graft taken from a genetically identical person is known as Isograft or Syngraft or Syngentic graft. This kind of transplantation is possible between two genetically identical twins. Since development of identical twins takes place from a single zygote, identical twins share same genes that are responsible for the production of antigens.

3. Allograft or Homograft: If the transplantation is carried between genetically different members of the same species then graft is called as "allograft". The allograft is formally named as "Homograft". The histo compartbility antigens of allograft are dissimilar with the host histo compartbility antigens. Hence immune system of recipient/ host identifies the graft as foreign and induces an immune response against to it, resulting rejection of graft.

4. Xenograft: If the transplantation between individuals of two different species is carried, for eg. transplanting monkey liver to human, the graft is referred as "Xenograft". Since the histocompatibility genes are quite different, hosts body rejects the graft more vigorously.

GENETICAL GROUND OF TRANSPLANTATION:-

As the antigens present on the nucleated cell act as identification marks of the cells, and play a key role in transplantation they are called as "hiscompatibility molecules" and the genes responsible for their production are referred as histocompatibility genes (Refer MHC).

Histocompatibility Test:

When tissue transplantation is anticipated, initially, donor and recipient are screened for ABO blood group compatibility. Later HLA Typing test using leukocytes can be accomplished. (Refer MHC)

TRANSPLANT REJECTION:

Since chance of rejection is very high in transplantation between genetically distinct individuals, transplantation is restricted to the donors of same species i.e. allograft. The rejection of allograft also very common due to incompatibility of MHC antigens, but the rate of rejection is different in different cases. Depending upon the percentage of match between donor and recipient, the rejection may be Acute rejection,or Hyper acute rejection or insidious rejection.

ACCUTE REJECTION: Acute rejection is due to stimulation of T lymphocytes and cell mediated immunity, it takes place subsequent to the establishment of blood vessel communication between recipient and implant. This kind of rejection is known as "early acute rejection reaction". If the recipient's immune system is suppressed with certain suppressive drugs, development of Abs against graft antigens takes place in due course time. Interaction of antibodies with the grafts antigens, results in the formation of immune complexes, followed by complement fixation and finally rejection of the graft. As this reaction is taking place after some time it is referred as "late acute rejection reactions".

HYPER ACUTE REJECTION: If antibodies for graft cells are already present in the host body rejection takes place very quickly, this quick rejection of graft is known as "Hyper acute rejection". Pre existence of antibodies in host is due to pre sensitization through previous pregnancies, or blood transfusion or through previous grafts.

INSIDIOUS REJECTION: Deposition of immune complexes on graft tissue leads to slow, silent and unexpressed or secret rejection of the graft. This silent rejection of graft is known as "insidious rejection". Irrespective to the type of rejection, the mechanism of rejection involves sensitized T cells and NK cells in the first set of reactions. Abs are believed to play an important role in chronic rejection. Hence the mechanism of graft rejection can be divided into first set and second set reactions.

(1) FIRST SET REACTIONS: Sensitization is the first step in these rejection reactions. Once the graft tissue is vascularized, the graft antigens travel to the lymph nodes through circulation and activate T Lymphocytes. Time required for T cell stimulation depends on the time taken for vascularization of the graft. For example rejection reactions take place very quickly in organ transplants, but delayed in skin grafts. In skin graft vascularization takes place in few days, but in case of organ graft, vascularization is established during the surgical process through direct anstomoses (connection of two structures), allowing passage of graft antigens to the lymph nodes, and activation of T cells.

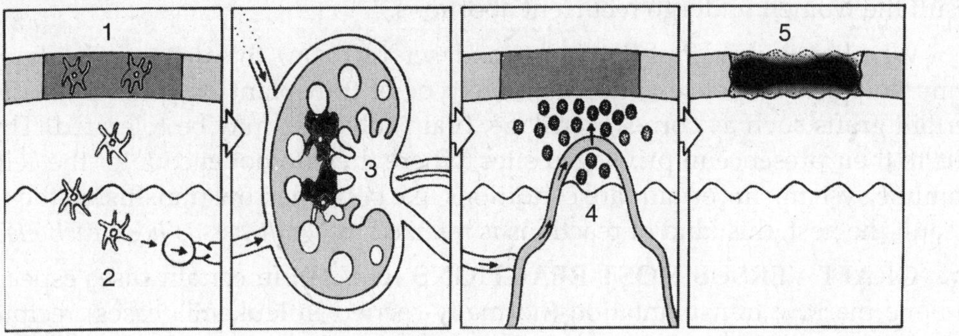

Fig. 16.1

When T lymphocytes are activated they proliferate to give clones of cells (Refer Chapter4). TC cells enter in to the circulation and reach the graft to destroy the implant tissue through cell-to-cell toxicity. Remaining T cells in the lymph nodes mobilize phagocytic leucocytes to the graft through their lymphokines. Since capillaries and vessels are composed of a single endothelial cell layer, the first sign of damage at the tissue level is seen in them. Damage of blood vessels results intravascular thrombosis, ischemia, hemorrhage, and blood coagulation. Histologically the reactions bear a resemblance to delayed type hypeı sensitive reactions.

(2) SECOND SET REACTIONS: The second set reaction can be compared to the secondary immune response to an antigen. It takes place when transplantation is repeated for the second time. Initially graft rejection reaction is brought abut by Tc cells, later Abs and NK cell involve in the reactions, hence in the second set reactions B cell are Important. Since the immune system is sensitized through previous graft and immune components are ready in the circulation, rejection of graft cells takes place soon after the establishment of circulation between host and graft. Infiltration of neutrophils, macrophages, and T_C cells to the site of inflammation serves to provide backup mechanism and ensure rapid and irreversible reactions. As the reactions are so quick vascularization does not take place and the graft tissue becomes pale yellow or whitish due to failure in blood supply. Hence the rejection of this whitish graft is referred as "white graft rejection".

The second set reactions are considered as hyper acute rejections reactions due to its rapid action. Second set reaction or hyper acute rejection can be seen rarely in the first attempt of transplantation. Repeated blood transfusions, or pregnancies, may root generation of Abs for foreign antigens; cross reactivity of this Abs may induce second set reactions even in first attempt of transplantation.

Study of this kind of rejection reaction suggests that there is a possibility of generation of sensitized cells and antibodies for allogenic antigens even in the absence of any graft. The basis for undiagnosed recurrent abortions in some women may be the same. Since MHC genes are co dominant in nature, fetus expresses both maternal and paternal antigens. If a woman carries Abs against her husbands

Ags, the fetus with paternal antigens may face the graft rejection reaction; as a result the women undergo recurrent abortions.

Whether it is a first set or second set reaction, the degree and type of immunological response varies with the type of transplant. In spite of mismatch certain grafts such as cornea, cartilage, brain cells etc., may be tolerated. This is due to their presence in privileged sites, where they do not encounter the cells of immune system. In certain rare conditions like bone marrow transfusion the graft assault the host, this kind of reactions is referred as *"graft-versus-host reactions"*.

GRAFT VERSUS HOST REACTIONS (G.V.H): In certain cases especially in bone marrow transplantation (normally carried in leukemia cases) recipients lymphocytes are destroyed prior to transplantation through irradiation, to prevent the graft rejection reactions. However the grafted bone marrow with its own lymphocytes perceives the host cells as foreign and starts destroying the recipient's cells. This kind of grafts reactions are referred as *"graft-versus-host reactions"* to highlight the problems raised by graft.

GVH reactions are not limited to bone marrow transplants; similar reactions can arise in other tissue or organ transplants. Study of G.V.H. reactions suggests that the G.V.H. reactions increase with age, because of latent infections such as viral, protozoan etc. If immune system of an aged recipient is suppressed prior to transplantation, the patient lost control over organisms of latent infection, and the organisms express their Ags in the absence of host resistance. The pathogen Ags can induce T cells of the graft, while reacting with pathogen Ags some of the graft T cells get sensitized to recipient Ags and carry GVH reactions.

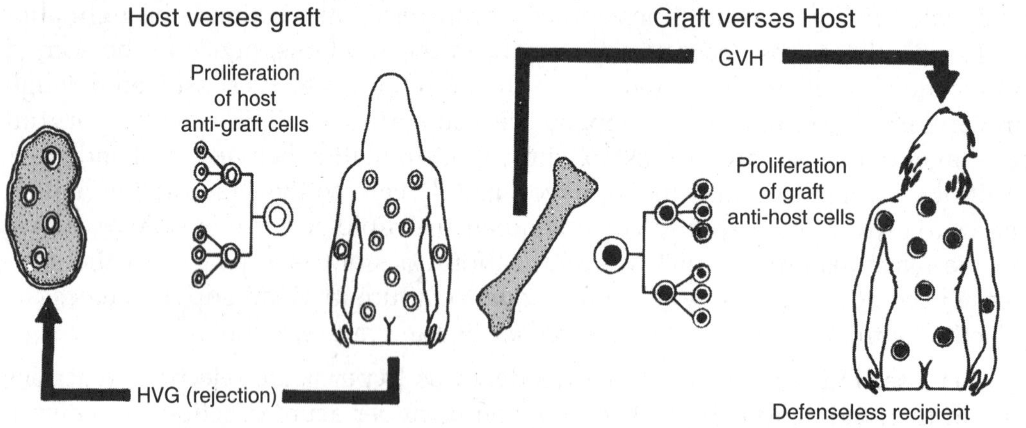

Fig. 16.2

MOLECULAR BASIS OF GRAFT REJECTION

CD4+ or T_H cells are responsible for inducing rejection reactions in host., CD4 cells even in the absence of CD8 or T_C cells can extend rejection reactions, but CD8 cells alone can't induce rejection reactions; they need stimulation from CD4 cells to execute their function. However once activated, CD8 cells can continue their action. The passenger leucocytes or interstitial dendritic cells of the donor cause direct activation of recipient TH cells. Other wise, antigen presenting cells of the host get hold of antigens shed from the transplant and present them to hosts TH cells to induce indirect activation (Direct activation is more powerful). Lymphokines such as growth and differentiation factor, TC cell activation factor, macrophage activation factor, B cell activation factor etc. released from the activated TH cells initiate rejection reactions. The antibodies produced by activated B cells cause damage to the vascular endothelium.

PREVENTION OF GRAFT REJECTION: Graft rejection can be prevented by using certain drugs such as Azathioprin, cyclophosphamide, methotexate cyclosporine, FK 506, Rampomycin etc. and slowly developing tolerance to the graft tissue. Since immune system is not specific for any particular region of the body, immunosuppressive drugs used to save the graft, suppress the whole immune system and the recipient becomes vulnerable to various other infections. In addition to immune suppression majority of immunosuppressive drugs are aimed to block proliferation of activated lymphocytes. As the drugs block proliferation, they block proliferation of certain normal cells such as RBC, epithelial cells of the gut etc. also, leading to serious and life threatening complications. A nonspecific immune suppression is also carried by X-irradiation and by using corticosteroids and cytotoxic drugs.

X-irradiation is highly toxic to actively replicating cells. Like immune suppressive drugs it also blocks cell division. Corticosteroids are anti inflammatory in function. The other treatments include use of anti lymphocyte serum to block activation of T cells alone. Even though this is some what better than the former treatments, chance of development of viral infections is there in the absence of T cells.

INDUCING TOLERANCE:-

Tolerance can be induced by using antidiotypic Abs against T cells. The antidiotypic Abs bind to T cells and prevent receiving stimulation from graft antigens. As there is no stimulation from graft, T cells remain calm with out inducing any reaction against the graft. This technique sounds good but not easy to apply practically, because maintenance of high levels of antibodies for an extended period of time in order to maintain tolerance to the transplanted tissue is not an easy task.

A treatment that is currently feasible and successful in some types of human transplantation is immune enhancement. Pre immunization with donor's antigens gradually raises tolerance to the graft. In this method the Abs raised through pre immunization might bind the passenger cells of the graft and destroy them before they can induce the recipient T ells or the Abs raised may be non compliment fixing, hence their binding to antigens block interaction of lymphocytes with graft antigens.

17

TUMOR IMMUNOLOGY

In spite of several check points in a cell cycle to check any modifications in DNA before its transfer to next generation, certain mutations takes place in DNA leading to loss of certain characters and control over its multiplication rate. The consequences of these modifications result in pathological over growth of modified tissues generally referred as **Tumor or Neoplasia** (meaning new formation) or "***cancer***". The altered character of tumor cells makes them immortal and they do not respond to the signals sent for regulation of growth. Even though rapid multiplication and uncontrolled growth are common characters for all tumors, certain tumors are less hazardous than the others. The hazardous character of tumors depends upon the metastasis nature of tumors. Metastasis is the ability of cells to separate from the mass and move through lymph or blood to invade the surrounding tissue. The tumors with metastasis are referred as "**Malignant tumors**" and the tumors with out metastasis are referred as "**Benign tumors**".

BENIGN TUMORS: Benign tumors are generally not harmful due to their well-defined growth with smooth boundaries that simply grow in diameter and restricted to one place but can be harmful if the tumor compresses the surrounding tissue against a hard surface in the body. The benign tumor usually grows at a relatively slow pace and may stop growing for a time when it reaches a certain size. A complete cure can usually be achieved by removing the abnormally grown tissue mass.

MALIGNANT TUMORS: The Malignant tumors are dreadful because their growth is not restricted to one place; their metastasis nature helps their spread from one place to other locations in the body via lymph or blood. Unlike benign tumor, it is very critical to locate and remove the malignant tumor. Generally malignant tumors are properly referred to as "Cancers". The origin of the word cancer is credited to the Greek physician Hippocrates (460-370 B.C.). In Greek, cancer refers to a crab. It is most likely applied to the disease to mind the shape of a crab, because of finger-like projections spreading from a cancer tissue mass resembles the structure of crab more over the spread of cancer can be in any direction just like the movement of a crab.

Cancers can affect all animals and people at all ages, even fetuses, but the risk for most varieties increases with age. Generally cancers form a tumor but some cancers, such as leukemia (blood cancer) does not form tumors and they are referred as "Liquid tumors". These liquid tumors that circulate in the blood may also form masses elsewhere in the body. Cancer causes about 13% of total deaths. According to the American Cancer Society, 7.6 million people died globally from cancer during 2007.

Altered biological properties of cancer cells

(1) Acquisition of self-sufficiency in growth signals.

(2) Loss of sensitivity to anti-growth signals.

(3) Loss of apoptosis, in order to allow growth despite genetic errors and external anti-growth signals.

(4) Loss of senescence, leading to limitless replicative potential (immortality).

(5) Acquisition of sustained "angiogenesis" (growth of new blood vessels from pre-existing vessels), allowing the tumor to grow beyond the limitations of passive nutrient diffusion.

(6) Acquisition of ability to invade neighbouring tissues, the defining property of invasive carcinoma.

(7) Acquisition of ability to metastases at distant sites, the classical property of malignant tumors (carcinomas or others).

Classification of Tumors:

Since development of tumor is possible in any region or organ of the body with dividing cell, tumors were broadly classified into 3 basic types based upon the embryonic origin of the tissues involved in the formation of tumor.

1. Carcinomas are the tumors developed from cells of ectodermal or endodermal origin. They invade surrounding tissues and organs and may metastasize, or spread, to lymph nodes and other sites. Based upon the histopathological appearance they can be differentiated into "Adenocarcinoma" and "squamous cell carcinoma" to reflect the involvement of glandular or squamous cells in tumor formation. Approximately 90%of human cancers are malignancies of epithelial cells.

2. Sarcomas (from the Greek 'sarx' meaning "flesh") are the tumors developed from connective tissue or mesoderm. Canaers of breast, colon, pancreas bones etc. comes under this type. Sarcomas are rare in humans; about 2% of human cancers come under this category.

3. Leukemia (Greek leukos "white"; aima "blood") is the tumour developed from bone marrow tissue or in blood. It is characterized by an abnormal proliferation of blood cells, usually white blood cells (leukocytes). Leukemia tumor is subdivided into lymphoblastic or lymphocytic leukemias and myeloid or myelogenous leukemias according to the blood cells affected.

To make it understandable to a common man, tumors were generally named after the organ or tissue from which it has been developed. For example, cancer developed in breast tissue is referred as breast cancer. Lung cancer, colon cancer, gastric cancer, skin cancer etc. are some more examples.

Different theories to explain cancer development: From the earliest times, physicians have wondered about the cause of cancer. The Egyptians blamed Gods for the development of cancers. Several theories were proposed by different scientists to explain the cause for cancers. Some of them are as follows.

Humoral theory: Hippocrates believed that the body contained four humors (body fluids) - blood, phlegm, yellow bile, and black bile. A balance of these fluids resulted in a state of health. Any excesses or deficiencies caused disease. An excess of black bile collecting in various body sites was thought to cause cancer. This theory of cancer was passed on by the Romans and was embraced by the influential doctor Galen's medical teaching, which remained unchallenged through the middle Ages for over 1300 years. During this period, the study of the body, including autopsies, was prohibited for religious reasons, thus limiting knowledge.

Lymph Theory: Among theories that replaced the humoral theory of cancer was cancer's formation by another fluid - lymph. Life was believed to consist of continuous and appropriate movement of the fluid parts through solids. Of all the fluids, the most important were blood and lymph. Stahl and Hofman theorized that the cancer was composed of fermenting and degenerating lymph varying in density, acidity and alkalinity. The lymph theory gained rapid support. John Hunter (1723-1792) agreed that tumors grow from lymph constantly thrown out by the blood.

Blastema Theory: In 1838, German pathologist Johannes Muller demonstrated that cancer is made up of cells and not lymph. But he was of the opinion that cancer cells did not arise from normal cells. Muller proposed that cancer cells arose from budding elements (blastema) between normal tissues. Muller's student Rudolph Virchow (1821-1902), the famous German pathologist, determined that all cells, including cancer cells, are derived from other cells.

Chronic Irritation Theory: Virchow proposed chronic irritation as the cause of cancer, but he falsely believed that cancers "spread like a liquid." A German surgeon, Karl Thiersch, showed that cancers metastasize through the spread of malignant cells and not through some unidentified fluid.

Trauma Theory: Despite advances in the understanding of cancer, from the late 1800s until the 1920s, cancer was thought by some to be caused by trauma. This belief was maintained despite the failure to cause cancer in experimental animals by injury.

Parasite Theory: In the 17th and 18th centuries, some believed that cancer was contagious. In fact, the first cancer hospital in France was forced to move from the city in 1779 because of the fear of the spread of cancer throughout the city.

A Nobel Prize was wrongly awarded in 1926 for scientific research documenting stomach cancer being caused by worms. With the inability to confirm this research, scientists lost interest in the parasite theory.

Reasons for tumor formation: Cancer is a genetic disease; it develops from mutations within the genes of cells. The "oncogenes" and "tumor suppressor genes" present in all individuals play a significant role in tumor formation. Oncogenes, activate cell division and influence embryonic development and tumor suppressor genes halt cell division. Since these two genes are typically found in normal human cells, certain mutations in them may transform their normal function resulting in the conversion of normal cells into tumor cells. Either inherited defects or acquired mutation due to exposure to carcinogens may cause conversion of normal cell into a tumor cell. Current evidence indicates that carcinogenesis results from a complex interaction of carcinogens and accumulated mutations in several genes.

How mutations cause Tumor: Due to mutations, some of the regular genes may fail to code proteins essential for regulation of cell cycle, Synthesis of proteins involved in the regulation of cell cycle are essential to stop access of defective or altered DNA to the daughter cells. Failure in regulation of cell cycle results in accumulation of mutations or abnormal characters in the daughter cells. The normal gene gradually lost its original characters and become a tumor gene and this modified tumor gene is known as "Proto-oncogene". After several divisions the cell with Proto-oncogene produces tumor. Mutations may also suppress the efficiency of certain tumor suppressor genes, as a result chances for tumor development increases.

Of the many known oncogenes some are derived from normal Proto-oncogenes. For example the **Ros** gene that encodes a protein essential for intracellular signal transduction in normal cells becomes an oncogene due to mutations and starts encoding a protein that acts as a signaling molecule for excessive or uncontrolled growth of cells. An oncoprotein encoded by an oncogene may be similar to the normal protein but excessive production i.e. higher than the normal levels may alter the character of normal cells and induces conversion of a normal cell into a tumor cell.

No one is sure exactly, what causes tumors to begin growing. There are, however, several things that can increase a person's risk of developing a tumor. Examples of substances that may damage DNA and induce carcinogenesis include:

1. Radiation: High-frequency radiation, such as ultraviolet and ionizing radiation, damages the genetic material DNA (deoxyribonucleic acid), possibly inducing genetically transferable abnormalities.

2. Viruses: Some human **retroviruses** and **papilloma** (DNA viruses) **viruses** exhibit carcinogenic gene sequence potential. Retrovirus may convert proto-oncogenes into oncogenes either by altering or condensing, to code proteins with abnormal activity or controlling with powerful regulators to induce the production in excess or in inappropriate circumstances.

3. Hormones: The role of hormones in carcinogenesis is still controversial, but it seems that, excessive use of some hormones, especially estrogen, produces cancer in animals.

4. Chemical substances: Some of the chemical substances that can induce carcinogenesis include:

Alkylating agents-leukemia,

Aromatic hydrocarbons and benzopyrene (from polluted air) - lung cancer,

Asbestos - mesothelioma of the lung,

Tobacco - cancer of the lung, oral cavity and upper airways, esophagus, pancreas, kidneys, and bladder,

Vinyl chloride - angiosarcoma of the liver

5. Diet: Diet has also been implicated, especially in the development of gastro intestinal cancer as a result of a high animal fat diet. Additives composed of nitrates and certain methods of food preparation particularly charboiling are also recognized factors.

5. Genetic predisposition: Genetic predisposition either directly (as in Wilms' tumor and retinoblastoma) or indirectly (in association with inherited conditions such as Down syndrome or immunodeficiency diseases) result in tumor formation.

6. Family history: A strong family history of tumors increases the chance that a person from that family will develop a tumor. The location of tumors is also thought to have a genetic basis in some people. For example, if mother, grandmother, and sister all had breast cancer, there is a very good chance of development of breast cancer in genetically related women of the family

IMMUNE SURVEILLANCE

Even though development of tumors is not common in all individuals, formation of tumor cells often takes place in almost all individuals. But the efficient surveillance of immune system identifies the abnormal cells whenever they develop inside the body and removes them before the formation of tumor. Tumor in certain individuals indicates either failure of defense mechanism or improper function of immune system. Chances of cancer development is high in patients with suppressed or week immune activity. Patients with AIDS are susceptible for various types of tumors.

In normal conditions immune response to tumors is similar to the immune response shown against foreign grafts. It may be specific like the response against a foreign cell, virus infected cell etc. or non-specific with the involvement of macrophages and natural killer cells like innate immune response to various foreign agents.

SPECIFIC IMMUNE RESPONSE:

T- Lymphocytes play a major role in destruction of the tumor cells. T-cell activation includes the production and activation of TH, TD and TC cells. Lymphokines released by the activated T-cells trigger and mobilize B-cells. The triggered B-cells produce plasma cells to secrete Abs against the tumor Ags (Refer antigens) developed on the newly formed tumor cells. Immune system engages all kinds of immune reactions such as cell mediated immune reactions, Ab dependent reactions, complement mediated reactions, phagocytization etc. to get rid of the tumor cells. Lymphokines such as B-cell growth factors, B-cell differential factors, migration inhibition factors etc. play an important role in immune surveillance of tumor cells. Sufficient quantities of IL-2 produced by Ag stimulated T-lymphocytes must be present in order to mount an effective counter attack against the tumor cell population.

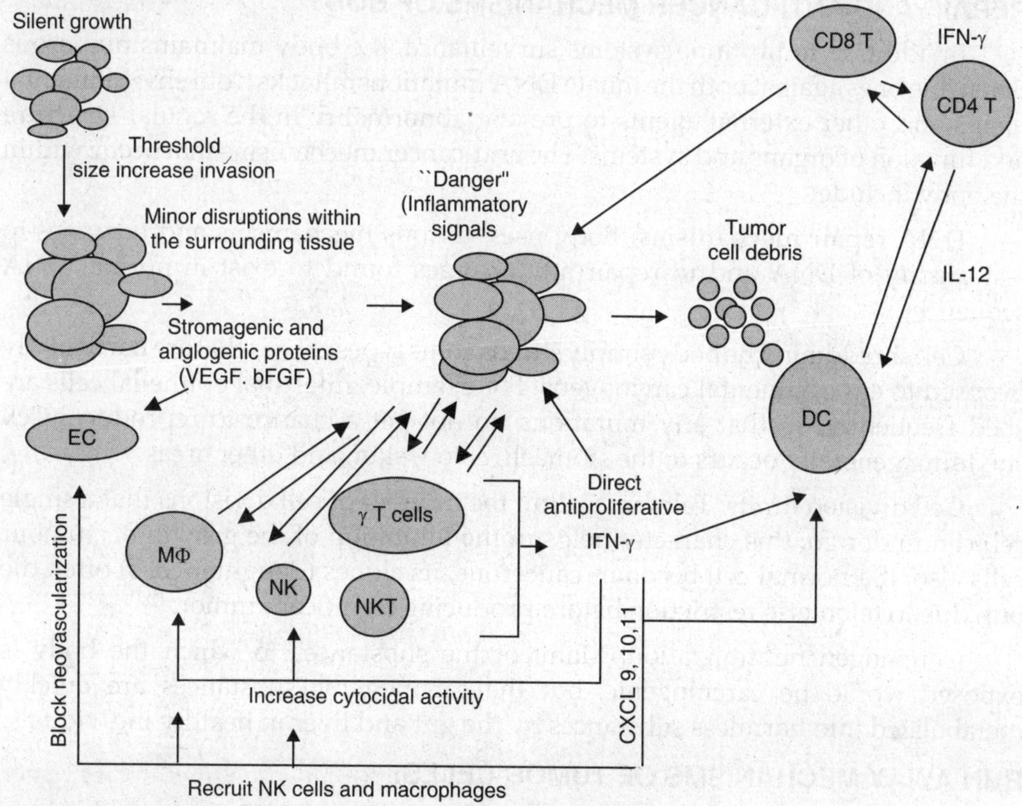

Fig. 17.1

NON-SPECIFIC IMMUNE RESPONSE:

Non-specific immune response against to any foreign agent is an innate character of animals, hence non-specific immune reactions also involved in the eradication of tumor cells with the help of macrophages and natural killer cells. Macrophages abolish tumor cells through cytolysis and phagocytosis. The activated lymphocytes and their secretions enhance the efficiency of macrophages in removal of tumor cells (The events leading to macrophage killing are still not very clear but if it is once revealed it may have potential role in cancer immunotherapy). Research article published in 197th volume of the journal "Science" suggests amended scrum and other environmental factors by "intrinsic cytotoxic effector system" of macrophages can enhance or suppress tumor killing activity of macrophages. The role of immune modulators in regulating NK-cell activity is still unclear, but the elucidation of protocols for sustained augmentation of NK-cell activity might lead to invention of more effective therapy of cancer. NK-cells with an unidentified NK target receptor seem to recognize the cancer cells. The tumor cells that express little or no MHC class-I Ags are more readily attacked by NK-cells than those that express greater amounts of class-I MHC. Although NK-cell killing is not MHC restricted, it appears to be influenced by MHC expression.

REPAIR AND ANTI-CANCER MECHANISMS OF BODY

In addition to immune systems surveillance, the body maintains numerous defensive lines against both the innate DNA mutations, attacks from environmental toxins and other external agents to prevent abnormality in the regular structure and function of organs and systems. The anti-cancer mechanisms that occur within the body include:

DNA repair mechanisms: Body uses various mechanisms and enzymes to test quality of DNA and to repair any changes found to exist in normal DNA sequences.

Cell shredding: The body simply shreds some types of cells that are particularly exposed to environmental carcinogens. For example, intestinal epithelial cells are shed frequently, so that any mutations do not get a chance to reproduce. Cell shedding generally occurs in the stomach, colon, skin, and other areas.

Cell division limits: Telomeres limit the number of cell divisions that a single cell can under go, this character helps in the inhibition of the growth of tumour cells also. If a normal cell becomes cancerous, its clones (daughter cells) often die out, due to telomeric restriction before producing significant tumor.

Carcinogen neutralization: Many of the substances to which the body is exposed would be carcinogenic, but the carcinogenic substances are quickly metabolized into harmless substances by the gut and liver in healthy individuals.

RUN AWAY MECHANISMS OF TUMOR CELLS:-

In spite of keen vigil of immune system and other body defense mechanisms tumor cells survive in some individuals and develop tumors. Various escape mechanisms such as sneaking through, modulating tumor antigens, masking of tumor Ags, inducing tolerance or production of blocking Abs and immuno suppressants etc. helps tumor cells in the escape and survival.

Sneaking Through: Newly formed tumor cells escape immune system's attack, by sneaking, till they increase their number to resist the immunological actions. Some tumors posses weak immunogenicity. This character helps in crashing immunological response till their number increases to a large extent. When the tumor cells increase in number they become strong enough to resist the attack of immune system and immune system fails to control the rapidly multiplying tumor cells.

Modulating Tumor Ags: To make invisible to immune surveillance certain tumor cells pull the newly formed Ags (Tumor Ags) to interior (cytoplasm) or stop expressing in surface Ags. Since tumor cells are the differentiated cells of their own, in the absence of expressed tumor Ags, immune system fail to enforce any action against the tumor cells. Redistribution of tumor antigens within the cell membrane also helps tumor cells in escaping immune surveillance.

Masking Tumor Ags: Certain tumor cells produce mucoproteins coat known as *Sialomucin* coat to hide their new Ags. Since sialomucin is a common component of the body, immune system fails to peep through this covering to attack the tumor cells.

Tumor induced tolerance: Certain tumor cells induce tolerance through synthesizing different immuno suppressants to suppress or activate TS-cells which in turn inhibit the activity of T_C, T_D and B-cells activity. Declined immunity is common feature in cancer patients.

Production of blocking agents: Certain tumor cells defend themselves from the action of immune system by producing auto antibodies known as "blocking antibodies" against their own antigens. When the blocking antibodies bind to their own surface antigens, they obstruct binding of other antibodies produced by the immune system against tumor cells. Since tumor antigens are bound with their own antibodies, immune system fails to identify and produce antibodies against the tumor antigens, even if immune system produces antibodies, the antibodies fail to get opportunity to bind with the tumor antigens due to the presence of blocking antigens. Unlike the regular antibodies the blocking antibodies fail to activate complement system, which is essential for the lysis or phagocytosis of target cells. More over in the presence of blocking antibodies, T_C-cells fail to bind with tumor cells to generate any lytic reactions.

Alteration of cell adhesion molecules: In addition to all, certain newly formed tumor cells alter their expression of cell adhesion molecules to reduce stable contact formation with cytotoxic cells of immune system to minimize their effect on their survival

Cell Adhesion Molecules (CAMs) are proteins located on the cell surface, that helps in binding with other cells or with the extracellular matrix (ECM) in the process called cell adhesion.

DIAGNOSIS:

Most cancers are initially recognized either by clinical and diagnostic tests or symptoms. Certain medical tests such as blood tests, X-rays, CT scans endoscopy etc help in identifying tumors. Biopsy, a histological examination is the definitive diagnosis for most malignancies. Study of immuno histochemistry and cytogenetical alterations are some of other tests practised by pathologists to diagnose tumors.

TREATMENT

Since "cancer" refers to a class of diseases, there is no single therapy to cure cancer. The choice of therapy depends upon the location of tumor, grade of the tumor, the juncture of the disease and general state of the patient (performance status).

SURGERY – cancers can be cured if removed entirely by surgery. This is possible only in the case of benign tumors, but in case of malignant tumors complete surgical excision is usually impossible because of their metastasis nature. A single cancer cell invisible to the naked eye may move to any new location of the body and develop tumor even after surgery.

CHEMOTHERAPY – Treating cancer through drugs is known as chemotherapy. Drugs used in chemotherapy are generally cytotoxic in nature; they interfere in cell division through various possible ways, such as in the duplication of DNA, in the separation of newly formed chromosomes etc. Chemotherapy cause potential harm to healthy tissue also. Today many of the tumors can be cured by appropriate combination of chemotherapy.

RADIATION THERAPY – Radiation therapy is the use of ionizing radiation to kill cells of tumor. It is also known as radiotherapy, X-ray therapy, or irradiation. Radiation therapy can be administered externally via external beam radiotherapy (EBRT) or internally via brachytherapy (a form of radiotherapy where a radioactive source is placed inside or next to the area requiring treatment). The effects of radiation therapy are localised and confined to the region being treated. Radiation damages both cancer cells and normal cells, but most normal cells can recover from the effects of radiation and function properly.

HORMONAL THERAPY The growth of some cancers can be inhibited by providing or blocking certain hormones. Common examples of hormone-sensitive tumors include certain types of breast and prostate cancers.

ANGIOGENESIS INHIBITORS - Angiogenesis inhibitors prevent the extensive growth of blood vessels (angiogenesis) required by the tumors to survive. "Bevacizumab" a monoclonal antibody against vascular endothelial growth factor, have been approved as an angiogenesis inhibitor and is in clinical use.

LIPOSOMAL THERAPY It is a new technique that uses chemotherapy drugs that have been packaged inside liposomes (synthetic fat globules). This liposome, or fatty coating, helps drugs in penetrate the cancer cells more selectively and decreases possible side effects (such as hair loss, nausea, and vomiting). Examples of liposomal medications are Doxil (the encapsulated form of doxorubicin) and Daunoxome (the encapsulated form of daunorubicin).

TARGETED THERAPY - It is a type of medication that blocks the growth of cancer cells by interfering with specific targeted molecules needed for carcinogenesis and tumor growth, rather than by simply interfering with rapidly dividing cells. Targeted cancer therapies may be more effective than current treatments and less harmful to normal cells. The main categories of targeted therapy are small molecules and monoclonal antibodies. Many oncologists believe that targeted therapies are the chemotherapy of the future.

IMMUNOTHERAPY OR BIOLOGIC THERAPY: - Immunotherapy is inducing patient's own immune system to work against the tumor cells. This can be achieved through immunization of the patient to train the patient's own immune system to recognize tumor cells as targets to be destroyed, or through the administration of therapeutic antibodies as drugs. Immunotherapy is the great hope for cancer treatment. While monoclonal antibodies, cytokines, and vaccines have individually shown some promise, a lot of research is going on to find some easy and effective therapy. Some of the therapies based on immune system are as follows.

(a) Antibody or monoclonal therapy: Antibody therapy can be used in a variety of ways to treat cancer. Monoclonal antibodies act through Antibody-Dependent Cell-Mediated Cytotoxicity (ADCC) or Complement-Dependent Cytotoxicity (CDC). Conjugated monoclonal antibodies with a toxin or a radioisotope (Radioimmunotherapy) can be used in the treatment because the antibody conjugate is absorbed into the cell itself; resulting in cell death. The chemotherapeutic agent can be taken directly into the targeted malignant cell, rather than being systemically absorbed with the help of antibodies. There are a number of antigens and corresponding monoclonal antibodies for the treatment of B cell malignancies. Some of the most active are listed in Table 9. Compared to hematologic malignancies, solid tumors do not have as many specific targets for monoclonal antibodies that are not cross-reactive with antigens on normal tissues. Two significant monoclonal antibodies used in solid tumors treatment are "**edrecolomab**" and "**trastuzumab**". Edrecolomab (trade name Panorex) is a chimeric mouse/human monoclonal antibody to the cell-surface glycoprotein expressed on epithelial tissues and on various carcinomas. Preliminary studies had shown promise of a possible use in patients with stage III colorectal carcinoma. Trastuzumab (Herceptin) is a monoclonal antibody that interferes with the HER2/new receptor. HER2/new receptor regulates cell growth, survival, adhesion, migration, and differentiation. The defective HER receptor proteins stuck in the "on" position in certain cancers, notably in some breast cancers. Trastuzumab antibody binds and blocks the receptor for receiving further signals to stop uncontrolled cell growth

Cytokines and Cancer Therapy: Cytokines are the messengers of the immune system. Cytokine therapy involves the administration of signaling molecules (usually proteins) that increase the maturation and growth of antigen presenting cells and T cells. IL-2 and interferon-alfa 2b are two cytokines approved for treatment of cancer. IL-2 has demonstrated activity against renal cell, melanoma, lymphoma, and leukemia. Interleukin-2 (IL-2) is a T cell growth factor that binds to a specific tripartite receptor on T cells. Interferon has activity in the same histology's but also in Kaposi's sarcoma, chronic myelogenous leukemia, and hairy cell leukemia. Interferon alfa has many roles. It upregulates genes like MHC class I, tumor antigens, and adhesion molecules. It is also an anti-angiogenic agent. It is extremely active in the immune system, promoting B and T cell activity. Interferon alfa can stimulate macrophages, even dendritic cells, and upregulates Fc receptors. Overall, cytokines are substances that appear to have application in the treatment of hematologic malignancies or immunogenic tumors.

Vaccine Approaches against Cancer

Efforts to treat cancer with vaccines date back to the origins of immunology.

Recent research has indicated that the vaccines are also useful in the prevention and treatment of cancer. Different types of vaccines are developed to treat different types of cancers. For example, new vaccines against the human papilloma virus (HPV) prevent women from getting cervical, vaginal, and vulvar cancer, and vaccines against hepatitis B virus (HBV) may lower risk of getting liver cancer in some people (Refer Chapter 18 for vaccines).

Advances in immunotherapy

The development and testing of second generation immunotherapies are already under way. Antibodies targeted to disease-causing antigens can be effective under certain circumstances, but in many cases their efficacy may be limited by other factors. To overcome this problem, cytokines are conjugated to them to trigger an immune response. Engineering the antibody in such a way that the conjugated cytokines get separated after entry into a cell by endocytosis can potentially increase the efficacy.

Therapeutic administration of certain conjugated cytokines may cause systemic inflammation, resulting in serious side effects and toxicity. Hens a new generation of chimeric molecules such as artificial T cell receptor, containig an immune-stimulatory cytokine attached to an antibody can target the cytokine's activity to a specific environment such as a tumor, and are able to generate a very effective yet localized immune response against the tumor tissue.

Use of immune cells cloned from patients immune system is a new immune therapy in cancer treatment. US doctors from the Clinical Research Division led by Cassian Yee at Fred Hutchinson Cancer Research Center in Seattle treated a skin cancer patient for the first time successfully by this method.

Table: 17.1

Cancer immunotherapy:Monoclonal antibodies

Antibody	Brand name	Approval date	**Type**	**Target**	**Approved treatments (S)**
Alemtuzumab	Campath	**2001**	Humanized	CD52	Chronic lymphocytic leukemia
Bevacizumab	Avastin	**2004**	Humanized	Vascular endothelial growth factor	Colorectal cancer
Cetuximab	Erbitux	**2004**	Chimeric	Epidermal growth factor receptor	Colorectal cancer

Gemtuzumab ozogamicin	Mylotarg	**2000**	Humanized	CD33	Acute myelogenous leukemia (with calicheamicin)
Ibritumomab tiuxetan	Zevalin	**200**	Murine	CD20	Non-Hodgkin lymphoma (with yttrium -90 or indium-111)
Panitumumab	Vectibix	**2006**	Human		Colorectal cancer
Rituximab	Rituxan, Mabthera	**1997**	Chimeric	CD20	Non Hodgkin Lymphoma
Trastuzumab	Herceptin	**1998**	Cumanized	ErbB2	Breast cancer

18

VACCINES

Immunity to a pathogen is not alike in every one. Various factors such as age, sex, nutrition, genetic back ground, and physiological status etc. influence imuune power. It has been recognized for centuries that certain diseases never reappear in the same individual after recovery. Since immune system acquires defense mechanism in the presence of a pathogen, an individual recovered from a disease develops resistance to that specific disease causing agent. Hence it is understood that resistance can be induced by the pathogen. Considering this fact, Chinese strived to prevent smallpox (a deadly disease characterized by pus filled blisters) by exposing uninfected individuals to substance of smallpox lesions. The process was named as "variolation" from the root word "**variola**" a synonym for smallpox. Variolation - the age old practice of inoculation took a variety of forms. One of it is removing pus and fluid from a smallpox lesion, and introducing it under the skin with a needle. Another method involved peeling scabs from lesions, drying and grinding them to a powder, and letting an uninfected person inhale this powder. An alternate to this is picking up a small amount of the scab powder with a needle and introducing it directly into the veins. Lady Mary Wortley Montagu, wife of the British ambassador to Turkey, observed this third method and introduced this practice into England in 1721. Although the effects of variolation varied, starting from mild illness in most individuals to death in a few, mortality and morbidity rates due to smallpox are certainly low in populations that used variolation than in those that did not.

In 1796 Edward Jenner, an English physician, used folk knowledge to find an alternative to variolation. He noticed dairy maids infected with cowpox are immune to small-pox. He then deliberately infected James Phipps, an eight year old boy, with cowpox and exposed him to smallpox virus. The small pox virus failed to generate disease in Phipps. After repeating the experiment on other children, including his own son, Jenner concluded that cowpox infection provided immunity to smallpox without the risks of variolation. He published the conclusions of his experiment in 1798. Consequently thousands of people protected themselves from the deadly smallpox disease by intentionally infecting themselves with cowpox. Jenner's work became popular as "vaccination," after "vacca," - the Latin word for cow, and the substance used for inoculation is referred as "vaccine."

Jenner in his experiment used a lancet to scratch some infected material from patient with cowpox and to introduce the same under the boy's skin. Fifty years after Jenner, the hypodermic syringe became available. In 1885, Louis Pasteur used one to vaccinate a young boy who had been bitten by a mad dog and was sure to die of rabies. The boy lived after immunization and immunization took another giant step forward. Since then, technological improvements included safety features, sharper and thinner needles. Even though, hypodermic injection remains the most common method of getting vaccine, it is not the only technology for immunization. Engineers and scientists continue to search for alternative routes such as mouth, nose etc. to introduce the vaccine.

The widespread vaccination technology has been marked a decrease in diseases, which once ravaged the world's population. An example of this is smallpox, once it is a major cause for death world-wide. Now the smallpox virus is found only in freezers, in high-containment laboratories the "Center for Disease Control and Prevention (CDC)" in Atlanta and the "Institute for Viral Preparations" in Moscow.

Vaccines are effective in preventing diseases, not only in individuals, but also in communities. This type of protection is called "herd immunity" or "community immunity." When a disease spreads from one individual to another, it requires both an infected individual to spread it and a susceptible individual to catch it. Herd immunity works by decreasing the numbers of susceptible people. When the number of susceptible people drops low enough, the disease disappear from the community because of non availability of enough people to carry on the catch-and-infect cycle. The greater the proportion of vaccinated members of a community, the faster the disease disappears. This is the reason that school children are often required to be vaccinated before attending school. Vaccination has resulted in marked decrease of many diseases including pertussis (whooping cough), polio, smallpox, and others.

Since vaccine tricks the body's immune system to produce antibodies to fight with a specific pathogen before the entry of effective pathogen, the vaccinated person is able to eradicate the pathogen immediately after its entry in to the body.

VACCINE

Vaccine is a preparation intended to produce immunity to a disease by stimulating the production of antibodies. Vaccines comprise substances such as suspensions of killed or attenuated microorganisms, or products or derivatives of microorganisms that can stimulate the immune system. In normal conditions disease causing organism induces an immune response in the host and by way of increase in immune response, the quantity of infectious agents gradually reduce due to gradual raise in immune response, ensuing recovery in physical condition. Immune response against the pathogen is multi-fold and includes the synthesis of proteins called "antibodies" and production of "memory cells". The antibodies binds to the disease causing organisms and lead to their eventual destruction. Memory cells remain in the blood stream for long time, some times they remain for the life time of the host. Memory cells mount a quick protective immune response when the same pathogen reenters in to the body. The response shown by the memory cells is often so rapid that infection doesn't develop. Vaccines initiate the production of antibodies and memory cells similar to the natural immune response but with out causing any harm to the individual. All the vaccines may not be very safe because of the presence of pathogens or their materials. The safety and effectiveness of a vaccine depends on how it is made and what it contains. There are six main types of vaccines:

1. Live virus vaccines.
2. Killed or inactivated virus vaccines.
3. Subunit vaccines (purified or recombinant viral antigen).
4. Recombinant virus vaccines.
5. Anti-idiotype antibodies.
6. DNA vaccines.

1. LIVE VACCINES: Live virus vaccines are prepared from attenuated strains that are completely or almost devoid of pathogenicity but are capable of inducing a protective immune response. Since a related virus from different host cannot cause disease in the new host it can also be used in live virus vaccines. Use of cowpox virus in the prevention of smallpox disease is one of the best examples for this. A pathogen can multiply in unnatural host (human) without any pathogenesis, but provide continuous antigenic stimulation over a period of time. Failure with these vaccines is rare but inadequate storage or administration may cause failure. Another possibility for the failure is interference of related viruses, as is suspected in the case of oral polio vaccine in developing countries.

Attenuation is a technique used for reducing the virulence of a virus, while using it in vaccine preparation. It is the counterpart of the vaccines produced by 'killing' the virus (inactivated vaccine). Several methods have been used to attenuate viruses for vaccine production. They are as follows:

a. Passage of the virus in "unnatural host" or host cell - Major vaccines for man and animals are developed in this way. After repeated passages in unnatural host, the virus loses its virulence; this virus can be administered to the natural host for immunization purpose. For example vaccine for yellow fever is developed by passing 17D strain of yellow fever virus in mice and then in chick embryos before using it for vaccination. In the same way Polio viruses are passed in monkey kidney cells and measles viruses are passed in chick embryo fibroblasts. Human diploid cells [aborted babies] such as the WI-38 and MRC-5 are now widely used for the same purpose.

b. Development of temperature sensitive mutants - This method may be used in combination with the above method for attenuation of pathogen. Variation in the temperature of the host helps in attenuation of the pathogen.

c. Use of an unnatural route - The virulence of the virus is often reduced when administered through an unnatural route. Hence administration of pathogenic or partially attenuated virus through an unnatural route also helps in immunization without any pathological activity in host. This principle is used in the immunization of military recruits against adult "Respiratory Distress Syndrome" using enterically coated live adenovirus.

POTENTIAL SAFETY PROBLEMS WITH LIVE VACCINES:

(1) Under attenuation. 2) Mutations leading to reversion of virulence. 3) Preparation instability 4) Contamination of viruses in cultured cells. 5) Heat liability 6) Not safe for pregnant women and immunocompromized patients such as AIDs patients, patents using immune suppressive drugs after transplantation etc.

(2) KILLED OR INACTIVATED WHOLE VIRUS VACCINES: These vaccines are prepared by simply inactivating the pathogens. Preparation of killed vaccines may take the route of heat or chemicals. The chemicals used include formaldehyde or beta- propiolactone. The traditional agent for inactivation of the virus is formalin. Excessive treatment can destroy immunogenicity, whereas insufficient treatment can leave infectious virus capable of causing disease. Soon after the distribution of inactivated polio vaccine, there was an outbreak of paralytic poliomyelitis in USA due to inadequate processing. This incident led to a review of the inactivation procedure.

Acute Respiratory Distress Syndrome ARDS is a clinical syndrome associated with a variety of pathological findings. These include pneumonia, eosinophilic pneumonia, cryptogenic organizing pneumonia, acute fibrinous organizing pneumonia, and diffuse alveolar damage (DAD). Of these, the pathology most commonly associated with ARDS is DAD.

Acute Respiratory Distress Syndrome or Acute respiratory disease (ARD) due to adenoviruses caused significant morbidity in military training populations. Since 1971 ARD has been controlled by the use of live, enteric-coated, adenovirus (ADV) types 4 and 7 vaccines.

Potential safety problems with Killed vaccines:

(1) Incomplete inactivation. 2) Increased risk of allergic reactions due to large amounts of antigen involved. 3) Live vaccines of certain viruses can induce reactivation, or become oncogenic in nature

(3) SUBUNIT VACCINES: Subunit vaccines are defined as those containing one or more pure or semi-pure antigens. Since the technology for growing viruses to high titers in cell cultures advanced, it became practicable to purify virus and viral antigens. It is now possible to identify the peptide sites encompassing the major antigenic sites of viral antigens, from which highly purified subunit vaccines can be produced. But some times increasing purification may lead to loss of immunogenicity and this may necessitate coupling to an immunogenic carrier protein or adjuvant, such as aluminum salt. In addition to using a whole protein as a vaccine, it is possible to identify individual epitopes within these protective proteins and develop peptide vaccines. The potential advantages of using subunits as vaccines are the increased safety and less antigenic competition, ability to target the vaccines and differentiation of vaccinated animals from infected animals is easy. Since only a few components are included in the vaccine ability to target the vaccines at the site where immunity is required is possible. Examples of purified subunit vaccines include the HA vaccines for influenza A and B, and hepatitis B surface antigens (HBs Ags) derived from the plasma of carriers.

Potential disadvantages of subunit vaccines

(1) The disadvantage of subunit vaccines is that they generally require strong adjuvants and these adjuvants often induce tissue reactions.

(2) Duration of immunity is generally shorter than the live vaccines.

(3) The major disadvantage of peptide vaccines is that they often need to be linked to carriers to enhance their immunogenicity.

(4) A pathogen can escape immune responses to a single epitope versus multiple epitope vaccines.

4. RECOMBINANT VIRAL PROTEINS: Virus proteins have been expressed in bacteria, yeast, mammalian cells, and viruses. *E.coli* cells are first to be used for this purpose but the expressed proteins are not glycosylated, which is a major drawback, as many of the immunogenic proteins of viruses are glycosylated. Recombinant hepatitis B vaccine is the only recombinant vaccine licensed at present.

5. LIVE GENETICALLY ENGINEERED VACCINES: Using molecular approaches (recombinant DNA technology), it is possible to identify specific virulent genes of different pathogens. The virulent gene can be deleted are modified by inducing multiple mutations through molecular technology. Using the pathogens with modified genes, it is possible to develop a safer vaccine than using conventional attenuation technologies. For example, the degree of attenuation can be controlled by deleting or mutating the appropriate gene or groups of genes. By deleting an entire gene or portion of a gene, the chances of reversion to virulence is dramatically reduced. The probability of reversion to virulence can further be reduced if two different genes separated by some space are deleted or mutated. Based on these factors, the newly engineered vaccines are much safer than the conventionally-produced live vaccines. In addition to that these vaccines can also be used as "marker vaccines" (A marker vaccines is a vaccine that helps to differentiate infected and vaccinated subjects). By deleting an essential gene, one can develop replication of incompetent viruses which are extremely safe, as they cannot be transmitted in the environment. A further advantage of live vaccines is that they can often be delivered via natural route of infection (mucosal route), thus inducing not only systemic immunity, but also mucosal immunity. By developing mucosal immunity, one can prevent the initiation of infection as well as preventing disease.

For example potential live vaccines using recombinant vaccinia viruses have been constructed for both hepatitis B and herpes simplex. These recombinant vaccinia viruses express cloned genes of the hepatitis B virus surface antigen (HBsAg) or the glycoprotein D from herpes simplex virus (HSV-gD). Inoculation of rabbits with the recombinant vaccinia virus that expresses the HBsAg or HSV-gD elicits the production of high-titered antibodies. Immunization of mice with the vaccinia recombinant expressing HSV-gD gave complete protection on subsequent challenge with lethal doses of live herpes simplex virus.

Hybrid virus vaccines are stable and stimulate both cellular and humoral immunity. They are relatively cheap and simple to produce. Being live vaccines, smaller quantities are enough for immunization.

Potential disadvantages of genetically engineered vaccines

The use of vaccinia also carries the risk of adverse reactions associated with the vaccine and the virus may spread to susceptible contacts. At present, efforts are being made to attenuate vaccinia virus further and the possibility of using other recombinant vectors is being explored, such as attenuated poliovirus and adenovirus.

5. SYNTHETIC PEPTIDES: The synthetic peptide approach to vaccine development arose in response to rapid DNA cloning and sequencing technology. This made it possible to quickly obtain primary sequences and construct various peptides. Major efforts were put into the development of a synthetic vaccine (a linear sequence of 20 amino acids) for foot-and-mouth disease virus (FMDV) for which even today no alternative exists besides the classical vaccine based on inactivated virus. Since synthetic peptide antigens are precisely defined and free from unnecessary components which may be associated with side effects, vaccines made with synthetic peptides have many advantages. They are stable and relatively cheap to manufacture. Furthermore, less quality assurance is required. Changes due to natural variation of the virus can be readily accommodated, which would be a great advantage for unstable viruses such as influenza.

It is generally assumed that, "synthetic peptides do not readily stimulate T cells because of their small size. It is now known that synthetic peptides can be highly immunogenic in their free form provided they contain T- cell epitopes, in addition to the B cell epitopes, to get recognized by T-helper cells. T-cell epitopes can be provided by carrier protein molecules, foreign antigens or within the synthetic peptide molecule itself. Synthetic peptides are not applicable to all viruses. This approach did not work in the case of polio viruses because; the important antigenic sites were made up of 2 or more different viral capsid proteins so that it is in a concise 3-D conformation.

Advantages of defined viral antigens or peptides include:

1. Production and quality control is simpler.
2. No nucleic acids or other viral or external proteins, therefore less toxic.
3. Safer in cases where viruses are oncogenic or establish a persistent infection.
4. Feasible even if virus cannot be cultivated.

Disadvantages:

1. May be less immunogenic than conventional inactivated whole-virus vaccines.
2. Requires adjuvant.
3. Requires primary course of injections followed by booster doses.
4. With out T cell epitopes they fail to elicit cell mediated immunity (CMI).

6. ANTI-IDIOTYPE ANTIBODIES: The ability of anti-idiotype antibodies to mimic foreign antigens has led to their development as vaccines to induce immunity against viruses, bacteria and protozoa in experimental animals. Anti-idiotypes have many potential uses as viral vaccines, particularly when the antigen is difficult to grow or hazardous. They have been used to induce immunity against a wide range of viruses, including HBV, rabies, Newcastle disease virus and FeLV, Reoviruses and Polioviruses.

7. DNA VACCINES: Recently, encouraging results are reported for DNA vaccines where by DNA coding for the foreign antigen is directly injected into the animal, so that the foreign antigen is directly produced by the host cells. In theory these vaccines would be extremely safe and devoid of side effects since the foreign antigens would be directly produced by the host animal. In addition, DNA is relatively inexpensive and easier to produce than conventional vaccines and thus this technology may one day increase the availability of vaccines to developing countries. Moreover, the time for development is relatively short, which may enable timely immunization against emerging infectious diseases. In addition, DNA vaccines can theoretically result in more long-term production of an antigenic protein when introduced into a relatively non dividing tissue, such as muscle.

Indeed some observers have already dubbed the new technology the "third revolution" in vaccine development on par with Pasteur's ground-breaking work with whole organisms and the development of subunit vaccines. The first clinical trials using injections of DNA to stimulate an immune response against a foreign protein began for HIV in 1995. Four other clinical trials using DNA vaccines against influenza, herpes simplex virus, T-cell lymphoma, and an additional trial for HIV were started in 1996.

The technique that is being tested in humans involves the direct injection of plasmids – (aditional DNA in bacteria) that contain genes for proteins to be produced by the organism being targeted for immunity. Once injected into the host's muscle tissue, the DNA is taken up by host cells, which then start expressing the foreign protein. The protein serves as an antigen,that stimulates an immune responses and protective immunological memory.

Enthusiasm for DNA vaccination in humans is tempered by the fact that delivery of the DNA to cells is still not optimal, particularly in larger animals. Another concern is the possibility, which exists with all gene therapy that is the vaccine's DNA may be integrated into host chromosomes and turn on oncogenes or turn off tumor suppressor genes. Another potential drawback is that extended immune stimulation by the foreign antigen could in theory provoke chronic inflammation or autoantibody production.

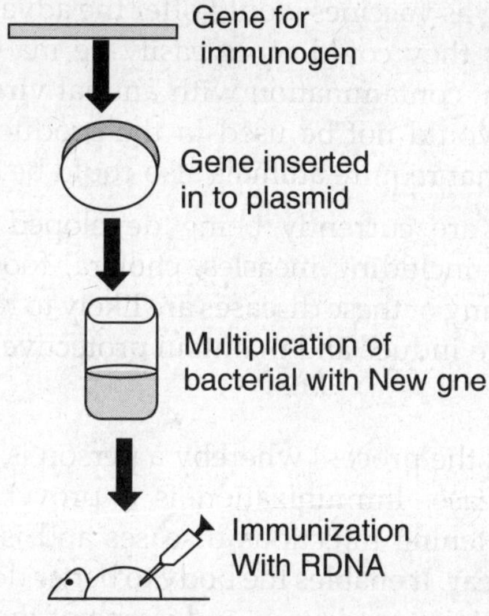

Fig. 18.1

Disadvantages:

- Limited to protein immunogens (not useful for non-protein based antigens such as bacterial polysaccharides).
- Risk of affecting genes, controlling cell growth.
- Possibility of inducing antibody production against DNA.
- Possibility of tolerance to the antigen (protein) produced.
- Potential for atypical processing of bacterial and parasite proteins.

Recent vaccinology

Polynucleotide vaccines: The most recent development in vaccinology is immunization with polynucleotides. This technology has been referred to as genetic immunization or DNA immunization. The basis for this approach to immunization is that, cells can take-up plasmid DNA and expresses the genes within the transfected cells. Thus, the animal acts as a bioreactor to produce the vaccine. This makes the vaccine relatively inexpensive to produce. Some of the advantages of polynucleotide immunization are (1) it is extremely safe, induces a broad range of immune response (cellular and humoral responses) (2) causes long-lived immunity(3) can induce immune responses in the presence of maternal antibodies. Most recently, it has also been used for immunizing fetuses. Thus, animals are born immune to the pathogens and at no time in the animal's life are they susceptible to these infectious agents. Although this is one of the most attractive developments in vaccinology, there is a great need to develop better delivery systems to improve the transfection efficiency in vivo.

Edible vaccines: Currently researchers are seeking to develop genetically altered plants that could provide immunity to infectious diseases. Studies have already shown that genetically engineered plants and their products can act as vaccines. Plants acting as vaccines would offer the advantage of being inexpensive to produce, and thus they could more easily be made available to developing countries. In addition, contamination with animal viruses would be eliminated, since cultured cells would not be used in the production process. Many of the quality control tests that require animals also could be eliminated.

Edible vaccines are currently being developed for a number of human and animal diseases, including measles, cholera, foot and mouth disease, and Hepatitis-B and C. Many of these diseases are likely to require booster vaccinations or multiple antigens to induce and maintain protective immunity.

IMMUNIZATION

Immunization is the process whereby a person is made immune or resistant to an infectious disease. Immunization is a proven tool for controlling and eliminating life-threatening infectious diseases and is estimated to avert over 2 million deaths each year. It enables the body to better defend itself against diseases caused by certain bacteria or viruses, and is one of the most cost-effective health investments, with proven strategies that make it accessible to even the most hard-to-reach and vulnerable populations. Immunization may occur on its own (when people are exposed to bacteria or viruses), or typically by the administration of a vaccine. When people are immunized against a disease by the administration of a vaccine, they do not get the disease or get only a mild form of it.

Vaccines stimulate the body's own immune system to protect the person against subsequent infection or disease. It has clearly defined target groups. It can be delivered effectively through outreach activities; and vaccination does not require any major lifestyle change.

There are two types of immunization - active and passive.

Active immunization: In active immunization, vaccines are used to stimulate the body's natural defense mechanisms. The body's immune system responds to a vaccine by producing appropriate immune cells and memory cells to recognize and attack the specific bacteria or virus contained in the vaccine. Then whenever the person is exposed to the specific bacteria or virus, the body automatically produces immune cells.

Passive immunization: In passive immunization, antibodies or activated immune cells against a specific infectious organism are given directly to a person. These antibodies and immune cells are obtained from several sources (Refer Chapter 12 for different types of immunity). Passive immunization is used for people whose immune system does not respond adequately to an infection or for people who acquire an infection before they can be vaccinated (for example, after exposure to the rabies virus). Passive immunization can also be used to prevent disease, when people are likely to be exposed and do not have time to get or complete a vaccination series. For example, a solution containing gamma globulin (a common type of antibody) is used to prevent hepatitis in people who travel to certain parts of the world. Passive immunization lasts for only a few days or weeks, until the body eliminates the injected antibodies.

Vaccines available today are highly reliable, and most people tolerate them well. They rarely have side effects, but they do not work in everyone. Some vaccines are routinely given to children for example polio vaccine, DPT, BCG etc.

Other vaccines are usually given mainly to specific groups of people. For example, the yellow fever vaccine is given only to people traveling to certain parts of Africa and South America. Still other vaccines are given following possible exposure to a specific disease. For example, the rabies vaccine may be given to a person who has been bitten by a dog.

Vaccines and antibodies are usually given by injection into a muscle (intramuscularly) or under the skin (subcutaneously). Antibodies are sometimes injected into a vein (intravenously) also.

Mode of immunization: Immunization can be given as prophylactic or therapeutic dose. Most vaccines are given prophylactically, i.e., prior to exposure to the pathogen. However, some vaccines can be administered therapeutically, i.e., post exposure (eg. rabies virus). The effectiveness of this mode of immunization depends on the rate of replication of the pathogen, incubation period and pathogenic mechanism. In a situation where pathogen has a short incubation period, the pathogenic mechanism is such that only a small amount of pathogenic molecules could be fatal (eg. tetanus and diphtheria) and/or bolus of infection is relatively large, both passive and active post exposure immunizations are essential. Passive prophylactic immunization is also needed in case of defects in immune system, such as hypo gamma globulinemia.

Table:18.1

National Immunization Schedule

Vaccine	Age				
	Birth	6 weeks	10 weeks	14 weeks	9-12 months
Primary vaccination					
BCG	+	–	–	–	–
Oral polio	+	+	+	+	–
DPT		+	+	+	–
Hepatitis B*		+	+	+	–
Measles				–	+
Booster Doses					
DPT + Oral Polio	16 to 24 months				
DT	5 years				

Tetanus toxoid (TT)	At 10 years and again at 16 years
Vitamin A*	9, 18, 24, 30 and 36 months
Pregnant women	
Tetanus toxoid (PW) : 1st does 2nd dose Booster	As early as possible during pregnancy (first contact) 1 month after 1st dose If previously vaccinated, within 3 years

- *Only in project areas

Table: 18.2

Adverse event occurring within 48 hours of DTP Vaccination

Event	Frequency
Local:	
Redness, swelling,pain	1 in 2-3 doses
Mild/Moderate systemic:	
Fever,drowsiness.fretfulness	1 in 2-3 doses
vomiting, anoxia	1 in 5-15 doses
More serious systemic:	
Persistent crying,fever	1 in 100-300 doses
convolutions	1in 1750 doses
Acute encephalopathy	1 in 100,000doses
permanent neurological defect	1 in 300.000 doses

PESSIMISTIC SIDE OF IMMUNIZATION: Active immunization may cause fever, malaise and discomfort. Some vaccines may also cause joint pains or arthritis (rubella), convulsions, sometimes fatal pertussis, or neurological disorders (influenza). Allergy to egg may develop as a consequence of viral vaccines produced in egg (measles, mumps, influenza, yellow fever). Booster shots result in more pronounced inflammatory effects than the primary immunization. The noticeable and serious side effects documented have been those following the DPT vaccine (Table 18.2). Most of these were attributable to the whole pertussis component of the vaccine and have been eliminated since the use of the acellular pertussis preparation.

19

IMMUNE DEFICIENCY DISEASES

We are constantly surrounded by a multitude of viruses, bacteria, microbes, parasites, and toxins that pose a potential threat to our health. Immune system enables the body to fight against these factors and helps in maintaining good health. Hence health of an individual depends upon the efficiency of immune system. Since the immune system is a complex network of cells, proteins, tissues, and organs that work together to fight off harmful substances and disease-causing microorganisms called pathogens, absence or abnormality or dysfunction of any segment of immune system can lead to immune deficiency. Immune deficiency typically leads to frequent infections and some times it may lead to additional medical problems, including cancers. Patients suffering from immune deficiencies often experience a variety of skin, respiratory, and bone problems as well, and they are more likely to have autoimmune diseases.

HOW DO IMMUNE DEFICIENCIES DEVELOP?

A large number of genes are required to generate the components of the immune system. Some immune deficiency diseases arise when one or more of these genes are defective. Immune system may be impaired during fetal development, resulting in congenital immune deficiency disorder. Immune deficiency may be hereditary or may be acquired. If immune deficiency is not inherited, various factors that affect the efficiency of immune system are as follows:

Illness or Infection or Injury: One of the common reasons for lowered immune functioning is illness or infection. Certain illnesses such as chicken pox, measles, tuberculosis, chronic hepatitis, and certain types of cancers weaken the immune system. Injuries such as burn trauma or surgery also tend to lower the immune system's first line of defense. Since the body has to split much of its energy and resources between healing and fighting off infections, immune system takes some time to recover from illness. During recovery period due to reduced efficiency of immune system, body becomes vulnerable to invasion of other pathogens. The second infection before the recovery of first infection, hits the immune system harder and recovery takes longer.

Lifestyle: Habits of individuals such as diet, sleep, hygiene, stress etc. also influence the efficiency of immune system. Malnutrition and unbalanced diet alo lower the function of immune system. Research has shown that poor nutrition compromises the lymphatic system, making the body more vulnerable to infection and disease. Even though the exact reason is not fully understood, it is found that people who suffer from sleep disturbances or poor quality sleep tend to have weaker immune functioning than those who sleep 7 and 8 hours each night. Many studies have shown that stress for prolonged period has a remarkable and powerful negative effect on the immune system. Simple hygienic habits such as washing hands regularly and keeping a clean living environment boost immune system efficiency.

Medication: Some medications, particularly immunosuppressant medications such as corticosteroids have an adverse effect on the immune system. Since suppression of the immune system is the purpose of these medications, they leave the body open to all sorts of other infections and illnesses by supressing immune system. Since chemotherapy reduces the white blood cell count, it often reduces the body's defenses for several months, both during and after treatment. By interfearing in the functioning of immune system regular use of antibiotics may also contribute to immune deficiency.

CLASSIFICATION OF IMMUNE DEFICIENCY

Considering the root cause, immune deficiency is classified into two types

1. Primary or inherited immune deficiency
2. Secondary or acquired, immune deficiency.

PRIMARY OR INHERITED IMMUNE DEFICIENCY:

The complex function of the immune system requires the cooperation of various organs, tissues, cells and proteins. A heritable abnormality in any of these factors of the complex immune system can lead to primary immune deficiency. The abnormality may be reflected in many forms such as, stem cell deficiency (defects in hemopoisis), B cell deficiency, T- cell deficiency, combined B and T cell deficiency, deficiency of phagocytes, complement deficiency etc. Immunodeficiencies range from very serious to very mild. The serious forms are often noticeable at birth or shortly thereafter. However, very mild forms may not be diagnosed until later in life, during adolescence or young adulthood. Since immune deficiency diseases are caused by hereditary or genetic defects they are not contagious, and can affect anyone, regardless of age or sex.

The World Health Organization (WHO) has identified nearly 150 primary immune deficiency diseases. The overall incidence of symptomatic primary immunodeficiency is estimated to be 1/10,000. Patients with primary immunodeficiency diseases commonly have an increased susceptibility to infection and require life-long therapies, such as intravenous immune globulin infusions, antibiotic therapies, bone marrow transplantations etc.

Primary immune deficiency diseases are generally grouped by the part of the immune system that is malfunctioning. They are sometimes classified according to which component is faulty (T cells, B cells, phagocytic cells or complement) or according to individual clinical syndromes. Four commonest primary immunodeficiencies seen apart from physiologic at hypogammaglobulinaemia of infancy, are transient hypogammaglobulinaemia of infancy (THI), IgG subclass deficiency, partial antibody deficiency with impaired polysaccharide responsiveness (IPR) and selective IgA deficiency.

Symptoms of primary immunodeficiency:

The most common problem for people with primary immunodeficiency disease is that they are more likely to get infections more often and the infections are more severe, longer lasting, and harder to cure than people with normal immune systems. In adition to opportunistic infections autoimmune problems are more common in primary immune deficiency.

Treatment for primary immunodeficiency

Even though no single treatment works in all cases of primary immunodeficiency, there are many treatment options that can even be combined to make it more likely to treat primary immunodeficiency. The basic treatment falls into three stages:

1. Clearing the current infection.
2. Avoiding germs and preventing exposure to new infections.
3. Correcting the immunodeficiency.

Prevention of primary immunodeficiency syndromes

Prevention of primary immunodeficiency depends on the identification and genetic counselling of likely carriers in families with a positive history. Prenatal diagnosis using such techniques as cultured amniotic cells or foetal blood may be possible for some disorders such as severe combined immunodeficiency. X-linked disorders may be excluded by sex determination.

Table: 19.1

Some Congenital Immunodeficiency Disorders

Factor responsible	Disorder
Problems with B cells (lymphocytes) and antibodies	X-linked agammaglobulinemia. Deficiency of a specific antibody (immunoglobulin), such as IgA deficiency, IgG sub class deficiency, immuno deficiency with increased IgM, Common variable immunodeficiency Transient hypogammaglobulinemia of infancy.
Problems with T cells (lymphocytes)	Chronic mucocutaneous candidiasis DiGeorge syndrome X-linked lymphoproliferative syndrome.
Problems with B and T cells	Ataxia-telangiectasia Hyperimmunoglobulinemia E syndrome Severe combined immunodeficiency Wiskott-Aldrich syndrome

Phagocytic defects	Neutropenia (Reduction in neutrophil count) Leukocyte adhesion deficiency Chemotactic defects Chronic granulomatous disease Chédiak-Higashi syndrome (rare)
Problems with complement proteins And MHC	Complement component 1 (C1) inhibitor deficiency (hereditary angioedema), C3 deficiency, C6 deficiency, C7 deficiency, C8 deficiency.

B cell deficiency syndrome: There are several types of B cell defects that lead to "hypogammaglobulinemia". Sever reduction in antibodies is a characteristic feature of hypogammaglobulinemia syndrome. This immune deficiency is an outcome of both inherited and developmental disorders. The common defects associated with B-cell function are (a) X-linked agammagloubulin anemia (b) IgA deficiency (c) IgG sub class deficiency (d) Immuno deficiency with increased IgM (e) Common variable immuno deficiency (f) Transient hypo gammaglobulin anemia of infancy.

a. X-linked agammaglobulinemia (X-LA): X-linked a-gamma globulinemia, is also called as Bruton's agammaglobulinemia or congenital agammaglobulinemia. It is a relatively rare inherited disease and was the first immunodeficiency disease ever identified. Failure of immunoglobulins (antibodies) production is responsible for this disease. Since the gene responsible for this disease is associated with X chromosome this disease is generally noticed in male infants' and is referred as "X-linked". In X-linked agammaglobulinemia, pre-B-lymphocytes fail to mature into B-lymphocytes (mature B-lymphocytes only produce antibodies). As a result antibodies production does not take place, and the child's body is unable to fight off bacterial and some viral infections. Right after they are born, babies are protected from infections by immunity transmitted to them by their mothers. The child receives maternal antibodies through placenta and breast milk. Within the next few months, their immune systems develop and begin to assume responsibility for fighting off infections. But sometimes, babies have immune deficiencies and they don't have the ability to fight off routine infections on their own. When the maternal antibodies are exhausted and supply is ceased, the child begins to suffer from severe recurrent infections. As they have normal T cells and cell mediated immunity, the child shows resistances to various diseases caused by intracellular pathogens, but fail to have humoral immunity. Close analysis shows that the children with X-linked agammaglobulinemia do have normal number of precursor B cells, but they fail to develop into functional cells due to unknown reason. Defective gene in long arm of X chromosome (X-LA) is found responsible for this disease in males.

b. Deficiency of IgA and IgG subclasses: It is the most common congenital immunodeficiency syndrome. When IgA-bearing B lymphocytes fail to mature into

IgA-secreting plasma cells, serum IgA levels are reduced ensuing IgA deficiency. Failure of terminal B-cell differentiation is attributed to (1) an intrinsic B-cell defect (2) inadequate or defective T-helper cells, (3) presence of or excessive IgA-specific T-cell suppressor cells, and (4) passage of maternal anti-IgA antibodies that suppress fetal IgA development. IgA antibody deficiency disease may be asymptomatic, but more commonly it leads to recurrent respiratory and digestive tract infections.

Since IgA antibodies present in mucosal layer gives protection to respiratory and digestive tracts, in the absence of IgA intact pathogens are able to penetrate mucosal surfaces and cause infections. Individuals with IgA deficiency tend to develop type II hypersensitivity (immune complex disease) problems. Unlike more generalized 'hypo-gamma-globulinemias'.IgA deficiency could not be treated with gama globulin therapy. Since the person with IgA deficiency is capable of producing normal amounts of other antibodies, their immune system may recognize injected IgA as foreign body and produce antibodies against the injected antibodies resulting in the formation of immune complex triggering 'immune complex syndrome'.

IgA antibody deficiency is associated with deficiencies of certain IgG subclasses. Because in intrinsic B-cell defect, the alpha one gene may be deleted along with other heavy-chain genes, homozygous deletions of large portions of the Ig heavy-chain locus may result in complete absence of 3 or more Ig classes (IgG2, IgG4, IgA1, and occasionally IgE). IgG2 subclass deficiency is most commonly associated with IgA deficiency.

c. Hyper IgM Syndrome (XHIGM): Patients with the X-linked Hyper IgM Syndrome show deficiency of a protein CD40 ligand found on the surface of T-lymphocytes. This primary immunodeficiency disease is inherited as an X linked recessive trait, and usually establish in boys only. As a consequence of the deficiency of this protein, T-lymphocytes are unable to instruct B lymphocytes to switch their gamaglobulins production from IgM to IgG and IgA. As a result, patients have decreased levels of IgG and IgA and normal or elevated levels of IgM. Since CD40 ligand is important to other functions of T-lymphocytes, they also have a defect in some of the protective functions of their T-lymphocytes. Most patients with the X-linked Hyper IgM (X-HIgM) syndrome develop clinical symptoms during their first year or second year of life. Increased susceptibility to infection is the most common problem in Hyper IgM syndrome.

This unusually produced IgM antibodies behave abnormally by binding to their self antigens present on neutrophils, platelets and other elements of the blood and tissue. In addition to immune deficiency problems contact of IgM antibodies to their self antigens results in auto immune diseases.

d. Common variable immune deficiency (CVID): It is characterized by low levels of antibodies in the blood stream and an increased susceptibility to infections. Both male and female are equally affected with this problem in the third or fourth decade of life. Patients with CVID develop recurrent infections of the sinuses, ears, nose lungs and gastrointestinal tract. They may also develop enlarged lymph nodes or an enlarged spleen. Individuals with CVID have an increased incidence of malignant lymphomas and autoimmune disorders such as lupus, rheumatoid arthritis, inflammatory bowel disease and autoimmune hemolytic anemia. The cause of this problem is not known but certain infections with viruses are suspected to be the culprits in causing this disease. Genetic factors do play a part in the development of common variable immunodeficiency. However, there is no single gene mutation that can be identified.

e. Transient hypogammagloubin of infancy: Transient hypogamma-globulinemia of infancy is a form of hypo-gamma-globulinemia that appears after birth and results in reduction in the IgG level and sometimes IgA and IgM also. Normally by three months of age babies' start synthesizing their own antibodies, as their maternal antibodies wane, but in transient hypogammagloubulinaemia the onset of normal immunoglobulin synthesis is delayed for as long as 36 months until then such infants are susceptible to pyogenic infections.

T cell deficiency: Since thymus is the organ for the development of T cells, failure of thymus development or its abnormal development results in the T cell production. The precursor T lymphocytes fail to populate in the thymus for further differentiation and multiplication to become immune competent T cells and the thymus does not become a lymphoid organ. Patients with no T cells or poor T cell function are susceptible to opportunistic infections. Since B cell function is dependent on T cells to certain extent, deficiency in T cells is associated with humoral immunity also. The following types of immune deficiencies are associated with T cells.

a. Chronic Mucocutaneous Candidiasis (CMC): Chronic mucocutaneous candidiasis is an immune deficiency disorder primarily due to T cell dysfunction characterized by persistent candidal infection of mucous membrane, skin, scalp and nails. Chronic mucous membrane candidiasis has an onset in infancy or childhood; the primary affected site is the oral cavity; however, lesions may occur on trunk, hands, feet and scalp. Although the initial lesions are identical to the ones seen in the general population, over time patients with CMC characteristically develop unique disfiguring lesions. The chronic infection and the large disfiguring nature of keratotic lesions are key characteristics of CMC.

b. Di george syndrome: It is a congenital defect in the organs (thymus, parathyroid) derived from the third and fourth pharyngeal pouches. DiGeorge syndrome is characterized by few specific cardiac malformations, a sub-set of facial attributes, and certain endocrine and immune anomalies. Some of the facial characteristics of DiGeorge syndrome are bifid uvula, high-arched palate, small mouth and wide set eyes, down-slanting eyes, hooded eyes, long face, cupped low set ears, bulbous nasal tip, and a dimpled or bifurcated nasal tip. Immune deficiency of varying severity, hypo calcemia (which may lead to seizures) and hypo parathyroidism are some of the most prominent features of DiGeorge syndrome.

The cause of Di George syndrome has been identified as a submicroscopic deletion in chromosome 22. Alcohol consumption during the early stages of fetal development may be one of the many environmental explanations for the micro deletion. The baby born with this disease may die by congestive heart failure within a day of birth. Since the heart is very sensitive to calcium levels, impaired calcium regulation caused by the absence or defective function of parathyroid glands is responsible for congestive heart failure. However patients, who crossed the neonatal period successfully, develop recurrent and chronic infections.

c. X-linked lymphoproliferative syndrome (XLP): It is an inherited disorder of the immune system that affects males. It is characterized by an abnormal immune response to infection by Epstein-Barr virus (EBV). Mutation in the gene that helps in controlling the immune response to an EBV results in an abnormal response. In addition to EBV infection patients are susceptibe to B-cell lymphomas and recurrent infections. X-linked lymphoproliferative syndrome occurs with a frequency of less than 1/million.

d. Ataxia –Telangiectasia: (ATI): An autosomal recessive trait is responsible for this disease. Affected children become wobbly due to ataxia (an uncontrolled muscle movement) at about 18 months of age. By six years of age dilated capillaries - i.e. Telangiectasia condition appears in the skin and eyes, severe sinus and lung infections are also common in children with this disease.

e. Hyperimmunoglobulin E syndrome: Hyperimmunoglobulin E syndrome is a rare inherited disease, associated with abnormalities of the skin, sinuses, lungs, bones, and teeth. It is caused by mutations in a gene on the X chromosome that encodes specific protein of T and Ntural killer cells (NK cells) called SAP. In the absence of SAP, lymphocytes proliferate unchecked in response to Epstein-Barr virus (EBV) infection, and NK cells do not function. Abnormal response of T-cells and natural killer cell to Epstein-Barr virus infection, leads to liver failure, immunodeficiency, lymphoma, fatal lymphoproliferative disease, or bone marrow aplasia. The syndrome is usually asymptomatic until EBV infection develops. About 75% of patients die by age 10, and all die by age 40 unless bone marrow transplantation is done.

SAP is a 15kDa protein associated with SLAM protein. SLAM (Signaling Lymphocyte-Activation Molecule) is a glycosylated type-I transmembrane protein which is present on the surface of B and T cells. SLAM is a high-affinity self-ligand which, when triggered, co-activated B or T lymphocyte responses and is considered to be important in bi-directional T - B cell stimulation.

f. Severe combined immunodeficiency (SCID): Severe Combined Immunodeficiency is a primary immune deficiency. It is actually a group of inherited disorders that cause severe abnormalities of the immune system. SCID is often called "bubble boy disease". SCID became widely known during the 1970's and 80's, when the world came to know about David Vetter, a boy who lived for 12 years in a plastic, germ-free bubble with X-linked SCID. The disorders lead to reduced or malfunctioning T- and B-lymphocytes.

SCID usually results in the onset of one or more serious infections within the first few months of life. These infections are usually serious, and may even be life threatening. They may include pneumonia, meningitis or bloodstream infections. The combined immune deficiency is a serious problem in infants and the infant may die with in the first two years by recurrent infections.

Several CSID case studies reveal that a gene on the X-chromosome is responsible for this disease in 50% of patients. And the remaining 50% are due to several autosomal recessive inheritance patterns or the result of spontaneous mutations in genes such as defective adenosine deaminase, and purine nucleoside phosphorylase (PNP) genes on other chromosomes. Deficiency of these enzymes results in the accumulation of metabolites that in turn inhibits the replication of lymphocytes. Bone marrow transplantation or gene therapy can help in saving the patient.

g. Combined Immune deficiency (CID): It is an inherited defect of immunity, including lack of immunoglobulin synthesis, absence of cell-mediated immunity, thymic hypoplasia and a marked reduction in the number of thymic, splenic and blood lymphocytes. It is inherited as an autosomal recessive trait. Various genetic defects are responsible for combined immune deficiency. Patients with CID disorder lack both B and T-cells, but have functional phagocytes. Defects in interaction of cell and cell signaling ensues immune deficiency. A survey of 108 infants with CID suggests that the impaired cell signalling function of common gama chains of the 1L - 2 receptors was the most prevalent defect. The next most common defect found in the infants was in the gene for the enzyme adenosine deaminase (ADA). Activity of ADA is high in lymphocyets, deficiency in adenosine deaminase results in accumulation of metabolic byproducts that are toxic to the cells. In the some way, deficiency of purine nucleoside phospharylase (PNP) also cause combined immune deficiency. Defects in ZAP-70, an important element in T-cell signal transduction causes depletion of CD8 cells. There are several other genetical defects responsible for combined immune deficiency. Combined immune deficiency syndrome (disease)

h. Wiskott-Aldrich syndrome: It is an immune deficiency disorder associated with irregularity in immunoglobulin M (IgM) production. A defective gene on the X chromosome is responsible for this disease. Hence females tend to be carriers of the syndrome while males with the defective gene develop symptoms. This rare immune deficiency leaves the body vulnerable to infection. It also causes low numbers of blood platelets. There may be serious infections such as pneumonia, meningitis, and blood poisoning (sepsis). Wiskott-Aldrich syndrome occurs in 4 per million live male births and affects people of all ethnic backgrounds. Eczema - a skin disorder develops in more than three-quarters of individuals with Wiskott-Aldrich syndrome. Individuals with the syndrome may be more allergy-prone and may develop asthma. As many as 40% of individuals with Wiskott-Aldrich syndrome may develop an autoimmune disorder, the most common are autoimmune hemolytic anemia, vasculitis, renal disease, arthritis, and Henoch-Schonlein purpura.

DEFECTS IN PHAGOCYTOSIS: Phagocytes (polymorpho nuclear cells, macrophages, monocytes) constitute an important part of the immune system. Since the function of phagocytes is phagocytosis, chemotaxis, extravasation, killing of pathogens etc., defects in any of these functions lead to immunodeficiency. The factors responsible for phagocytic disorders may be extrinsic or intrinsic. Susceptibility to infections owing to phagocytic dysfunction ranges from mild recurrent skin infections to overwhelming fatal systemic infections. Affected patients are more susceptible to bacterial and fungal infections, but have a normal resistance to viral infections. Extrinsic defects include opsonic abnormalities secondary to deficiencies of antibody and complement factors. Intrinsic disorders of phagocytes may be defects in granulocyte killing ability and chemotaxis (cell movement).

a. Neutropenia (Reduction in neutrophil count): When the peripheral blood neutrophil count goes below 1500 /mm/cube or totally nil, the condition is called neutrepenia or a granulocytopenia. This condition is associated with a number of primary disorders including congenital neutropenia (Kostmann's syndrome), cyclic neutropenia, and myelokathexis or failure of release of neutrophils from the bone marrow. Genetic defects in the progenitor cells results in neutropenia condition. Experimental evidence indicates that this genetic defect causes decrease in the production of granulocyte colony stimulating factors that in turn results in reduced or nil neutrophils. In addition to genetic factors certain outside factors such as radiation and drugs also affect the proliferation of granulocytes.

Neutropenia is also common in several primary immune deficiencies, including X-linked hyper-IgM, X-linked agammaglobulinemia, and reticular dysgenesis. Acquired autoimmune and isoimmune neutropenia result from antibodies directed against neutrophils. Increased neutrophil destruction is also common in chronic splenomegaly and in certain autoimmune diseases such as Felty's syndrome, lupus erythematosus etc.

b. Leukocyte adhesion deficiency (LAD) syndrome: Leukocyte adhesion deficiency (LAD) a rare primary immunodeficiency is due to defects in the leucocyte adhesion process. The phagocytes reach the site of inflammation to remove the pathogen. A sequence of events such as marginalization, extravasation and movement to the site of inflammation through chemotaxis take place before the final action of phagocytes. Defect in any one or more of these events affect the whole function of phagocytes. LAD is a failure to express CD18 a surface marker which forms the complement receptor protein for C3b on lymphocytes, macrophages, and neutrophils. Complement receptor protein is essential in adhesion for different lymphocytes. An autosomal genetic defect results in defective production and also functions of this protein molecule. Since the adhesion of phagocytes to the capillary endothelial cells near the site of infection is necessary to develop effective inflammatory response, failure in the adhesion results in impaired function of not only phagocytes but also NK cells and T cells.

c. Chemotatic defects: In some patients functional defect of phagocytes occur through their failure in reaching the area of infection due to defect in chemotaxis.

Defect in the factors of complement system, such as C3a, C5a, C6, C7 is responsible for this failure in chemotaxis. This kind of disorder of neutrophils is also referred as "Lazy leucocyte syndrome".

d. Chronic granulomatous disease (CGD): Intracellular killing and digestion of phagocytosed pathogen is the last but most important step in the function of phagocytes but, in patients with chronic granulomatus diseases intracellular killing does not take place due to a defective gene. In 70% of patients the culprit is X-linked gene but in others an autosomal recessive gene is responsible. Chronic granulomatous disease is characterized by white blood cells (WBCs) that cannot produce activated O2 compounds and defective microbicidal function of phagocytes. Manifestations include recurrent infections; multiple granulomatous lesions of the lungs, liver, lymph nodes, gastro intestinal and urinogenital tracts; abscesses; lymphadenitis; hypergammaglobulinemia; elevated erythrocyte sedimentation rate (ESR); and anemia. More than 50% of cases of chronic granulomatous disease (CGD) are inherited as an X-linked recessive trait and thus occur only in males; in the rest, inheritance is autosomal recessive.

e. Chediak Higashi Syndrome (CHS): Chédiak-Higashi syndrome is a rare childhood autosomal recessive disorder that affects multiple systems of the body. The underlying defect in Chédiak-Higashi syndrome remains elusive, but the disorder can be considered a model for defects in vesicle formation, fusion, or trafficking. The Chédiak-Higashi syndrome locus on human chromosome 1 encodes a lysosomal trafficking regulator, formerly termed LYST (currently termed CHS1), which is defective in patients with CHS. The CHS protein is expressed in the cytoplasm of cells of a variety of tissues. Defects in CHS protein may cause an abnormality of organellar protein trafficking. Hence Patients with Chédiak-Higashi syndrome exhibit alterations in neutrophils. These alterations include neutropenia, which may be profound; decreased deformability, resulting in impaired chemotaxis; and delayed phagolysosomal fusion. This results in impaired bactericidal activity. The disease is often fatal in childhood as a result of infection or an accelerated lymphoma like phase; therefore, few patients live to adulthood. Recurrent bacterial infections, partial albinism, and aggressive but non malignant infiltration of organs by lymphoid cells are common in this disease. Phagocytes of the patient show giant granules formed by ingested pathogens, as they lost ability of killing the engulfed pathogen.

Complement Deficiency : Enzymes of complement system are essential in immunological reactions. Deficiency of the complement enzymes ensue an increased susceptibility to infections. Deficiencies of the classical complement pathway have been strongly linked to the development of autoimmune disorders, especially those in which excessive immune complexes are formed. Patients may develop collagen vascular disorders, mainly systematic lupus erythmatosus (SLE). This may result from the combination of impaired complement-dependent B-cell tolerance and impaired clearance of immune complex and apoptotic cells. Recurrent bacterial infection is common in patients with C2 deficiency. Atherosclerosis also appears to occur at a higher frequency in individuals with

C2 deficiency. Complement deficiency can be acquired or inherited. Acquired deficiency may be acutely caused by infection or it may occur in conjunction with chronic rheumatological or autoimmune disorders. Inherited deficiency is rare in the general population, with an estimated frequency of 0.03%, excluding MBL (manose binding lectin) deficiency. MBL deficiency is thought to be fairly common, with a 3% frequency in general population. Likewise, MASP-2 (manose binding lectin associated serine protease) deficiency may also be very common.

Among C1-C9 components, C2 deficiency is the most common, with an incidence rate of 1 case per 10,000 populations. Most complement deficiencies equally affect males and females; however, properdin deficiency is X-linked recessive

C1 deficiency generally leads to severe immune complex disease with features of SLE and glomerulonephritis. C2 deficiency has been the most commonly reported classical pathway defect. Skin and joint manifestations are common, and renal disease is relatively rare. Patients with C2 deficiency are also reported to have recurrent or invasive infections. C3 deficiency is rare. Because of its importance as a convergence point of the three complement pathways; all patients with C3 deficiency develop recurrent, severe, pyrogenic infections early in life. Some patients may also develop membranoproliferative glomerulonephritis. C3 deficiency leads to an inability to formulate membrane attack complex (MAC), thus markedly compromising chemotactic and bactericidal activities of the complement cascade. Even though complete C4 deficiency is rare, almost all patients with complete C4 deficiency have discoid or SLE, with or without associated glomerulonephritis.

Heriditary Angio Neurotic edema: (HAE): Inherited autosomal dominant trait is responsible for this disease. Deficiency of complement enzyme "C1" inhibitor results in the development of angio neurotic edema - a recurrent circumscribed swelling of various parts of the body. The pathology and symptoms depends on the region where the swelling is generated. For example angeo edema of the upper airway presents a serious condition due to obstruction in respiration. The edema is mediated by two abnormally generated peptides by compliment system. The peptides disturb the contact of endothelial cells of capillary venules and build gaps between them. The gaps in the capillary venules allow leakage of plasma resulting in the development of edema.

MHC Class 2 molecules: An inappropriate function of a defective gene, present on the autosomes results in MHC class II deficiency. Failure in expression of class II MHC molecule on antigen presenting cells blocks antigen presentation to T cells. In the absence of antigen presentation, T cells fail to develop in to TH or (CD4) T cells. Lack of TH cells lead to deficiency in antibodies and the affected person obviously suffer with recurrent infections.

SECONDARY IMMUNE DEFICIENCY: Secondary immune deficiency is acquired, rather than inherited, disorders. It refers to the depression of the immune responses due to the influence of certain non genetic factors. For example most of the drugs used in cancer chemotherapy are cytotoxic for T cells, and the immune suppressive drugs used at the time of transplantation also affect the efficiency of immune system. Certain viral infections such as *German measles, rubella, Epstein-Barr virus, cytomegalovirus, felin leukemia, human immunodeficiency virus* (HIV) etc. cause damage to the immune system, resulting in secondary immune deficiency.

Where do Immunodeficiency Diseases come from?

Primary immunodeficiency diseases are usually inherited. Like anything that is inherited, these diseases are the result of altered or mutated genes that can be passed on from parent to child or can arise as genes are being copied. One or both parents, usually healthy themselves, may carry a gene (or genes) that is somehow defective or mutated, so that it no longer produces the right protein product. If their child inherits a defective gene and does not have a normal gene to compensate, the child may show signs of immunodeficiency. Loss of just one small molecule (if it is an important one) can impair the body's immune system. Sometimes close relatives - brothers, sisters, cousins - also inherit the defective gene. If they do not inherit a normal gene copy they may also have immunodeficiency. In some immunodeficiency diseases, some may have only mild symptoms, while others may have no symptoms at all.

It is also possible to develop, or acquire, an immunodeficiency disorder during one's lifetime. This can be the result of immune system damage due to an infection, as is the case with AIDS - the acquired immune deficiency syndrome. An immunodeficiency can also develop as the unintended side-effect of certain drug or radiation treatments, such as those given to cancer or transplant patients.

In addition to that many environmental toxins such as polychlorinated biphenyls, iodine, lead, cadmium, smoke, cigarettes, and pesticides like DDT etc. have a suppressive effect on the immune system as do deficiencies of copper zinc vitamin E and selenium. Malnutrition also causes secondary immune deficiency. For example protein deficiency due to malnutrition leads to reduced immunoglobulin synthesis.

Lifc style and habits of an individual also interfere in immune functions. Since normal immune functions including both T and B lymphocytes activities decline with age, aging is also one of the factors for secondary immune deficiency. As there is normal decline in immune functions, the incidence of infections, autoimmune and immune complex diseases and cancers increases with age. The progress of this acquired secondary immune deficiency disease can be reversed if the underlying cause is treatable. Since various factors are influencing immune response secondary or acquired immunodeficiency is more common than primary immunodeficiency. The immunodeficiency disorder that tops the list in its severity of damage to the body is AIDS. It is characterized by a variety of unusual infections and otherwise rare cancers.

AIDs: (Refer Chapter 22 for details on AIDS).

Diabetes: Diabetes is a metabolic disorder due to loss of blood glucose homeostasis. Human body has to maintain the blood glucose level at a very narrow range, which is done with insulin and glucagon. In the presence of insulin about two-thirds of the body's cells absorb glucose from the blood for use as fuel, for conversion to other needed molecules, or for storage. Insulin is also the principal control signal for conversion of excess glucose to glycogen for internal storage in liver and muscle cells. Lowered glucose levels result both in the reduced release of insulin from the beta cells and in the reverse conversion of glycogen to glucose when glucose levels fall. If body does not produce or properly uses insulin, blood glucose is not utilized properly leading to loss of homeostasis in blood glucose. When blood sugar level is constantly high it leads to kidney failure, cardiovascular problems and neuropathy.

Patients with diabetes are 4 times more likely to have coronary heart disease and stroke. In addition, Gestational diabetes is more dangerous for pregnant women and their fetus. Hypoglycemia (low glucose levels) when there are frequent episodes of hypoglycemia, an ignorance develops in the body to react to low blood glucose levels. Body stops releasing the hormone epinephrine and other stress hormones when blood glucose drops too low. The loss of the body's ability to release stress hormones after repeated episodes of hypoglycemia is called hypoglycemia-associated autonomic failure, or HAAF.

The increase in incidence of diabetes in developing countries follows the trend of urbanization and lifestyle changes, perhaps most importantly a "Western-style" diet. This has suggested an environmental (i.e., dietary) effect.

Chronic liver disease – cirrhosis: The liver has many functions. Some of the functions are: to produce substances that break down fats, convert glucose to glycogen, produce urea, make certain amino acids, filter harmful substances from the blood (such as alcohol), storage of vitamins and minerals (vitamins A, D, K and B12) and maintain a proper level of glucose in the blood. The destruction of the normal architecture and the loss of liver cells prevent the liver from functioning normally. Excess Alcohol, chronic viral hepatitis, primary biliary cirrhosis, autoimmune chronic active hepatitis, drugs and chemicals, metabolic and inherited disorders etc. cause destruction of liver. Some of the diseases affecting the liver function are hepatitis, liver cancer, and cirrhosis (a chronic inflammation that progresses ultimately to organ failure).

Cirrhosis is a serious condition. Only 30 per cent of patients with this problem survive five years after diagnosis and the outlook is worse if the cause is alcohol and the patient continues to drink. Cirrhosis leads to edema and ascites (accumulation of fluid in abdomen).

Chronic renal disease – especially nephrotic syndrome: The main function of the kidney is to separate urea, mineral salts, toxins, and other waste products from the blood. The kidney also plays a major role in regulating levels of various minerals such as calcium, sodium, and potassium in the blood and conservation of water, salts, and electrolytes. If the kidneys' ability to remove and regulate water and chemicals is seriously damaged by disease, waste products and excess fluid build up occur, causing severe swelling and symptoms of uremia (kidney failure). There are many different types and causes of kidney disease. These can be characterized as hereditary, congenital or acquired. Kidney diseases are numerous; nephritis is the general term to describe kidney diseases. The most common type of nephritis is glomerulonephritis. Lupus nephritis is an inflammation of the kidney caused by systemic lupus erythematosus (SLE), a disease of the immune system. Diabetic Nephropathy is a kidney condition that occurs only in people with diabetes mellitus. It results in progressive damage of the small filtering units of the kidney (glomeruli). About 20-30% of people with diabetes develop diabetic nephropathy. Glomerulonephritis is a type of kidney disease caused by inflammation of the internal kidney structures. As a result, large amount of protein is found in the urine.

There are a number of people who are considered to be at high risk for developing chronic acquired kidney disease. The high risk individuals are those with hypertension, diabetes mellitus, cardiovascular disease and first degree relatives of patients with hypertension, diabetes mellitus or renal disease. Certain medications, toxins, pesticides and "street" drugs (i.e., heroin) can also produce kidney damage

Immune suppression due to radiation, cytotoxic and/or steroid therapy: Chemotherapy (chemo) and radiation are two of only three sanctioned medical procedures (surgery is the third) utilized in the treatment of cancer. Chemo involves antimetabolites that attempt to disrupt cancer cell growth and reproduction and cytotoxic (cell poisoning) drugs to kill cancer cells. Chemo and radiation are also utilized to shrink the cancer tumor size prior to surgery, with an objective to make removal both less invasive to the patient and more effective in removing the cancerous tumor or tumors. Chemotherapy causes the barrier of the intestine to become permeable and leaky, allowing detrimental bacteria and fungi to enter the bloodstream and impaired nutrient digestion. Chemotherapy suppresses the immune response while severely depleting Taurine, a key ingredient of bile needed for fat-soluble vitamin absorption, cell membrane integrity and calcium/ sodium balance. Most forms of chemotherapy cause depletion of Vitamin A and interfere with intestinal absorption of Vitamin K, needed for proper blood density. Dermatitis on the skin is common, while haemoglobin (red blood cell) levels are lowered after chemotherapy.

Radiation therapy damages bone marrow by X-ray or Gamma-ray emission, while causing a severe decline in needed vitamin C concentration in the bone marrow and the body's sodium/potassium balance. Further, radiation therapy shrinks the spleen and thymus gland, while causing a reduction in white blood cell counts known as lycopenia. Regarding the immune response, both helper T-cells and suppressor T-cells are reduced.

Malnutrition, vitamin and mineral deficiency: Malnutrition is the insufficient, excessive or imbalanced consumption of nutrients. Deficiency diseases are diseases in humans that are directly or indirectly caused by a lack of essential nutrients in the diet. Deficiency diseases are commonly associated with chronic malnutrition. A number of different nutrition disorders may arise, depending on which nutrients are under or overabundant in the diet. According a study by the International Agency for Research on Cancer, in the developing world, cancers of the liver, stomach and esophagus are often linked to consumption of carcinogenic preserved foods, such as smoked or salted food, and parasitic infections that attack organs. Malnutrition, in the form of iodine deficiency, is the most common preventable cause of mental impairment worldwide.

Malnutrition increases the risk of infection and infectious diseases; for example, vitamin C deficiency cause dental cavities, low infection resistance (colds), anemia, bleeding gums, breath shortness, capillary wall ruptures (bruise easily), muscle degeneration, nosebleeds, poor digestion, stress, weakened cartilages, blood clots, and slow healing wounds.

Autoimmune disorders, e.g. systemic lupus erythematosus: Refer auto immune diseases.

Environmental exposure to chemicals and 'xenobiotics': Xenobiotics are chemical components both natural and synthetic foreign to the organisms. They produce immunosupression effect on living beings.more specifically these include changes in leucocyte cellularity, lymphocyte sub population, imunosupression with increased susceptibility to infection and tumor development.

Thymoma with hypogammaglobulinaemia – Good's syndrome: Refer to Auto immune diseases.

20

IMMUNOHAEMATOLOGY

Blood transfusion is the best and immediate solution for protecting a patient suffering with chronic health problems due to reduced blood or blood components in circulation. Replacement of total blood or its components such as blood cells, fluids etc. through intravenous administration is the best and most effective therapeutic tool when judiciously applied. Transformation of total blood allows transfer of all components of blood such as blood cells platelets, serum proteins etc.

Until 1901 blood transfusion was not very safe, many patients died due to incompatible blood transfusion. German immunologist *Landsteiner* in 1901 identified the existence of blood group antigens on human red blood cells, and presence of natural antigens in serum during his experiments with different red cells and plasma factors. He discovered that blood clumping was an immunological reaction, which occurs when the receiver of blood transfusion has antibodies against the donor's blood cells. Karl Landsteiner's work made it possible to determine blood groups and thus paved the way for blood transfusions to be carried out safely. For this discovery he was awarded Nobel Prize in Physiology / Medicine in 1930.

The disparity in human blood is due to the presence or absence of certain protein molecules called antigens and antibodies. The antigens are located on the surface of the red blood cells and the antibodies are in the blood plasma. Different types and combinations of these molecules are present in different individuals. Blood group is inherited from parents. The blood group antigens are inherited according to a simple Mendelian system. There are more than 20 genetically determined blood group systems known today, but the ABO and Rh systems are the most important ones used for blood transfusions. Not all blood groups are compatible with each other. Mixing incompatible blood groups leads to clumping or agglutination of RBCs which is hazardous for individuals.

According to the ABO blood group system, there are four different kinds of blood groups: A, B, AB and O involving three allelic genes called A, B and O genes. The genes for O antigen are not expressed where as A and B genes are dominant and expressed in the form of antigens on the surface of RBCs. Since both A and B genes are co dominant in the presence of both the genes RBCs express both A and B antigens on their surface. Thus a person with "AB" blood group is heterozygous with both A and B genes but "O" group person is homogenous genetically with two recessive O genes. A person with "A" or "B" group may be homozygous (AA or BB) or heterozygous (AO or BO).

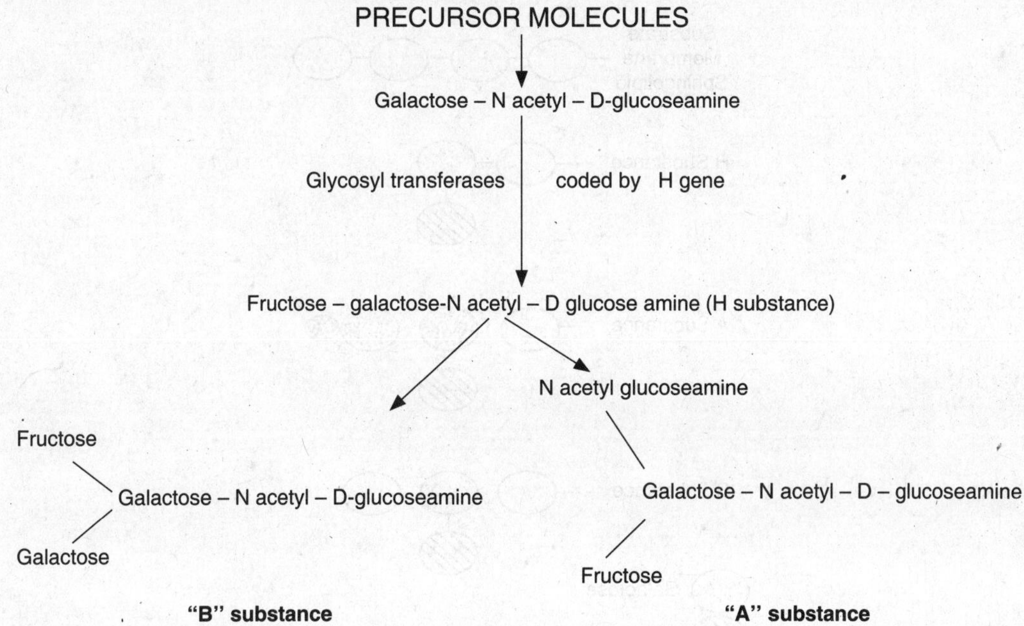

Fig. 20.1

Table : 20.1

Blood Group	Antigens	Antibodies	Can give blood to	Can receive blood from
AB	A and B	None	AB	AB, A, B, O
A	A	B	A and AB	A and O
B	B	A	B and AB	B and O
O	None	A and B	AB, A, B, O	O

In fact O blood group individuals produce a substance called "H antigen", that acts as a precursor for A and B substances. The H locus is located on chromosome 19. It contains 3 exons and it encodes a fucosyltransferase that produces the H antigen on RBCs. In the presence of A or B genes the precursor is converted into A, B or AB substances and in the absence of A or B genes H substance alone is expressed on the RBC's of the blood of the 'O' blood group. In addition to A, B and H substances/ antigens Lea (Lewis a) and Leb (Lewis b) antigens, present on different locus also can be inherited. All the genes code different glycosyl transferases to act on precursor molecules of antigens. If glycosyl transferase adds a fucose molecule to the terminal glucose residue, the precursor becomes H substance and presence of H substance alone on the RBC's makes the blood group as 'O". In blood group A glycosyl transferase links N-acetyl-D-galactosamine to the terminal galactose of H substance. But in blood group B glycosyl transferase enzyme adds one more galactose to the terminal galactose of H substance. In the presence of both A and B genes glycosyl transferase act in both ways on the precursor molecules, and results in the production of both A and B substances.

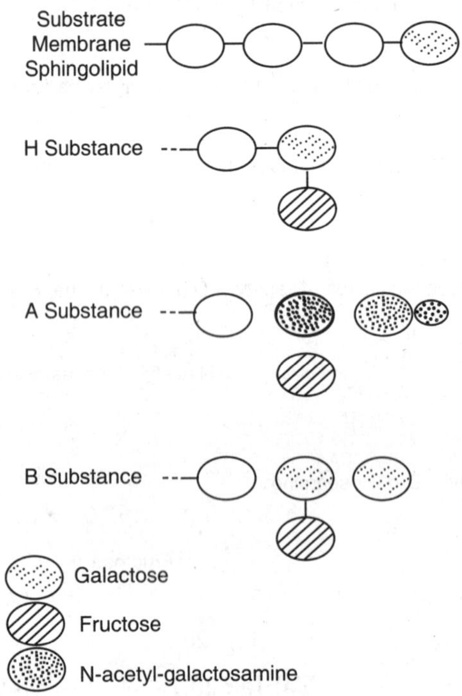

Fig. 20.2

Landsteiner and Wiener in 1937 identified another important agglutinogen "Rh" on RBCs. They are expressed as part of a protein complex in the RBC membrane. This complex is only expressed in cells of the erythroid line, and therefore Rh antigens are only expressed in RBCs. Since antibodies raised against the Rh antigens reacted with RBC's of Rhesus monkey, the newly discovered RBC antigens are refered as "Rhesus antigens" The blood with Rh antigens on RBCs is referred as the Rh+ (Rh positive) blood group and the blood without the Rh antigens on RBCs is considered as Rh- (Rh negative) Unlike A, B antigens Rh antigens do not have any natural antibodies. Hence development of Rh antibodies in Rh- individuals occur only after interaction with Rh+ antigens. Being the main cause of hemolytic disease of the newborn (HDN) it has remained of primary importance in obstetrics. In general majority (about 85%) of people are Rh+. Significance of the Rh blood group is related to the fact that the Rh antigens are highly immunogenic. The complexity of the Rh blood group antigens begins with the highly polymorphic genes that encode them. There are two genes, RHD and RHCE that are closely linked. They are 97% identical, and are located next to each other on chromosome 1. Numerous genetic rearrangements between them has produced hybrid Rh genes that encode a myriad of distinct Rh antigens. The most important antigen produced by one of the dominant genes D is "antigen D". Antigens produced by RHCE are not much important immunologically. Rh- blood group shows the presence of homozygous condition (dd) for receive gene.

The Rh⁻ factor is widely studied in reproduction immunology because; in normal conditions Rh factor does not have any natural antibodies. Hence there may not be any transfusion reactions if Rh⁺ blood is transferred to Rh⁻ individual. After interaction with the Rh⁺ antigens, the Rh⁻ person's immune system starts producing antibodies against Rh⁺ antigens. Majority of antibodies formed against the Rh antigens are of the IgG type. Since the production of antibodies takes time, delayed type transfusion reactions may develop in the recipient. If the same individual receives Rh+ blood again, an immediate transfusion reaction develops due to the presence of antibodies produced following the previous exposure to Rh + antigens.

In women Rh⁻ factor plays a very important role during pregnancy. The second baby of Rh⁻ mother and Rh⁺ father face several complications due to the formation of antibodies against Rh+ antigens of first baby. (Since Rh⁺ genes are dominant in nature, most probably babies of Rh⁻ mother and Rh⁺ father get Rh⁺ blood group) The complications due to the presence of Rh⁺ antibodies may sometimes be severe resulting miscarriage or death of the baby through "erythroblastosis fetalis" (Refer Hypersensitivity) Development of Coombs test in 1945, the advent of transfusion medicine, and understanding of hemolytic disease of the newborn led to the discovery of more blood groups.

Besides A, B, O system other groups such as Kidd, Kell, Duffy, MNS and Lewis groups have been identified. But these groups are of no importance for blood transfusion, but have got medical importance. A total of 30 human blood group systems are now recognized by the International Society of Blood Transfusion (ISBT). A complete blood type would describe a full set of 30 substances on the surface of RBCs, and an individual's blood type is one of the many possible combinations of blood-group antigens. Continuity of work in blood transfusion immunology suggests the presence of about 300 different antigens on the RBCs that are ignored during transfusion due to the absence of natural antibodies and their poor antigenicity.

Delayed transfusion reactions even with compatible blood transfusion occur in patients who have under gone several transfusions. These delayed reactions are due to the presence of minor blood group antigens. The antibodies that are produced after exposure to minor blood group antigens are of IgG type. IgG antibodies are not very good in complement fixation, hence complement mediated RBC lysis is incomplete and the completion of RBC destruction takes place in extravascular sites. Phagocytes and macrophages help in the completion of RBC lysis. The extravascular lysis of RBCs prevents release of haemoglobin into the circulation or plasma. The pre transfusion testing (cross matching) helps to detect potentially harmful antibodies in a patient before transfusion and to select red cell units that will not react with them.

The natural antibodies of A, B blood group antigens are mostly IgM type. Binding of IgM antibodies with the antigens present on the surface of RBCs leads to activation of compliment system and destruction of the target cell. Hence release of haemoglobin into the circulation takes place leading to various health problems such as jaundice, haemoglobinuria, renal failure, fever or even death in severe conditions.

Table : 20.2

BLOOD GROUPS

PHENOTYPE (Groups)	GENOTYPE (Genes)	ANTIGEN	ANTIBODIES
O	0, 0	H	Anti A, anti B
A	AA, AO	A	Anti B
B	BO, BB	B	Anti A
AB	AB	AB	None
Rh^{+ve}	DO, DD	D	None
Rh^{-ve}	Dd	None	None

Development of blood group antigens and antibodies:

Development of blood group antigens begins in the sixth week of fetal life. Their concentration gradually increases and at the time of birth their quantity reaches to one fourth of the adult level. The adult level is reached at about puberty.

Natural anti A and anti B antibodies are IgM type and their development takes place during childhood from exposure to colon bacteria that normally inhabits the lower gastro intestinal tract. Since the antigens of colon bacteria are similar to the blood group antigens, the antibodies developed against the colon bacteria cross react with the antigens of foreign red blood cells. Immune systems tolerance to self antigens prevents development of antibodies against the antigens present on their own RBC. Absence of antibodies in AB blood group and presence of anti A and anti B antibodies in O blood group indicates the tolerent nature of immune system to their self antigens.

Time of Appearance

Anti-A and anti-B production generally begins after the first few months of life. Occasionally infants can be found with already produced antibodies at the time of birth. Antibody production remains fairly constant until late in adult life. In elderly people, anti-A and anti-B levels may be lower than those seen in young adults. Since antibody production normally begins after birth, results that are obtained with the sera of newborns or infants of about 4-6 months of age cannot be considered valid because, the antibodies may have been acquired through the placental transfer from mother.

Table : 20.3

SOME OF THE BLOOD GROUP SYSTEMS STUDIED AND THE TOTAL NO OF RECOGNIZED ANTIGENS

BLOOD GROUP SYSTEM	NO OF ALLELS RECOGNIZED	CORRESPONDING ANTIGENS
Rh	38	Cc, D, E, e
MNS	29	M, N, S
Lutherani	20	Lu^a, Lu^b
Kell	19	K, K, Kpa, Kpb, Jsa, Jsb
ABO	9	A, B
Duffy	5	Xg^a
I	5	I, I
Lewis	4	Le^a, Ie^b
P	3	PiP
Kidd (J^k)	2	Jk^a, Jk^b
Diego (di)	2	Di^a, Di^b
Cartright (y^t)	2	Yt^a, Yt^b
Xg	1	Xg^a

Reactivity of Anti-A and Anti-B

Anti-A and anti-B antibodies are usually IgM and do not pass through the placenta, but some mothers "naturally" have IgG anti-A or IgG anti-B antibodies, which can pass through the placenta. Maternal IgG antibodies with specificity for the ABO blood group system when passed through the placenta to the fetal circulation can cause hemolysis of fetal red blood cells, leading to fetal anemia and ABO hemolytic disease of the newborn. Although very uncommon, cases of ABO hemolytic disease of the newborn (also known as ABO HDN) have been reported in infants born to mothers with blood groups Aand B. Some mothers may be sensitized by fetal-maternal transfusion of ABO incompatible red blood and produce immune IgG antibodies against the antigen they do not have and their baby does. For example, when a mother of genotype OO (blood group O) carries a fetus of genotype AO (blood group A) she may produce IgG anti-A antibodies. The father will either have blood group A, with genotype AA or AO, or more rarely, have blood group AB, with genotype AB.

Table: 20.4

Blood Compatibility

Patient blood Type	Compatible Red Cell Types	Compatible Plasma Types (FFP & Cryoprecipitate)
A	A, O	A, AB
B	B, O	B, AB
O	O	O, A, B, AB

AB	AB, A, B, O	AB
Rh Positive	RhPositive Rh Negative	RhPositive Rh Negative
Rh Negative	Rh Negative	RhPositive Rh Negative

Almost always, blood group of an individual is constant for life time, but very rarely an individual's blood type changes through addition or suppression of an antigen by infection, malignancy, or autoimmune disease.

An example of this rare phenomenon is the case of Demi-Lee Brennan, an Australian citizen, whose blood group changed after a liver transplant. Another more common cause in blood-type change is a bone-marrow transplant. Bone-marrow transplants are performed for many having leukemia and lymphoma, among other diseases. If a person receives bone marrow from someone who is of a different ABO type (eg, if type A patient receives a type O bone marrow), the patient's blood type will eventually convert to the donor's type.

Some blood types are associated with inheritance of certain diseases; for example, the Kell antigen is sometimes associated with McLeod syndrome.

Certain blood types may affect susceptibility to infections, for example resistance to specific malaria species is seen in individuals lacking the Duffy antigen. The Duffy antigen, presumably a result of natural selection, is less common in ethnic groups from areas with a high incidence of malaria.

Importance of blood group immunology

It is important and useful for blood transfusion, Identifying blood diseases, for paternity tests in medico legal cases and also in anthropological studies

Selection of blood for safe transfusion: - It is preferable for patients to receive blood and plasma of the same ABO and Rh group. However if the required blood type is unavailable, a patient may be given a product of an alternative but compatible group as shown below.

Since O Rh Negative (O-) red cells have neither ABO nor Rh antigens on their surface, O Rh Negative red cells can be used in emergency situations. When life saving transfusion is required prior to completion of cross match, O Rh negative red cells can be used.

Group O is often referred to as the universal red cell donor due to the absence of antigens on its surface. Group AB individuals have neither anti-A nor anti-B antibodies in their plasma therefore group AB plasma can be given to patients of any ABO blood group and AB blood group is often referred to as the universal plasma donor.

Transfusion Reactions

Each blood product transfused carries a small risk of acute or delayed adverse effect.

Some of the Immediate Adverse Effects of Transfusion are as follows:

Febrile Reactions: Fever and chills during transfusion are thought to be caused by recipient antibodies reacting with white cell antigens or white cell fragments in the blood product or due to cytokines which accumulate in the blood product during storage. Fever occurs more commonly with platelet transfusion than red cell transfusion. Fever may be the initial symptom in a more serious transfusion reaction such as bacterial contamination or haemolytic reaction and should be taken seriously.

Prevention: A proportion of patients who have febrile reactions will have similar reactions to subsequent transfusions. Many are prevented by leucocyte filtration (either bedside or pre-storage).

Urticarial (Allergic) Reactions: These are seen in approximately 1% of recipients and caused by foreign plasma proteins. On rare occasions they may be associated with laryngeal oedema and bronchospasm.

Management: If urticaria occurs in isolation (without fever and other signs), the solution for the problem is slowing the rate of transfusion or stopping transfusion temporarily. If symptoms are bothersome, administering an antihistamine before restarting the transfusion is advisable. If associated with other symptoms, transfusion should be stoped till further investigations are carried to confirm the safety.

Anaphylactic (Severe Allergic) Reactions: In some cases patients with IgA deficiency, who have anti-IgA antibodies can have these reactions. Anaphylactic reactions have signs of cardiovascular instability including hypotension, tachycardia, loss of consciousness, cardiac arrhythmia, shock and cardiac arrest. Sometimes respiratory involvement with dyspnoea and stridor are prominent.

Management: Patients with anti-IgA antibodies deficiency require special blood products such as washed red blood cells and plasma products prepared from IgA deficient donors. Stopping the transfusion immediately, supportive care including airway management may be required for managing the conditions. Adrenaline usually given as 1:1000 solution, 0.01mg/kg s.c./i.m. may be useful. For further transfusion haematologist supervision is advised.

Acute Haemolytic Reactions: Majority of haemolytic reactions are caused by transfusion of A,B,O incompatible blood, Most haemolytic reactions are the result of human error such as the transfusion of properly labeled blood to the wrong patient, or improper identification of pre transfused blood samples. Chills, fever, pain (along IV line, back, chest), hypotension, dark urine, uncontrolled bleeding due to disseminated vascular coagulation (DIC) are the symptoms of haemolytic reactions.

Management: Immediate discontinuity of transfusion is the only solution for this problem.

Bacterial Contamination: Very high fever, rigors, profound hypotension, nausea and/or diarrhea may develop if the blood used for transfusion is contaminated with bacteria.

Management: Immediate discontinuity of transfusion is the only solution for this problem.

Transfusion-Related Acute Lung Injury: Transfusion related acute Lung Injury (TRALI) is a clinical diagnosis of exclusion, characterized by acute respiratory distress and bilaterally symmetrical pulmonary oedema with hypoxaemia that develops within 2 to 8 hours after a transfusion. Pulmonary vascular effects occur due to the cytokines present in the transfused product or from interaction between patient white cell antigens and donor antibodies (or vice versa).

Volume Overload: Patients with cardiopulmonary disease and infants are at the risk of volume overload especially during rapid transfusion.

Hypothermia: Rapid infusion of large volumes of stored blood contributes to hypothermia. Infants are particularly at risk during exchange or massive transfusion.

Citrate toxicity: Citrate is the anticoagulant used in blood products. Usually citrate is metabolised rapidly by the liver. Rapid administration of large quantities of stored blood may cause hypocalcaemia and hypomagnesaemia when citrate binds to calcium and magnesium. This can result in myocardial depression or coagulopathy. Patients most at risk are those with liver dysfunction or neonates with immature liver function having rapid large volume transfusion.

Potassium Effects: Stored red cells leak potassium proportionately throughout their storage life. Irradiation of red cells increases the rate of potassium leakage. Clinically significant hyperkalaemia can occur during rapid, large volume transfusion of older red cell units in small infants and children.

DELAYED AND LONG TERM ADVERSE EFFECTS OF TRANSFUSION

Delayed Haemolysis: Patients may develop antibodies to red cell antigens. Antibodies can occur naturally, or may arise as a consequence of previous transfusion or pregnancy. A delayed haemolytic reaction occurs when a patient develops an antibody directed against an antigen on transfused red cells. The antibody may cause shortened red cell survival, with clinical features of fever, jaundice and lower than expected haemoglobin following transfusion. Most delayed haemolytic reactions produce few symptoms and may go unrecognized; however there are reports of serious consequences in critically ill patients.

Alloimmunisation: If patients with sickle cell disease or major haemoglobinopathy syndromes are chronically transfused, they face greatest risk of alloantibody formation. Alloantibody formation is asymptomatic. Alloimmunisation to the D and K (Kell) antigens is prevented by the provision of Rh(D) negative and Kell negative blood for Rh(D) negative, Kell negative patients. This is important for females with child-bearing potential as these antibodies can cause severe haemolytic disease of the newborn during pregnancy.

Platelets refractory: When thrombocytopenic patients do not achieve the expected post-transfusion platelet count increment, they are said to be refractory. This usually occurs in patients receiving frequent platelet transfusions due to development of antibodies to leucocyte antigens (HLA) or human platelet antigens (HPA). This condition can be managed by the provision of HLA or HPA matched platelets.

Additional information about blood groups and transfusion :

(1) Glycoprotein molecule that contains sialic acid is known to be attached to the lipid and project from the surface as rod like structures. Thus red cell antigens may be glycolipids or glycoproteins.

(2) It has been suggested that the weak A and B antigen reactions in neonatal red cells are due to lack of the substrate on the red cells.

(3) The antigens of Rh, K, FY, JK, MNs, Di, Do and Se system as well as coa and Lua appear to be fully developed at birth.

(4) Several red cell antigens like A, A1, B, H, Rh, MNs, P, Lu, K, Le, Fy, Jk and I system have been demonstrated on erythroblasts.

(5) Occasionally the expected iso agglutinins cannot be demonstrated in serum samples, especially if the serum is collected from an elderly patient.

(6) In conditions such as hypo or agamma globulinemia and leukemia the iso agglutinins may be absent.

(7) Although large number of subgroups is identified they may occasionally generate transfusion problems. Since the antigens are so weak they were not recognized and the red cells are mistyped as 'O group'. If this happens in the case of donor's blood group identification, it may lead to delayed transfusion reactions when large quantities of RBC's were transfused.

(8) In an obstetrical patient anti A is unimportant as it does not cause hemolytic disease of the newborn.

(9) Unusual Inheritance of the ABO genes: In extremely rare conditions, parent with A group can have a child with 'AB group' or an AB parent can have 'O group' child. The families in which this has occurred have been thoroughly studied to rule out non paternity or non maternity. In these cases it is believed that the AB individual inherits both A and B genes on a single chromosomes from one parent and "O gene" from the other parent. In one family A and B were shown to have been transmitted together through four generations.

Exception to the rules of inheritance provides geneticists with material for speculation about the complexity of genes.

(10) There are two kinds of H antigens. The more common anti H is a cold agglutinin (that reacts below room temperature). This antibody reacts more strongly with cells of group O, A2 and A1 B cells. Because H antigen of A1 and A/B seems to be well hidden, hence anti H is occasionally found in the serum of A1 and A1B people. High tittered anti H may react at room temperature.

(11) H-gene constitutes to the expression of the A and B genes. H antigen found in greatest concentration in O group persons. The gene H is very common and most of the people are homozygous for H gene.

12) Inheritance of H is independent of ABO, but ABH antigens are all formed from the basic material. The basic material of H has a protein or lipid back bone to which sugars are attached. Addition of one more sugars to the chain creates a new antigen. The type of sugar and the position in which it is attached determine specificity of the antigen. The H, A and B genes each control the attachment of a different sugar. H gene acts first and attaches a sugar (fructose) to the basic material. The resultant molecule is recognizable as antigen H and is capable of reacting with anti H antibody.

13) Although the antigen I, i and the corresponding antibodies are not part of the ABO system, they seem to be related to it. The nature of the relationship is still obscure. Anti I react with the red cells of almost all the adults. Since they are cold agglutinins they rarely react above 300 C but react at room temperature 22-250C. They bind compliment to donor cells in room temperature.

14) Not all cases of erythroblastosis fetalis /haemolytic disease of the fetus and new born could be explained by the presence of anti Rh in the maternal serum. Even in the absence of anti Rh antibodies some babies are born with haemolytic disease. This is due to the presence of antibodies. The antibodies are referred as "incomplete antibodies" by Race, "blocking antibodies" by Weiner. Another antibody that gives reaction similar to Rh but not identical to anti D is found when the search for better methods to identify anti Rh antigen is attempted.

15) The Rh antigens have definite molecular configurations that are repeated in many places on the red cell surface. There may be as many as 30 000D sites on each red cell.

16) D antigen is clinically the most important antigen of the Rh system because it is the most immunogenic antigen.

17) It is not possible to prevent foetal cells from reaching the mother but the formation of anti D can be suppressed by proper treatment immediately post partum.

18) A blood type is classified as rare when more than 200 donors have to be screened to find one compatible donor with blood of that type. Existence of other blood groups does not have much importance in blood transfusion but they may cause difficulties during cross matching for blood transfusion. MN system, Duffy system, Kell system, Lewis system, p system, Luthern system, Kidd system, Diego etc are some of the other blood groups noticed in humans.

19) Anti A, anti B, are capable of fixing complement but the antibodies other than ABO system cause extra vascular haemolysis and usually produce milder signs and symptoms such as fever, anemia and jaundice.

20) Primary immune response to Rhesus antigen is weak. Low titer of antibodies may be found after 6-8 weeks of delivery. In many cases primary sensitization may not lead to detectable antibody response but during second and

subsequent pregnancies with Rh+ foetus detectable levels of antibodies appear due to second immune response. The antibody most frequently responsible for the disease is anti D that is of IgG type immunoglobulin. It crosses placenta, coats D positive cells of foetus which are then destroyed by spleen.

20) Sensitization to the D antigen can be prevented by administration of Rh immunoglobulin to mother at 28 weeks gestation and again within 72 hours of delivery of Rh+ baby as well as after spontaneous or induced abortion and after amniocentesis. WHO has recommended following doses of ant Rh antibody.

(1) Abortion less than 12 weeks - 050µg.

(2) Termination of pregnancy 12 weeks – 200-300 µg.

(3) Mismatched Rh blood transfusion- 25 µg/ml of red cells.

21

IMMUNOPARASITOLOGY

Immunoparasitology is "the study of the immunology of host-parasite relationships". Parasites are pathogens that simultaneously injure and derive sustenance from its host. They are skilled evaders of host immunity. Parasites are the organisms that complete part or all of their life cycle within a host organism. Infections of humans caused by parasites number in billions and range from relatively innocuous to fatal. The diseases caused by these parasites constitute major human health problems throughout the world. The incidence of many parasitic diseases (eg. schistosomiasis, malaria) have increased rather than decreased in recent years. Other parasitic illnesses have increased in importance as a result of the AIDS epidemic (eg., cryptosporidiosis, Pneumocystis carinii pneumonia, and strongyloidiasis).

Like other pathogens, parasites must survive in the face of a highly potent immune system. Over millions of years of evolution, they succeed in this through a great diversity of strategies for avoiding immune detection, suppressing cellular immunity and deflecting immune attack mechanisms. Similarly hosts have evolved resistance in various ways to overcome their entry and existence. Host-parasite interactions provide fascinating examples of evolutionary 'arms-races' in which the immune system plays a key role.

The different mechanisms of resistance established by host can be divided into two main types

(1) Nonspecific mechanism (innate immunity) carried by different factors.

(2) Specific mechanism (Acquired immunity) carried by the immune system.

NONSPECIFIC MECHANISM

The first line of defense against parasites, as with other pathogens, is the innate immune system, which is 'hardwired' and primed even in the absence of infection. In addition to various factors providing innate immunity, the best studied nonspecific mechanism involves in parasite resistance is expressed by the red blood cells to invasion or growth of plasmodia (malaria parasite). Individuals heterozygous or homozygous for the sickle cell haemoglobin trait are considerably more resistant to *Plasmodium falciparum* than the individuals with normal haemoglobin. Similarly individuals' lacking Duffy factor in their red blood cells are not susceptible to *P. vivax*. Possibly both deficiency of the Duffy factor and the sickle cell haemoglobin trait have become established in malaria-endemic populations as a result of selective pressure exerted by malaria. Epidemiologic evidence suggests that other inherited red blood cell abnormalities, such as thalassanemia and glucose-6-phosphate dehydrogenase deficiency, may contribute to survival of individuals in various malaria-endemic geographical regions. A second well-documented example for nonspecific resistance mechanism is the resistance expressed by the *trypanolytic factor* of human serum against *Trypanosoma brucei* brucei, an agent of trypanosomiasis (sleeping sickness). There is evidence that several other factors, such as nutrition, age, sex of the host etc. may also contribute to the host's resistance to various parasites. Although nonspecific factors can play a key role in resistance, usually they work in conjunction with the host's Specific mechanism.

SPECIFIC MECHANISM

The interaction of immune system with infectious organisms is a dynamic interplay of host mechanisms aimed at eliminating parasites and infections. The development of immunity is a complex process arising from the interactions of many different kinds of cells over a period of time. The resistance of individual hosts to infectious parasites varies. Effects of specific mechanism are often local and many cell types secreting several different mediators may be present at sites of immune rejection. Moreover, the processes involved in controlling the multiplication of parasites in an infected individual may differ from those responsible for the ultimate development of resistance to further infection. Modern research in immunoparasitology is directed towards understanding and exploiting the capacity to develop effective anti-parasite immunity.

IMMUNE RESPONSE TO PROTOZOANS:

Protozoa are one-celled animals found worldwide in most habitats. Most species are free living, but all higher animals are infected with one or more species of protozoa. Infections range from asymptomatic to life threatening, depending on the species and strain of the parasite and the resistance of the host.

When protozoa enter the blood stream or tissues they can often survive and replicate because they adapt to the resisting natural host defenses. Protozoa cause chronic and persistent infections, because natural immunity against them is weak and because protozoa have evolved multiple mechanisms for evading and resisting specific immunity. Since they evolved multiple mechanisms for evading and resisting specific immunity and natural immunity, they cause chronic and persistent infections. They stimulate distinct patterns of immune responses due to diversity in their structural and biochemical properties.

NATURAL AND SPECIFIC IMMUNE RESPONSE TO PROTOZOA:

Resistance to the protozoan parasites involves nonspecific factors as well as specific factors such as humoral and cellular mechanisms. Cellular immunity is believed to be the most important defense mechanism in diseases such as leishmaniasis and toxoplasmosis. Macrophages play an important role in animals infected with *Toxoplasma*. Cytokines are involved in the control of both the immune response and pathology. The cytokines produced by T cells and other immune cell types do not act directly on the parasites but influence other cell types of host, to control both immune response and pathology. The response of immune cells to cytokines includes a variety of physiological changes, such as changes in glucose, fatty acid and protein metabolism that usually influence all phases of immune response. Unlike most viral and bacterial infections, protozoan diseases are often chronic, lasting months or years. Protozoan disease when associated with a strong host immune response, the chronic infection is apt to result in a high incidence of immunopathology. The extra cellular stay of protozoans can elicit humoral responses. Antigen-antibody complexes in the region of antibody excess activate hageman blood coagulation factor (Factor XII), which in turn activates the coagulation, fibrinolytic, kinin and complement systems. This type of immediate hypersensitivity is responsible for various clinical syndromes including hyperviscosity of blood, edema, and hypotension etc. in *African trypanosomiasis.* Similar disease mechanisms involving a strong humoral immune response would be expected in other infections by protozoans.

In general antibodies serve to control the level of parasites existing in the blood stream and tissue fluids, whereas cell mediated immune responses are directed largely against intracellular parasites. Serum antibodies directed against protozoan surface antigens may opsonize, agglutinate or immobilize them to kill with the help of complement and cytotoxic cells. The immune complexes circulating in serum get deposited in the kidneys and other tissues of humans and animals infected with protozoans. If inflammatory cell infiltrates accompanied these deposits, it causes glomerulonephritis.

Kinin System

The plasma kinin system is an enzymatic system that is triggered by activated factor XII.

The activation of prekallikrein into kallikrein by the activated factor XII occurs on the surface of biomaterials and in the fluid phase (Figure 4).

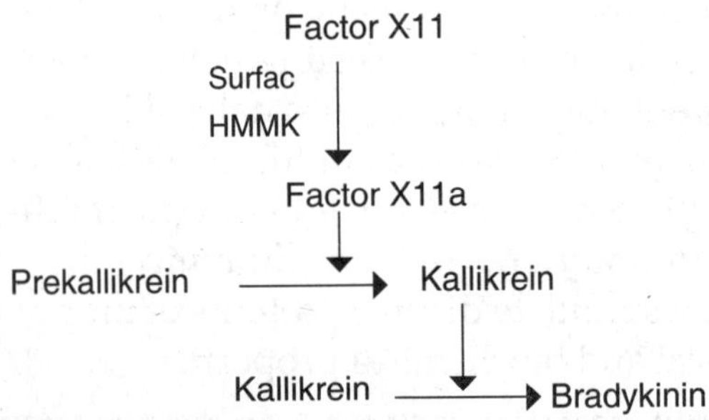

Simplified schematic represents kinin system

Fibrinolytic mechanism: It is an ordered sequence of interactions between an enzyme and a cofactor on a specific substrate; the components of the process include plasminogen, tissue plasminogen activator, urokinase and kallikrein.

Some of the antibodies may act to inhibit protozoan enzymes in such a away that the pathogens replication is prevented. For example T. brucei gambiense lives within the bloodstream (bloodstream form) to reenter its vector through blood. Its presence in the blood induce humoral immune response and the protozoan's may be phagocytyzed by macrophages. But many protozoans are resistant to phagocytic process and may even replicate within macrophages. In infections by Leishmania species, cellular defense mechanisms depends upon CD_4^+ T-lymphocytes and activated macrophages as effector cells that are regulated by cytokines of Th1 subset. But many protozoans are resistant to humoral and cell mediated immune responses due to the defense mechanisms adopted by them.

IMMUNE EVASION MECHANISMS OF PROTOZOA:

In spite of immune surveillance certain protozoans often enter the blood stream, become resistant to immune effector mechanisms. Some of the remarkably effective ways developed by protozoans to resist specific immunity are as follows:

1. *Antigenic Masking*: Antigenic masking is the ability of a parasite to escape immune detection by covering itself with host antigens. Some protozoans become non immunogenic/ non antigenic by masking themselves with host antigens eg. Trypanosoma theileri in cattle, *Trypanosoma lewisi* in rat.

2. *Blocking of Serum Factors*: Some parasites acquire a coating of antigen-antibody complexes or noncytotoxic antibodies that sterically blocks the binding of specific antibody or lymphocytes to the parasite surface antigens.

3. *Intracellular Location*: The anatomic sequestration (intracellular habitat) of some protozoan parasites protects them from the direct effects of the host's immune response. Their intra cellular habitat conceals the parasite antigens and delays detection by the immune system. This is commonly observed with *Plasmodium and T. gondi*

4. *Antigenic Variation*: Some protozoan parasites change their surface antigens during the course of an infection. Parasites carrying the new antigens escape the immune response to the original antigens.

5. *Antigen shedding*: Some protozoans shed their antigen coats either spontaneously or after binding with specific antibodies eg. *E. histolytica.*

6. *Hypo immunogenic:* Some protozoa become hypo immunogenic at certain stages of their life for example cyst stage of *T.gondi* will not stimulate host response.

7. *Immunosuppression:* Parasitic protozoan infections generally produce some degree of host immunosuppression. This reduced immune response may delay detection of antigenic variants. It may also reduce the ability of the immune system to inhibit the growth of and/or to kill the parasites. Sometimes immune suppression is caused directly by parasite products and sometimes involves antigenic mimicry, which often appears in association with parasitic diseases (abnormalities in cytokine production, deficient T cell activation) eg. *Trypanosoma, Leishmania, Toxoplasma, Entamoeba.*

Table: 21.1

SOME PROPOSED IMMUNE ESCAPE MECHANISMS USED BY PROTOZOANS

SNo	Mechanisms	Posible Examples
1.	Antigen Variation	African Trypanosomes, *Plasmodium, Giardia*
2.	Masked or Shared host antigens	African Trypanosomes
3.	Blocking	No documented example
4.	Intracellular	American Trypanosomes, *Plasmodium, Leishmania, Toxoplasma*
5.	Immunosuppression	African Trypanosomes, *American* Trypanosomes

BACTERIA

Bacteria enters the host either through natural openings/routes such as respiratory tract, gastrointestinal tract , urinary tract etc. or through damaged natural barriers such as skin and mucosa layer. The immune response to bacteria depends on the size, number, virulence etc. of the pathogen entered in to the body. The common response to extra cellular bacteria is antibody mediated (humoral response), but delayed type hypersensitivity is employed in case of intracellular bacteria. Pathogenic mechanisms of bacteria may be direct through cell rupture or by causing inflammation, or by means of exotoxins (soluble molecules released by bacteria to trigger pathological change in host) or by endotoxins such as lipopolysaccharides that can trigger inflammation. Immune responses to pathogens can be carried by inflammation for lysis of infected cells; killing of uninfected cells also takes place resulting in tissue damage and resulting disease. Rheumatic fever is the best example for this kind of disease. Innate immunity prevails initially, with the activation of macrophages and inflammatory cells.

Extracellular bacteria are first (0-4hrs) handled by the innate immune response. Macrophages and other cells secrete cytokines and chemokines that attract inflammatory cells to the site of infection. Alternate complement pathway is also activated to eradicate the pathogens. This causes an immediate inflammatory response that keeps the bacteria in check before other processes take over. In the later period the adaptive immune response takes over, and involves specific antibody production.

Antibodies prevent infection by blocking the ability of attachment of microbes to the host cells for invasion. In addition to that antibodies neutralize infectivity and pathogenicity of released toxins by binding to them and interfering with their functions. Antibodies opsonize microbes to promote their phagocytosis and activate the classical complement pathway.

Certain bacteria such as *Clostridia or B. anthracis* releases toxic products in to the host body and the toxic products are responsible for pathogenesis. Neutralization of toxic products such as Clostridium botulinum type B, anthrax toxin etc. is essential to save the body and regulate normal metabolic activities. Hence the immune system neutralizes the toxic products in addition to killing/ removing parasites with the help of antibodies. Neutralization occurs as a result of blocking of the union of the toxin and its receptor on the host cell. IgG antibodies are totally responsible for toxin neutralization.

Cell mediated immune response takes control of intracellular bacteria. The bacteria can be located within vesicles in cells, or within the cytoplasm itself. Intracellular bacteria residing in vesicles within phagocytes are removed by activated phagocytes. This activation is provided by CD_4^+ cells, cytokines etc. CD_8^+ T cells on the other hand differentiate into cytotoxic cells and directly kill the infected cell (bacteria within cytoplasm of cell) thus eliminating the infection.

IMMUNOLOGICAL TOLERANCE TO A BACTERIAL ANTIGEN

Tolerance is a property of the host in which there is an immunologically-specific reduction in the immune response to a given antigen. Tolerance to an Antigen can arise in a number of ways, but three are possibly relevant to bacterial infections.

1. Fetal exposure to Antigens: In the early stages of the development of an immunesystem, cells expressing molecules that bind tightly to self-molecules are destroyed or silenced, whereas cells expressing molecules that do not bind strongly to self-molecules and have potential for binding strongly to foreign molecules are preserved. Hence if a fetus is infected at very early stages of immunological development, the microbial antigen may be seen as "self", thus inducing tolerance (failure to undergo an immunological response) to the antigen which may persist even after birth.

2. High persistent doses of circulating Antigens. When immunological system becomes overwhelmed, tolerance to bacterium or one of its products might arise due to large amounts of circulating bacterial antigens in the blood.

3. Molecular mimicry. If bacterial antigens are very similar to normal host "antigens", immune system consider them as their own and does not respond to them. This kind of rtesemblance between bacterial antigens and host antigens is referred to as molecular mimicry. In this case the antigenic determinants of the bacterium are so closely related chemically to host tissue components that the immunological cells cannot distinguish between the two to raise immune response. For eg. bacterial capsules polysaccharides hyaluronic acid, sialic acids are very similar to host tissue polysaccharides.

4. Antigenic Disguises: Some pathogens can hide their unique antigens from opsonizing antibodies or complement. Bacteria may be able to coat themselves with host proteins such as fibrin, fibronectin, or even immunolobulin molecules. In this way they are able to hide their own antigenic surface components from the immunological system. For eg. *S. aureus* produces cell-bound coagulase and clumping factor that cause fibrin to clot and to deposit on the cell surface. This disguises the bacteria immunologically so that they are not readily identified as antigens and targeted for an immunological response. Protein A produced by *S. aureus*, and the analogous protein G produced by *Streptococcus pyogenes*, bind to the Fc portion of immunoglobulins, thus coating the bacteria with antibodies and canceling their opsonizing capacity by the disorientation. *E. coli K1*, that causes meningitis in newborns, has a capsule composed predominantly of sialic acid providing an antigenic disguise, as does the hyaluronic acid capsule of *Streptococcus pyogenes*.

5. Immune suppression: Some pathogens cause immune suppression in their infected host. Under the influence of pathogens the host shows depressed immune responses to antigens in general, including those of the infecting pathogen. Suppressed immune responses are occasionally observed during chronic bacterial infections such as leprosy and tuberculosis. In extreme forms of leprosy, caused by *Mycobacterium leprae*, there is a poor response to pathogen antigens, as well as unrelated antigens. After patients have been successfully treated, immunological reactivity reappears suggesting that, general immunosuppression is in fact due to the disease. In mild cases of leprosy there is an associated immunological suppression that is specific for *M. leprae* antigens. This is different from tolerance, since unique antigens (proteins) of *M. leprae* have been associated as the cause of this immunosuppression. This could be explained by (1) lack of costimulatory signals (interference with cytokine secretion); (2) activation of suppressor T cells; (3) disturbances in TH1/TH2 cell activities.

6. Not exposing themselves to immune forces. Intracellular pathogens can evade host immunological responses as long as they stay inside the infected cells and they do not allow microbial antigen to form on the cell surface. This is seen in macrophages infected with *Brucella, Listeria* or *M. leprae.* The macrophages support the growth of the bacteria and at the same time gives them protection from immune responses. Some intracellular pathogens (*Yersinia, Shigella, Listeria, E. coli*) may take up shelter in cells that are neither phagocytes nor APC's and their antigens are not displayed on the infected cell's surface. They are virtually unseen by cells of the immune system.

7. Not inducing an inflammatory response: Some pathogens persist on the luminal surfaces of the gastro intestinal tract, oral cavity and the urinary tract, or the lumen of the salivary gland, mammary gland or the kidney tubule. In the absence of host cells destruction, the pathogen may avoid inducing an inflammatory response, and there is no way in which sensitized lymphocytes or circulating antibodies can reach the site to eliminate the infection. Secretary IgA could react with surface antigens on bacterial cells, but the complement sequence fails to get activated and the cells would not be destroyed. Conceivably, IgA antibodies could immobilize bacteria by agglutination of cells or block adherence of bacteria to tissue or cell surfaces, but it is unlikely that IgA would kill bacteria directly or inhibit their growth.

8. Inaccessible to the forces of immune system: In the carrier state, *S. typhi* is able to colonize the biliary tract (gall bladder) away from the immune forces, and be shed into urine and feces. Bacteria causing infections of the hair follicles, such as acne, seldom encounter the immunological tissues. Streptococcus mutans can initiate dental caries at any time after the eruption of the teeth, regardless of the immune status of the host. The carrier state of typhoid fever results from a persistent infection by the typhoid bacillus, Salmonella typhi. The organism is not eliminated during the initial infection and persists in the host for months, years or a life time.

9. Induction of Ineffective Antibody: Many types of antibodies are formed against a given antigen. If antibodies formed against a bacterial antigen are of low avidity, or if they are directed against unimportant antigenic determinants, they may have only weak anti bacterial action or even aid a pathogen in blocking the attachment of any functional antibodies that might be present. In the case of Neisseria gonorrhoeae the presence of antibody to an outer membrane protein called rmp interferes with the serum bactericidal reaction and in some way compromises the surface defenses of the female urinogenital tract. Increased susceptibility to reinfection is highly correlated with the presence of circulating rmp antibodies.

10. Antibodies Absorbed by Soluble Bacterial Antigens: Some bacteria can liberate antigenic surface components in a soluble form into the tissue fluids. These soluble antigens are able to combine with and "neutralize" antibodies before they reach the bacterial cells. For example, small amounts of endotoxin may be released into surrounding fluids by Gram-negative bacteria. *Streptococcus pneumoniae* and Neisseria meningitidis are known to release capsular polysaccharides during growth in tissues. They are found in the serum of patients with pneumococcas pneumonia and in the cerebrospinal fluid of patients with meningitis. Theoretically, these released surface antigens could "mop up" antibody before it reaches the bacterial surface which should be an advantage to the pathogen. *Neisseria gonorrhoeae, N. meningitidis, Haemophilus influenzae, Streptococcus pneumoniae and Streptococcus mutans,* which can grow on the surfaces of the body, produce IgA proteases that inactivate secretory IgA by cleaving the molecule at the hinge region, detaching the Fc region of the immunoglobulin.

11. Antigenic Variation: One way bacteria can trick forces of the immunological response is to periodically change antigens, i.e., to undergo antigenic variation. Antigens may vary or change in the host during the course of an infection, or an organism can exist in nature as multiple antigenic types (serotypes or serovars). Antigenic variation is an important mechanism used by pathogenic microorganisms for escaping the neutralizing activities of antibodies. *Neisseria gonorrhoeae* can change fimbrial antigens during the course of an infection. During initial stages of an infection, adherence to epithelial cells of the cervix or urethra is mediated by pili (fimbriae). *N. gonorrhoeae* is capable of undergoing of "pili switching" or phase variation and increases resistance to phagocytosis and immune lysis.

The "relapses" of relapsing fever caused by the spirochete, *Borrelia recurrentis,* isa result of antigenic variation by the organism. After infection, the bacteria multiplies in tissues and cause a febrile illness until the onset of an immunological response a week or so later. Bacteria then disappear from the blood because of antibody mediated phagocytosis, lysis, agglutination, etc., and the fever falls. Then an antigenically distinct mutant arises in the infected individual, multiplies, and in 4-10 days reappears in the blood and there is another febrile attack. The immunological system is stimulated and responds by conquering the new antigenic variant, but the cycle continues such that there may be up to 10 febrile episodes before final recovery. With each attack a new antigenic variant of the spirochete appears and a new set of antibodies is formed in the host.

12. Multiple antigenic types or serotypes: Many pathogenic bacteria exist in nature as multiple antigenic types or serotypes meaning that they are variant strains of the same pathogenic species. For example, there are multiple serotypes of *Salmonella enterica* based on differences in cell wall (O) antigens and/or flagellar (H) antigens. There are 80 different antigenic types of Streptococcus pyogenes based on M-proteins on the cell surface. There are over one hundred strains of Streptococcus pneumoniae depending on their capsular polysaccharide antigens. Based on minor differences in surface structure chemistry there are multiple serotypes of *Vibrio cholerae, Staphylococcus aureus, Escherichia coli, Neisseria gonorrhoeae* and an assortment of other bacterial pathogens.

13. Capable of shedding old antigens and present new ones: If the immunological response is a critical defense against a pathogen, then being able to shed old antigens and present new ones to the immune system might allow infection or continued invasion by the pathogen to occur. Furthermore, the infected host would seem to be the ideal selective environment for the emergence of new antigenic variants of bacteria, providing the organism's other virulence determinants remains intact. Perhaps this explains why many successful bacterial pathogens exist in a great variety of antigenic types.

VIRUSES

Viruses are small, obligate intracellular parasites which cause infection by invading cells of the body and multiplying within them. Within their life cycle they have a relatively short extracellular period, prior to infecting the cells, and a longer intracellular period during which they undergo replication. The immune system has mechanisms which can attack the virus in both these phases of its life cycle, and this involve both non-specific and specific effector mechanisms.

Non-Specific Mechanisms

Interferons: Viral infection of cells directly stimulates the production of Type I interferons. Type I interferons lead to the induction of an "antiviral state" in the cells that is characterized by inhibition of both viral replication and cell proliferation, and also enhancement of the ability of natural killer cells to lyse virally infected cells.

Natural Killer Cells: Natural killer (NK) cells lyse virally infected cells. Even though they are not antigen specific, they clearly exhibit some degree of selectivity in targeting "abnormal" cells for lysis. Thus NK cells may be effective early in the course of viral infection, and may limit the spread of infection during the early stage, while antigen-specific lymphocytes are being recruited and clonally expanded.

Specific Mechanisms

Both humoral and cell mediated arms of the immune response play a role as specific effector mechanisms in antiviral immunity.

Antibody: Specific antibodies are important in defence mechanism to provide protection against viral infections. The most effective type of antiviral antibody is "neutralizing" antibody - this antibody binds to the virus (usually to the viral envelope), and blocks the virus from binding and gaining entry in to the host cell. It also acts as opsonin in enhancing phagocytosis of virus particles.

Cytotoxic T Cells: The principal effector cells which are involved in clearing established viral infections are the virus specific CD_8^+ cytotoxic T lymphocytes (CTL). These cells recognise (viral) antigens which have been synthesised within cell's nucleus or cytosol, and which have been degraded.

Although the host has a variety of defenses to protect against viral infections, sometimes it is the immune response to the infection that is the direct cause of tissue injury. For example, infants infected with cytomegalovirus have circulating immune complexes that are deposited in the kidneys and joints resulting in pathology such as arthritis and glomerular nephritis.

Viruses have evolved a variety of strategies to evade immune recognition and persist unmolested in the host. Many viruses are able to suppress immune responses and thereby overcome or minimize host defenses. The evasion of virus is accomplished by several mechanisms. They are as follows

Antigenic drift and shift: Viruses show an antigenic drift, as mutation and selection gradually change the aminoacid sequence of the surface antigens. For example Influenza virus in human population shows great antigenic variation within each subtype. This permits the parasite to persist in a population for many years. The antigenic shift in Influenza virus results in development of new strains.

Rapid turnover: The rapid turn over of population ensures the persistence of Influenza virus with out antigenic drift in horse.

Antigen presentation: Viral interference with antigen presentation via MHC class I is observed during infection with numerous viruses and is interpreted as a mechanism for viral escape from cytotoxic T (Tc) cell recognition. Interference is exerted at diverse stages of the MHC class I antigen processing and presentation pathway.

Inhibition of apoptosis: The phosphatidylinositol 3-kinase (PI3K) - Akt pathway is utilized by many cell types for inhibition of apoptosis and cellular survival. Virus modulation of this pathway provides an alternative to the expression of viral oncogenes or the direct inhibition of pro-apoptotic proteins.

Inability of host antibodies to neutralize virus: The best example is HIV which infects the CD_4^+ cells thereby destroying the specific immune system. Other viruses for eg. measles virus can also infect lymphocytes and affect their replication and differentiation. Some of the mechanisms by which viruses can evade host defenses are illustrated in

Table: 21.2
Viral Products that Interfere with Host Defenses

Host Defense Affected	Virus	Virus Product	Mechanism
Interferon	EBV	EBERS (small RNAs)	Blocks protein kinase activation
	Vaccinia	eIF- 2alpha homolog	Prevents phosphorylation of eIF-2alpha by protein kinase
Complement	Vaccinia	Homologues of complement control proteins	Blocks complement activation
Antibody	HSV-1	gE/gI	Binds Fc-gamma and blocks function
Cytokines	Myxoma	IFN-gamma receptor homolog	Competes for IFN-gamma and blocks function
	Shope fibroma virus	TNF receptor	Competes for TNF and blocks function
	EBV	**IL-10 homolog**	Reduces IFN-gamma function
MHC Class I	**CMV**	Early protein	Prevents transport of peptide-loaded MHC
	Adenovirus	E3	Blocks transport of MHC to surface
Apoptosis	Adenovirus	14.7 K	Inhibits capsases
	EBV	Bcl-2 homolog	Anti-apoptotic
NK cells	HCMV	UL-18	MHC homolog inhibits NK cells

Helminth parasites

Helminths are worm-like parasites characterized by elongated, flat or round bodies. Many helminth parasites are long-lived and cause chronic infections. Within their mammalian hosts they often undergo extensive growth and differentiation with the ultimate goal of producing stages intended for transmission to the next intermediate host. Usually, the life stage responsible for infecting the mammalian host is the larva, and the larva must migrate within the host to its appropriate niche where it can grow and reproduce. To smooth the progress helminth parasites have evolved diverse molecular mechanisms that facilitate their establishment, growth and reproduction inside an immunologically hostile environment.

Tissue-dwelling parasites, parasites localized in the lumen of ducts are able to produce immunomodulatory substances to escape to the host immune responses.

For example, *Necator americanus* secretes a metalloprotease which cleaves eotaxin, a chemotactic factor for eosinophils. Gastrointestinal nematodes also produce superoxide dismutase and glutathione S-transferase which neutralize toxic oxide radicals. A cystatin produced by *H. contortus* and *N. brasiliensis* modulates the antigen presentation to T cells by inhibiting cysteine proteases of antigen presenting cells, involved in the processing of the antigen. Certain Juveniles get covered by IgM antibodies. Since eosinophils do not express Fc receptor, IgM deposition on Juveniles could inhibit eosinophil adhesion and destruction by them. *F. hepatica* releases cathepsin L-protease which cleaves IgE and IgG involved in the antibody dependent cyto toxicity.

Immunomodulation induced by filarial parasites has been shown to act on different arms of the immune system including lymphocytes and antigen presenting cells. T cells from filarial patients exhibit an impaired production of IL-2, IFN- , and IL-5, as well as decreased Ag-specific proliferation. Lymphatic filariasis and schistosomiasis are associated with diminished antigen -specific immune responsiveness.

B cells exhibit diminished precursor frequencies and in vitro unresponsiveness to the helminth parasites. In addition, parasites have been shown to induce a profound dysfunction in multiple types of antigen presenting cells including dendritic cells, macrophages and Langerhans cells. A dysfunction occurs at the level of gene transcription, in the induction of cytokines and chemokines also. Above all pathogen induced antigen presenting cell exhibit a diminished capacity to stimulate CD4+ T cells.

The down-regulation of T cell receptor expression on B cells and monocytes could be a direct effect of parasites antigens on B cells and monocytes. Helminth parasites cause diminished cytokine/chemokine production by antigen presenting cells.

The evolved mechanisms help the pathogens to overcome host immune responses to thrive in immune-exposed locations such as lymphatics, bloodstream, and gastrointestinal tract. Hence most helminth infections induce relatively little disease despite extraordinarily high loads of infection.

22

AIDS

"Acquired Immune Deficiency Syndrome" or AIDS in short is a medical condition. The word "Acquired" means that the disease is not hereditary but develops after birth from contact with a disease causing agent (in this case, HIV). Immunodeficiency - means that the disease is characterized by a weakening of the immune system and the last word "Syndrome" refers to a group of symptoms that collectively indicate or characterize a disease. The term AIDS refers to an advanced stage of HIV infection. It is a new epidemic disease caused by human immunodeficiency virus (HIV) infection. It describes the whole group of symptoms and diseases associated with the damage, HIV causes, to the immune system.

How HIV Cause AIDS

HIV destroys CD_4 positive (CD_4^+) T cells, which are white blood cells crucial to maintaining the function of the human immune system. As the HIV infection progresses, there is ongoing damage to immune defense cells and the body becomes increasingly less able to fight off infection. Individuals with advanced HIV disease become susceptible to opportunistic infections that don't show up in people with healthy immune systems.

Not everyone who has HIV infection develops AIDS. Most people who are infected with HIV can carry the virus for years before developing any serious symptoms. But over time, HIV levels increase in the blood while the number of CD_4^+ T cells decline. Experts estimate that about half the people with HIV will develop AIDS within 10 years after becoming infected. This time varies greatly from person to person, however, and depends on many factors, including a person's health status and health-related behaviour. People are said to have AIDS when they have certain signs or symptoms specified in guidelines formulated by the U.S. Centers for Disease Control and Prevention (CDC).

The definition of AIDS given by CDC's includes:

1. HIV-infected people with fewer than 200 CD_4^+ T cells per cubic millimeter of blood (compared with CD_4^+ T cell counts of about 1,000 for healthy people)

2. People with HIV infection have at least one of more than two dozen AIDS-associated conditions, due to HIV's attack on the immune system

AIDS-associated conditions include opportunistic infections by bacteria, fungi, and viruses. Opportunistic infections are caused by germs that are around us all the time but normally they can be fought off by a healthy immune system. Once the immune system is sufficiently weakened, such infections will develop and produce a wide range of symptoms. Some of these symptoms can be very severe. When the immune system is weakened certain cancers also become more common.

Examples of opportunistic infections and cancers

The table below shows examples of common opportunistic infections and cancers and the body systems that they occur in.

Table: 22.1

System	Examples of Infection/Cancer
Respiratory system	Pneumocystis jirovecii Pneumonia (PCP) Tuberculosis (TB) Kaposi's Sarcoma (KS)
Gastro-intestinal system	Cryptosporidiosis Candida Cytomegolavirus (CMV) Isosporiasis Kaposi's Sarcoma
Central/peripheral Nervous system	Cytomegolavirus Toxoplasmosis Cryptococcosis Non Hodgkin's lymphoma Varicella Zoster Herpes simplex
Skin	Herpes simplex Kaposi's sarcoma Varicella Zoster

Most AIDS-associated conditions are rarely serious in healthy individuals. In people with AIDS, however, these infections are often severe and sometimes fatal because the immune system is so damaged by HIV that the body cannot fight them off.

Human Immunodeficiency Virus (HIV):

HIV is a lentivirus, and like all viruses of this type, it attacks the immune system. Lentiviruses are in turn part of a larger group of viruses known as retroviruses. The name 'lentivirus' literally means 'slow virus' because they take such a long time to produce any adverse effects in the body. This is why there are many people who are unaware of their HIV infection, and unfortunately, can spread the virus to others. HIV multiplies in the CD4+ T cells of human immune system's and kills vast number of the cells it infects causing imune deficiency in the host.

Retroviruses are viruses that contain RNA (ribonucleic acid) as their genetic material. After infecting a cell, retroviruses convert their RNA into DNA with the help of an enzyme called reverse transcriptase and then proceeds to replicate it self using the cell's machinery.

Structure of HIV: Unlike most bacteria, HIV particles are too small to be seen through an ordinary microscope. However they can be seen clearly with an electron microscope. Outside of a human cell, HIV exists as roughly spherical particles. HIV is spherical in shape and has a diameter of 0.1 microns (1/10,000 of a millimeter). The outer coat of the virus, known as the viral envelope, is composed of two layers of fatty molecules taken from the membrane of a human cell. When a newly formed virus particle buds from the cell it covers itsef with the cell membrane(envelope is a common feature in animal viruses but uncommon in plant viruses). Along with the proteins of host cell viral envelope, caries about 72 copies (on average) of a complex HIV protein known as Env. These Env copies protrude or spike through the surface of the virus particle. Env consists of a cap made of three molecules called glycoprotein 120 (gp120), and a stem consisting of three molecules called gyclycoprotein 41 (gp41) that anchor the structure in the viral envelope.

Within the viral envelope is a bullet-shaped core or capsid, made up of 2,000 copies of the viral protein - p24. The capsid surrounds two single strands of HIV RNA, each of which has a complete copy of the virus's genes. HIV has three structural genes - gag, pol, and env, that contain information needed to make structural proteins for new virus particles. The env gene, for example, codes for a protein called gp160 that is broken down by a viral enzyme to form gp120 and gp41, the components of the env protein.

The remaining six genes of HIV are regulatory genes (tat, rev, nef, vif, vpr, and vpu) that contain information needed to produce proteins that control the ability of HIV to infect a cell, produce new copies of virus, or cause disease. For instance the protein encoded by nef is apparently necessary for the virus to replicate efficiently, and the vpu-encoded protein influences the release of new virus particles from infected cells. Recently, researchers discovered that vif (the protein encoded by the vif gene) interacts with an antiviral defense protein in host cells (APOBEC3G), causing inactivation of the antiviral effect and enhancing HIV replication. This interaction may serve as a new target for antiviral drugs.

The ends of each strand of HIV RNA contain an RNA sequence called the long terminal repeat (LTR). Regions in the LTR act as switches to control production of new viruses and can be triggered by proteins from either HIV or the host cell.

HIV's core also includes a protein called p7, the HIV nucleocapsid protein. Three enzymes carry out later steps in the life cycle of virus. They are reverse transcriptase, integrase, and protease. Another HIV protein called p17, or the HIV matrix protein, lies between the viral core and the viral envelope.

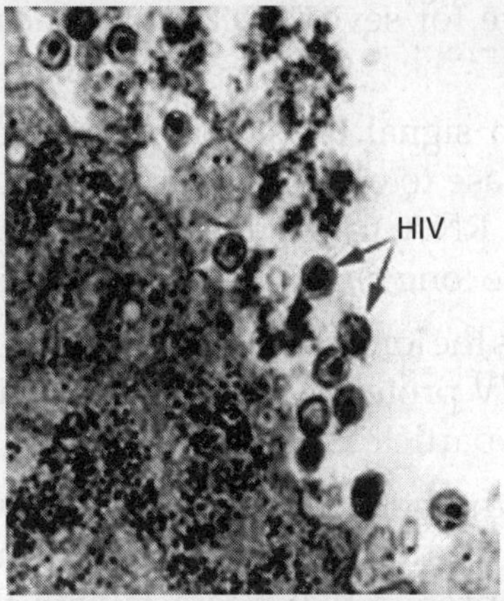

Fig. 22.1. This transmission electron micrographic image shows mature forms of the human immunodeficiency virus (HIV) in a tissue sample.
(Source CDC)

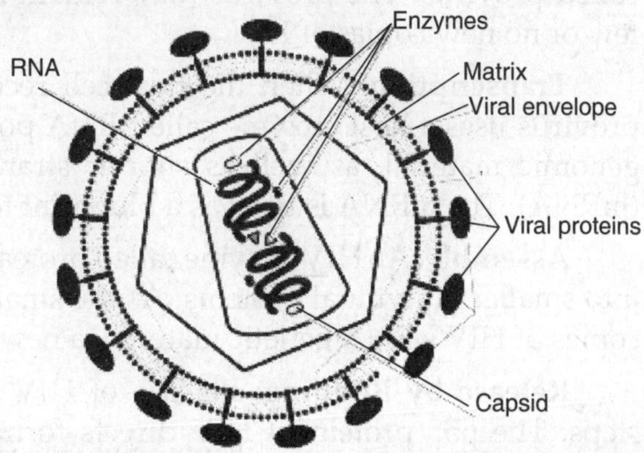

Fig. 22.2 Structure of Human Immunodeficiency virus (HIV)

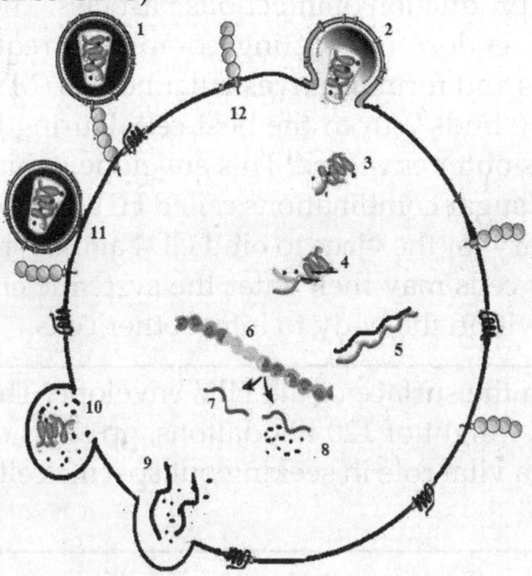

Fig: 22.3 HIV Replication

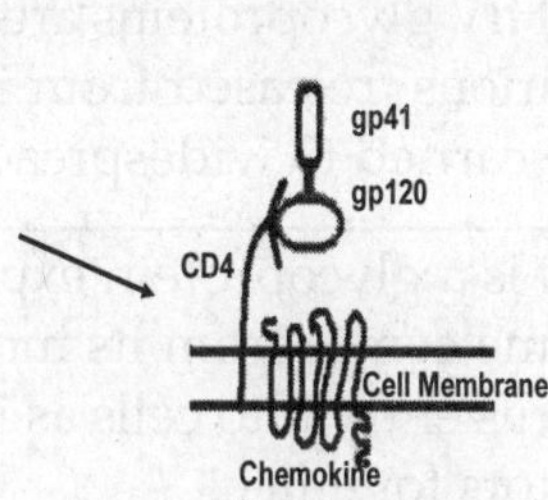

Fig. 22.4

Binding and Fusion: HIV entry into a host cell begins with gp120 binding to CD4 receptor, which induces a conformational change in gp120, exposing co receptor binding sites. After the chemokine coreceptor is engaged, the gp41 on the HIV surface undergoes a conformational change. Conformational change in gp41 leads to formation of a stable structure that allows fusion of HIV and host cell membranes with a fusion pore, through which the viral core enters the host cell. These cores can utilize host cell microtubules to move toward the cell nucleus.

Reverse Transcription: Once within the cell, the enzyme product of the pol gene, reverse transcriptase synthesizes linear double-stranded cDNA.

Integration: The newly formed HIV DNA is then inserted into the host cell genomic DNA by the integrase enzyme of the HIV. The integrated HIV DNA is called provirus. The provirus may remain inactive for several years, producing few or no new copies of HIV.

Transcription: When the host cell receives a signal to become active, the provirus uses a host enzyme called RNA polymerase to create copies of the HIV genomic material, as well as shorter strands of RNA called messenger RNA (mRNA). The mRNA is used as a blueprint to make long chains of HIV proteins.

Assembly: An HIV enzyme called protease cuts the long chains of HIV proteins into smaller individual proteins. As the smaller HIV proteins come together with copies of HIV's RNA genetic material, a new virus particle is assembled.

Release by Budding: Release of HIV from the host cell occurs in several steps. The p55 protein of HIV directs formation of a capsid (CA) protein that surrounds the RNA of HIV, a nucleocapsid (NC) protein that interacts with the RNA within the capsid, and matrix (MA) protein that surrounds the capsid and lies just beneath the viral envelope. A protease enzyme encoded by the pol gene of HIV cleaves the large precursor proteins to produce the MA, CA, and NC proteins. Budding virions utilize host cell membrane to form the outer virion envelope of the budding virion that is necessary for production of infectious particles. The process of viral budding relies on cellular endosomal sorting complexes required for transport (ESCRT), that sort proteins and form multivesicular bodies (MVBs). The newly assembled virus pushes out ("buds") from the host cell. During budding, the new virus steals part of the cell's outer envelope. This envelope, which acts as a covering, is studded with protein/sugar combinations called HIV glycoproteins. These HIV glycoproteins are necessary for the virus to bind CD4 and co- receptors. HIV virions released from infected cells may then enter the systemic circulation and be carried to widespread sites within the body to infect other cells.

gp120 is a glycoprotein exposed on the surface of the HIV envelope. The 120 in its name comes from its molecular weight of 120 kilodaltons. gp120 is essential for virus entry into cells as it plays a vital role in seeking out specific cell surface receptors for entry.

Types of HIV

One of the obstacles to treatment of the Human Immunodeficiency Virus is its high genetic variability. HIV mutates very readily resulting in the formation of many different strains of HIV, even within the body of a single infected person. Based on genetic similarities, the numerous virus strains may be classified into types, groups and subtypes.

There are two types of HIV: HIV-1 and HIV-2. Both types are transmitted by sexual contact, through blood, and from mother to child, and they appear to cause clinically indistinguishable AIDS. HIV-1 is related to viruses found in chimpanzees and gorillas living in western Africa, while HIV-2 viruses are related to viruses found in sooty mangabeys. HIV-2 seems to be less easily transmitted, and the period between initial infection and illness is longer in the case of HIV-2. The relatively uncommon HIV-2 type is concentrated in West Africa and it is rarely found elsewhere.

HIV-1 is predominant virus all over the world. When people refer to HIV without specifying the type of virus they will be referring to HIV-1. The strains of HIV-1 can be classified into four groups: the "major" group M, the "outlier" group O and two new groups, N and P. These four groups may represent four separate introductions of simian immunodeficiency virus into humans.

Group M: With 'M' for "major", this is by far the most common type of HIV, with more than 90% of HIV/AIDS cases deriving from infection with HIV-1 group M. Group M can be further subdivided into subtypes based on genetic sequence data. Some of the subtypes are known to be more virulent or resistant to different medications. The subtypes are as follows:

Subtype A - Subtype A and CRF A/G predominate in west and central Africa, also causing much of the Russian epidemic.

Subtype B - subtype B has been the most common subtype/CRF in Europe, America, Japan and Australia. Although this remains the case, other subtypes are becoming more frequent and now account for at least 25% of new infections in Europe.

Subtype C - largely predominant in southern and eastern Africa, India and Nepal. It has caused the world's worst HIV epidemics and is responsible for around half of all infections.

Subtype D - generally seen in Eastern and central Africa only.

Subtype F - found in central Africa, South America and Eastern Europe.

Subtype G - found in Africa and central Europe.

Subtype H - limited to central Africa.

Subtype J - primarily found in North, Central and West Africa, and the Caribbean, Subtype K - limited to the Democratic Republic of Congo and Cameroon.

Subtype E has never been identified as a nonrecombinant only recombined with subtype A as CRF01_AE.

Group N: The 'N' stands for "non-M, non-O". This group was discovered in 1998 and has only been seen in Cameroon. As of 2006, only 10 Group N infections had been identified.

Group O: The O ("Outlier") group is not usually seen outside of West-central Africa. It is reportedly most common in Cameroon. The group caused some concern because it could not be detected by early versions of the HIV-1 test kits. More advanced HIV tests have now been developed to detect both Group O and

Group N.

Group P: In 2009, a newly-analyzed HIV sequence was reported to have greater similarity to a simian immunodeficiency virus discovered in wild gorillas (SIVgor) than to SIVs from chimpanzees (SIVcpz). The virus had been isolated from a Cameroonian woman residing in France who was diagnosed with HIV-1 infection in 2004. The scientists reporting this sequence placed it in a proposed Group P "pending the identification of further human cases".

Occasionally, two viruses of different subtypes can meet in the cell of an infected person and mix together their genetic material to create a new hybrid virus. Many of these new strains do not survive for long, but those that infect more than one person are known as "circulating recombinant forms" or CRFs. For example, the CRF A/B is a mixture of subtypes A and B. It is almost certain that new HIV genetic subtypes and CRFs will be discovered in the future, and indeed that new ones will develop as virus recombination and mutation continue to occur. The current subtypes and CRFs will also continue to spread to new areas as the global epidemic continues.

SYMPTOMS OF HIV INFECTION: As the immune system fails, symptoms develop. Initially many of the symptoms are mild, but as the immune system deteriorates the symptoms worsen. HIV infection can generally be broken down into four distinct stages: primary infection, clinically asymptomatic stage, symptomatic HIV infection, and progression from HIV to AIDS.

STAGE 1: Primary HIV infection

This stage of infection lasts for a few weeks and is often accompanied by a short flu-like illness. In about 20% of people the symptoms are serious enough to consult a doctor, but the diagnosis of HIV infection is frequently missed. During this stage there is a large amount of HIV in the peripheral blood and the immune system begins to respond to the virus by producing HIV antibodies and cytotoxic lymphocytes. This process is known as seroconversion. If an HIV antibody test is done before seroconversion is complete then it may not be positive.

STAGE 2: Clinically asymptomatic stage:

This stage lasts for an average of ten years and, as its name suggests, it is free from major symptoms, although there may be swollen glands. The level of HIV in the peripheral blood drops to very low levels but people remain infectious and HIV antibodies are detectable in the blood, so antibody tests will show a positive result.

Research has shown that HIV is not dormant during this stage, but is very active in the lymph nodes. A test which measures HIV RNA (HIV genetic material) is viral load test, and it has an important role in the treatment of HIV infection.

STAGE 3: Symptomatic HIV infection:

Over time the immune system becomes severely damaged by HIV. The lymph nodes and tissues become damaged because of the years of activity. HIV mutates and becomes more pathogenic. The body fails to keep up with replacing the T helper cells that are lost.

As the immune system fails, symptoms develop. Initially many of the symptoms are mild, but as the immune system deteriorates the symptoms worsen. Symptomatic HIV infection is mainly caused by the emergence of opportunistic infections and cancers that the immune system would normally prevent. This stage of HIV infection is often characterised by multi-system disease and infections can occur in almost all body systems.

STAGE 4: Progression from HIV to AIDS:

As the immune system becomes more and more damaged the illnesses that occur become more and more severe leading eventually to an AIDS diagnosis.

Symptoms of HIV vary according to the stage of the infection.

WHO clinical staging of HIV disease in adults and adolescents (2006 revision)

In resource-poor communities, medical facilities are sometimes poorly equipped, and it is not possible to use CD4 and viral load test results to determine the right time to begin antiretroviral treatment. The World Health Organisation (WHO) has therefore developed a staging system for HIV disease, based on clinical symptoms, which may be used to guide medical decision making.

Clinical Stage I:

Asymptomatic

Persistent generalized lymphadenopathy

Clinical Stage II:

Moderate unexplained weight loss (under 10% of presumed or measured body weight)

Recurrent respiratory tract infections (sinusitis, tonsillitis, otitis media, pharyngitis)

Herpes zoster

Angular chelitis

Recurrent oral ulceration

Papular pruritic eruptions

Seborrhoeic dermatitis

Fungal nail infections

Clinical Stage III:

Unexplained severe weight loss (over 10% of presumed or measured body weight)

Unexplained chronic diarrhoea for longer than one month

Unexplained persistent fever (intermittent or constant for longer than one month)

Persistent oral candidiasis

Oral hairy leukoplakia

Pulmonary tuberculosis

Severe bacterial infections (e.g. pneumonia, empyema, pyomyositis, bone or joint infection, meningitis, bacteraemia)

Acute necrotizing ulcerative stomatitis, gingivitis or periodontitis

Unexplained anaemia (below 8 g/dl), neutropenia (below 0.5 billion/l) and/or chronic thrombocytopenia (below 50 billion/l)

Clinical Stage IV:

HIV wasting syndrome

Pneumocystis pneumonia

Recurrent severe bacterial pneumonia

Chronic herpes simplex infection (orolabial, genital or anorectal of more than one month's duration or visceral at any site).

Oesophageal candidiasis (or candidiasis of trachea, bronchi or lungs).

Extrapulmonary tuberculosis.

Kaposi sarcoma.

Cytomegalovirus infection (retinitis or infection of other organs).

Central nervous system toxoplasmosis.

HIV encephalopathy .

Extrapulmonary cryptococcosis including meningitis.

Disseminated non-tuberculous mycobacteria infection.

Progressive multifocal leukoencephalopathy.

Chronic cryptosporidiosis.

Chronic isosporiasis .

Disseminated mycosis (extrapulmonary histoplasmosis, coccidiomycosis).

Recurrent septicaemia (including non-typhoidal Salmonella).

Lymphoma (cerebral or B cell non-Hodgkin).

Invasive cervical carcinoma.

Atypical disseminated leishmaniasis.

Symptomatic HIV-associated nephropathy or HIV-associated cardiomyopathy.

TRANSMISSION OF HIV:

HIV is present to variable degrees in the blood and genital secretions of almost all individuals infected with HIV, regardless of whether they have symptoms or not. The spread of HIV can occur when these secretions come in contact with tissues such as those lining the vagina, anal area, mouth, or eyes (the mucus membranes), or with a break in the skin, such as from a cut or puncture by a needle. The most common ways in which HIV is spreading throughout the world include sexual contact, sharing needles, and by transmission from infected mothers to their newborns during pregnancy, labor, or breastfeeding. How ever HIV-2 is transmitted less frequently from pregnant mother to her child and sexual route than HIV-1. The different modes of transmission of HIV are:

Sexual:

Sexual transmission of HIV is most common means of transmission of HIV and unprotected sexual relationship is the most common reason for HIV transmission. Transmission occurs when infected secretions of one person come into contact with the genital, oral, or rectal mucous membranes of other person.

Blood or blood product:

Transmission through this route is common in intravenous drug users, hemophiliacs and those who receive blood transfusions and blood products. Health care workers like nurses, doctors, tattooing, piercing etc. are high risk behavior and can lead to infection by HIV. The spread of HIV by exposure to infected blood usually results from sharing needles, as in those used for illicit drugs. HIV can also spread by sharing needles for anabolic steroids to increase muscle, tattooing, and body piercing.

Pregnant mother to child:

The transmission of the HIV from the mother to the child can occur during pregnancy, during childbirth or through breast milk. The risk of transmission to the child is high in absence of treatment. With treatment the rate and extent of transmission of the infection in newborn and fetus reduces dramatically. For prophylaxis antiretroviral drugs are prescribed to infants also.

Other routes:

HIV can also be transmitted by saliva, tears and urine of infected individuals but at present no data is available. This is because saliva, in contrast to genital secretions, has been shown to contain very little HIV. Still, theoretical risks are associated with the sharing of toothbrushes and shaving razors because they can cause bleeding, and blood can contain large amounts of HIV. Consequently, these items should not be shared with infected people. Similarly, without sexual exposure or direct contact with blood, there is little if any risk of HIV infection.

FACTS ABOUT HIV TRANSMISSION:

- HIV cannot survive for very long outside of the body.
- HIV cannot be transmitted through routine daily activities such as using a toilet seat, sharing food utensils or drinking glasses, shaking hands, or through kissing.
- The virus can only be transmitted from person to person, not through animals or insect bites.

- People infected with HIV who are taking antiretroviral therapy can still infect others through unprotected sex and needle-sharing.
- HIV is not transmitted by insects. No evidence of HIV transmission through insects -even in areas where there are many cases of AIDS and large populations of insects such as mosquitoes.

THE START OF AIDS

The history of AIDS is a short one. As recently as the 1970s, no one was aware of this deadly illness. Since then the global AIDS epidemic has become one of the greatest threats to human health and development. AIDS first came to light in the early 1980s. The first recognised cases of AIDS occurred in USA in the early 1980s. A number of gay men in New York and California suddenly began to develop rare opportunistic infections and cancers that seemed stubbornly resistant to any treatment. At that time, AIDS did not yet have a name, but it quickly became obvious that all the men were suffering from a common syndrome and it was referred as 'Gay men's immune deficiency Syndrome'. The discovery of HIV, the Human Immunodeficiency Virus, was made soon after.

Since certain strains of SIVs bear a very close resemblance to the two types of HIV it is now generally accepted that HIV is a descendant of a Simian Immunodeficiency Virus. In February 1999 a group of researchers from the University of Alabama announced that they had found a type of SIVcpz that was almost identical to HIV-1. This particular strain was identified in a frozen sample taken from a captive member of the sub-group of chimpanzees known as Pan troglodytes troglodytes (P. t. troglodytes), which were once common in west-central Africa. They claimed that this sample proved that chimpanzees were the source of HIV-1, and that the virus had at some point crossed species from chimps to humans.

Four of the earliest known instances of HIV infection are as follows:

1. A plasma sample taken in 1959 from an adult male living in the Democratic Republic of the Congo.
2. A lymph node sample taken in 1960 from an adult female, also from the Democratic Republic of the Congo.
3. HIV found in tissue samples from an American teenager who died in St. Louis in 1969.
4. HIV found in tissue samples from a Norwegian sailor who died around 1976.

A 1998 analysis of the plasma sample from 1959 suggested that HIV-1 infected the humans around the 1940s or the early 1950s.

In January 2000, the results of a new study suggested that the first case of HIV-1 infection occurred around 1931 in West Africa. This estimate (which had a 15 year margin of error) was based on a complex computer model of HIV's evolution.

However, a study in 2008 dated the origin of HIV between 1884 and 1924, much earlier than previous estimates. The researchers compared the viral sequence from 1959 (the oldest known HIV-1 specimen) to the newly discovered sequence from 1960. They found a significant genetic difference between them; demonstrating diversification of HIV-1 occurred long before the AIDS pandemic was recognised.

Transmission by bloodsucking insects:

The results of experiments and observations of insect biting behavior indicate that when an insect bites a person, it does not inject its own or a previously bitten person's or animal's blood into the next person bitten. Rather, it injects saliva, which acts as a lubricant or anticoagulant so the insect can feed efficiently. Since the pathogens that can cause diseases such as yellow fever and malaria exist in saliva they are transmitted through the saliva during feeding process of bloodsucking insects. However, HIV lives for only a short time inside an insect and, unlike organisms that are transmitted via insect bites; HIV does not survive and reproduce in insects. Thus, even if the virus enters a mosquito or another sucking or biting insect, the insect does not become infected and cannot transmit HIV to the next human it feeds on or bites. Hence there is no reason to fear about the biting or bloodsucking insects in case of HIV transmission.

There is also no reason to fear that biting or bloodsucking insects, such as a mosquito, testees fly etc.could transmit HIV from one person to another through HIV-infected blood left on its mouth parts. Two factors serve to explain why this is so--first, infected people do not have constant, high levels of HIV in their bloodstreams and, second, insect mouth parts do not retain large amounts of blood on their surfaces. Further, scientists who study insects have determined that biting insects normally do not travel from one person to the next.

Origin of HIV:

In recent times it has being generally accepted that some viruses can be transferred from animals to human through the process know as Zoonosis. Indeed, the very fact that chimpanzees obtained SIV from two other species of primate shows just how easily this crossover can occur. However, it has now been proved that HIV (Human immune virus) only affect human being and as such can not reside in chimpanzees.Several theories were proposed by different scientists to explain the origin of HIV. Below are some of the most common theories about how this 'zoonosis' took place, and how SIV became HIV in humans:

The 'Hunter' Theory: The most commonly accepted theory is that of the 'hunter'. As per this theory SIVcpz might be transferred to humans as a result of chimps being killed and eaten or their blood getting into cuts or wounds of the hunter.

The Oral Polio Vaccine (OPV) theory: As per this theory HIV might have transferred iatrogenically (i.e. via medical interventions). Edward Hooper suggests that the polio vaccine prepared from the virus cultivated in kidney cells taken from local chimps infected with SIVcmz might be contaminated with chimp SIV.

Mutations of SIV might have resulted in the production of HIV.

The Contaminated Needle Theory: This is an extension of the original 'hunter' theory. Use of disposable plastic syringes became commonplace around the world as a cheap, sterile way to administer medicines. The huge quantities of syringes needed would have been very costly therefore one single syringe might have been used to inject multiple patients without any sterilisation in between. This would rapidly have transferred any viral particles (with a hunter's blood for example) from one person to another, creating huge potential for the virus to mutate and replicate in each new individual it entered, even if the SIV within the original person infected had not yet converted to HIV.

The Colonialism Theory: It is one of the more recent theories based on the basic 'hunter theory. It was first proposed in 2000 by Jim Moore. During the late 19th and early 20th century, much of Africa was ruled by colonial forces. Colonial rule was particularly harsh and many Africans were forced into labour camps where sanitation was poor, food was scarce and physical demands were extreme. A stray and perhaps sick chimpanzee with SIV would have made a welcome extra source of food for the workers. Moore also believes that many of the labourers would have been inoculated with unsterile needles against diseases such as smallpox (to keep them alive and working), and that many of the camps actively employed prostitutes to keep the workers happy, creating numerous possibilities for onward transmission.

The Conspiracy Theory: Some say that HIV is a 'conspiracy theory' or that it is 'man-made'. A significant number of African Americans who believe HIV were manufactured as part of a biological warfare programme, designed to wipe out large numbers of black and homosexual people.

Spread of the Epidemic: It is likely that we will never know who the first person was to be infected with HIV, or exactly how it spread from that initial person. Scientists investigating the possibilities often become very attached to their individual 'pet' theories and insist that theirs is the only true answer, but the spread of AIDS could quite conceivably have been induced by a combination of many different events. Whether through injections, travel, wars, colonial practices or genetic engineering, the realities of the 20th Century have undoubtedly had a major role to play.

HIV EVASION:

HIV replicates rapidly with several billion new viruses made every day in a person infected with HIV. Its ability to mutate and evolve makes HIV so difficult to stop. Reverse transcriptase, the enzyme that makes DNA copies of HIV's RNA, often makes random mistakes. As a result, new types or strains of HIV develop in a person infected with HIV. Some strains are harder to kill because of their ability to infect and kill other types of cells, while other strains replicate at faster rates. The more virulent and infectious strains of HIV are typically found in people who are in the late stages of infection. Different strains of HIV can also recombine to produce an even wider range of strains. The constant changes in HIV help to evade the surveillance of immune system. Its ability to evolve rapidly is one of the major reasons why HIV is such a deadly virus. Above all antiretroviral drugs are capable of suppressing HIV, even to undetectable levels in the blood, but they cannot eliminate the virus hiding in these latent reservoirs.

DIAGNOSTIC TESTS

AIDS tests cover a number of different procedures used to diagnose and treat HIV patients. Some AIDS tests are used to diagnose patients or confirm a diagnosis; others are used to measure the progression of the disease or the effectiveness of specific treatment regimens. Some AIDS tests can also be used to screen blood donations for safe use in transfusions.

Diagnostic blood tests for AIDS are usually given to persons in high-risk populations who have been exposed to HIV or who have the early symptoms of AIDS.Most persons infected with HIV will develop a detectable level of antibody within three months of infection.

It is possible to diagnose HIV infection by isolating the virus itself from ablood sample or by demonstrating the presence of HIV antigen in the blood. Isolating the virus itself is expensive, not widely available, and slow. More common are blood tests that works by detecting the presence of antibodies to the HIV virus.They are as follows:

Enzyme-linked immunosorbent assay (ELISA): ELISA (also sometimes called EIA) is often used as the first screening tool for HIV. HIV antibody tests are the most appropriate test for routine diagnosis of HIV among adults. It is inexpensive and very sensitive for detecting the presence of HIV antibodies. In most cases, a blood sample is tested, but other types of ELISAs that use saliva and urine have also been developed. The actual ELISA takes 3.5 to 4 hours.

ELISA test involves HIV antigens that are attached to a plastic surface. A sample of the patient's blood serum is added. If there are any HIV antibodies in the blood, they will attach to the HIV antigens. After rinsing off excess blood factors, a second antibody is added. This antibody binds with any HIV antibodies that are attached to the HIVantigens. The second antibody also contains a chemical that changes color, indicating the presence of HIV antibodies in the patient's blood.

Occasionally the result may be a false positive. Western blot or immunoblot test is used to confirm the diagnosis of AIDS.

Western blot (WB) testing: It is only performed if an ELISA or rapid test is positive. The WB can be positive, negative, or indeterminate. Indeterminate tests are neither positive nor negative. An indeterminate result usually means that a person has just begun to seroconvert at the time of their test. In the rare cases in which this occurs, the person will need to be retested, usually about one month later. False positive results are extremely rare with the WB, so it confirms (proves) that HIV antibodies are present.

In Western blot testing procedure HIV antigens are suspended in a flat slab of gel. An electric current run through the gel causes the proteins to separate from one another and move varying distances depending on their molecular size. Afterwards, the gel is pressed against a nylon or nitrocellulose filter, transferring the proteins to the filter. The patient's blood is made to react against the filter, followed by treatment with developing chemicals. If HIV antibodies are present,they show up as a colored patch or blot on the filter.

Immunofluorescent assay (IFA): The IFA can be used instead of the WB to confirm ELISA results. Like the WB, IFA tests for the presence of antibodies in a blood sample. The exact strategy is slightly different in that it uses a microscope. It can be faster than a WB. Instead of Western blotting sometimes this test is used to confirm ELISA results.An IFA test detects the presence of HIV antibody in a sample of the patient's serum by mixing HIV antigen with a fluorescent chemical. If antibodies are present in the test sample their binding with HIV antigens can be observed under a microscope with ultraviolet light.

Polymerase chain reaction (PCR): A PCR test is used to evaluate the very small number of AIDS patients with false-negative ELISA and Western blot tests. PCR testing is based on present knowledge of the genetic sequences in HIV. It can detect the genetic material of HIV rather than the antibodies to the virus, and so can identify HIV in the blood within two or three weeks of infection. This test works by amplifying the presence of HIV nucleic acids in a blood sample. Numerous copies of a gene are made by separating the two strands of DNA containing the gene segment, marking its location, using DNA polymerase to make a copy, and then continuously replicating the copies. The test is also known as a viral load test and HIV NAAT (nucleic acid amplification testing). Since the virus is continually generating new variants, PCR testing could yield a false negative in patients with these new variants.

Antigen test (P24 test): The antigen on HIV that most commonly provokes an antibody response is the protein P24. Early in HIV infection, P24 is produced in excess and can be detected in the blood serum (although as HIV becomes fully established in the body it will fade to undetectable levels). P24 antigen tests are not usually used for general HIV diagnostic purposes, as they have a very low sensitivity and they only work before antibodies are produced in the period immediately after HIV infection. They are now most often used as a component of 'fourth generation' tests. Some of the most modern HIV tests combine P24 antigen tests with standard antibody tests to reduce the 'diagnostic window'. Testing for antibodies and P24 antigen simultaneously has the advantage of enabling earlier and more accurate HIV detection.

PROGNOSTIC TESTS

Blood tests to evaluate patients already diagnosed with HIV infection are as important as the diagnostic tests. Because AIDS has a long latency period, some persons may be infected with the virus for 10 years or longer before they develop symptoms of AIDS. These patients are sometimes called antibody-positive asymptomatic carriers. Prognostic tests also help drug researchers evaluate the usefulness of new medications in treating AIDS.

BLOOD CELL COUNTS. Doctors can measure the number or proportion of certain types of cells in an AIDS patient's blood to see whether and how rapidly the disease is progressing, or whether certain treatments are helping the patient. These cell count tests include:

Complete blood count (CBC): A CBC is a routine analysis performed on a sample of blood taken from the patients. The measurements taken in a CBC include a white blood cell count (WBC), a red blood cell count (RBC), the red cell distribution width, the hematocrit and the amount of haemoglobin. Specific AIDS-related signs in a CBC include a low hematocrit, a sharp decrease in the number of blood platelets, and a low level of a neutrophils.

Absolute CD4+ lymphocytes: Since HIV targets CD_4^+ lymphocytes, their number in the patient's blood can be used to track the course of the infection. This blood cell count is considered the most accurate indicator for the presence of an opportunistic infection in an AIDS patient. An absolute count below 200-300 CD_4^+ lymphocytes in 1 cubic millimeter (mm3) of blood indicates that the patient is vulnerable to some opportunistic infections.

CD4+ lymphocyte percentage: Some doctors think that this is a more accurate test than the absolute count because the percentage does not depend on a manual calculation of the number of types of different white blood cells.

HIV Viral load Tests. Another type of blood test for monitoring AIDS patients is the viral load test. It supplements the CD_4^+ count, which can tell the doctor the extent of the patient's loss of immune function, but not the speed of HIV replication in the body. The viral load test is based on PCR techniques and can measure the number of copies of HIV nucleic acids.

Oral HIV Tests. Scientists have developed oral HIV tests that can be conducted with saliva samples. It is considered as an excellent alternative to blood sample testing.

Rapid HIV Tests. A finger-stick test that can be read quickly from a whole blood sample had shown promising results in the fall of 2003. Another test, called the VScan test kit, requires no refrigeration or electricity and can safely be stored at room temperature. Even if the positive results must be confirmed by ELISA or Western blotting, an accurate initial rapid test can help screen populations for HIV antibodies.

Beta 2-Microglobulin (BETA2M): Beta-microglobulin is a protein found on the surface of all human cells with a nucleus. It is released into the blood when a cell dies. Although rising blood levels of β2M are found in patients with cancer and other serious diseases, a rising β2M blood level can be used to measure the progression of AIDS.

Genotypic drug resistance Test. Genotypic testing can help determine whether specific gene mutations, common in people with HIV, are causing drug resistance and drug failure. The test looks for specific genetic mutations within the virus that are known to cause resistance to certain drugs used in HIV treatment.

For example the drug 3TC, also known as lamivudine (Epivir), is not effective against strains of HIV that have a mutation at a particular position on the reverse transcriptase protein - amino acid 184 - known as M184V (M→V, methionine to valine). So if the genotypic resistance test shows a mutation at position M184V, it is likely the person is resistant to 3TC and not likely to respond to 3TC treatment. Genotypic tests are only effective if the person is already taking antiviral medication and if the viral load is greater than 1,000 copies per milliliter (ml) of blood.

Phenotypic drug resistance Testing. Phenotypic testing directly measures the sensitivity of a patient's HIV to particular drugs and drug combinations. Phenotypic testing is a more direct measurement of resistance than genotypic testing. Unlike genotypic testing, phenotypic testing does not require a high viral load but it is recommended that persons already be taking antiretroviral drugs.

AIDS SEROLOGY IN CHILDREN

Children born to HIV-infected mothers may acquire the infection through the mother's placenta or during the birth process. Younger infants can be diagnosed by direct culture of the HIV virus, PCR testing, and p24 antigen testing. These techniques allow a pediatrician to identify 50% of infected children at or near birth.

TREATMENT/ MEDICATION:

Currently there is no cure for AIDS. Over the past 10 years, however, therapies have been developed to fight both HIV infection and its associated health problems (infections and cancers) to help them stay healthier and live longer. Some medications used today target HIV itself, to reduce the virus's assault on the immune system, or to even prevent the virus from entering human immune cells. Other treatments are used to treat or prevent specific opportunistic infections that threaten the health of people with HIV-damaged immune systems.

HIV treatment has 4 major goals they are:

1. Extend patients' life expectancy and quality of life.
2. Prevent HIV from progressing by reducing the viral load to undetectable levels.
3. Restore and preserve the immune system to normal.
4. Reduce the risk of transmitting HIV to others.

Treatments that Suppress HIV

Drugs that interfere with the activity of a retrovirus such as HIV are generally known as antiretrovirals. Nearly all antiretroviral medications currently approved to treat HIV infection target reverse transcriptase and protease that are involved in different stages of viral replication. A new treatment approved in the past year works in a completely new way by preventing the virus from entering the human immune cells.

Four classes of antiretroviral drugs have been developed to interfere with the activity of these viral enzymes and slow down the multiplication of the virus. These are:

- Nucleoside analog reverse transcriptase inhibitors (NRTIs): NRTIs interrupt at an early stage of HIV replication by interfering with the activity of reverse transcriptase. AZT (zidovudine) is the first drug approved for treating HIV infection,
- Non-nucleoside reverse transcriptase inhibitors (NNRTIs): NNRTIs also work by hindering the action of reverse transcriptase. This class of drugs includes delavirdine, nevirapine, and efavirenz.
- Protease inhibitors: Protease inhibitors interrupt a later stage of viral replication. This class of drugs includes saquinavir, indinavir, ritonavir, nelfinavir, and amprenavir.
- Fusion inhibitors: Fusion inhibitors prevent HIV from entering human immune cells. The only fusion inhibitor approved to date is enfuvirtide.

Studies have found that various combinations of antiretroviral drugs are more effective in suppressing HIV than antiretroviral drugs used alone. Experts refer to one common treatment approach, usually involving a protease inhibitor combined with two other antiretroviral drugs, as "highly active antiretroviral therapy" or "HAART".

Drug combinations, or drug "cocktails," also can help reduce the risk that drug-resistant HIV will develop. When drug resistance occurs, medications that initially succeeded in suppressing the replication of HIV in the patient's body, loose their effectiveness. Antiretroviral drugs have side effects that can limit their use in some people. AZT, for example, may result in a loss of blood cells and protease inhibitors can cause nausea, diarrhea, and other symptoms.

Treating AIDS-Related Conditions

Since opportunistic infections are common in HIV patients, several drugs and therapies are used to prevent or treat opportunistic infections and other AIDS-related conditions. Some of the drugs used to treat opportunistic infections are as follows:

- **Pneumocystis carinii pneumonia:** People who develop this lung infection are generally treated with TMP/SMX (a combination of antibiotic drugs) or pentamidine. Doctors also prescribe these medications as preventive therapy for adult patients whose CD4+ T cell counts fall below 200.
- **Yeast infections in women:** Physicians often prescribe a drug called fluconazole to treat yeast and other fungal infections. Fluconazole also can safely prevent vaginal and esophageal candidiasis without development of drug resistance.
- **Pelvic inflammatory disease:** PID is treated with antibiotics. Women with mild cases may be treated on an outpatient basis. HIV-positive pregnant women suspected of having PID are usually hospitalized, treated with intravenous antibiotics approved for use during pregnancy, and monitored closely.

- **HIV-related wasting:** Megestrol acetate (Megace) is often prescribed for HIV-associated wasting, but it can cause significant irregular vaginal bleeding in women. Another drug, nandrolone, may not have these side effects and is currently undergoing drug trials.
- **Kaposi's sarcoma and other cancers:** Cancers are treated with radiation, chemotherapy, or injections of alpha interferon, a genetically engineered, naturally occurring protein.
- **CMV Retinitis:** Improvements in anti-HIV treatments as well as preventive and therapeutic approaches to managing CMV have resulted in a decreased incidence of CMV retinitis. Today, the incidence of CMV retinitis is about one quarter what it was previous to the introduction of HAART. While early CMV retinitis therapies were delivered intravenously, current treatments include medications in pill form for all stages of CMV retinitis.

PROBLEMS WITH AIDS DRUG THERAPY:

AIDS drugs do not cure the condition, but they help to manage it and postpone life-threatening complications. However, there are problems with AIDS drug therapy:

Side effects of drugs are a major concern in treatment. Another major problem is the cost of the drugs used in treating AIDS.

Since antiviral drugs have so far not been curative, the hope is to find a vaccine. The technology for vaccine development is present, and serious efforts are being made to find one.

23

REPRODUCTIVE IMMUNOLOGY

Most multicellular animals mount allogeneic immune responses to protect themselves from invasion by foreign organisms. But in natural pregnancies, the embryo/fetus genetically different from the mother survives despite the presence of maternal T cells specific for paternally inherited histocompatibility antigens. If immune system is functional during pregnancy, the fetus carrying both maternal and paternal genes has to be rejected like that of a graft. It is a wonder of pregnancy that the fetus is not rejected by the mother's immune system. This situation comprises one of the major paradoxes of contemporary immunology, raising the question of how the genetically different embryo/fetus and mother co-exist during gestation.

Immunology of reproduction and tolerance of the genetically distinct embryo and its symbiotic existence with in the mother is one of the most essential and intriguing paradoxes of life. Since successful pregnancy of placental mammals depends on adaptation of the woman's immune system to tolerate a genetically foreign fetus, the adaptive immune system of placental mammals has evolved to tolerate the fetus. Rejection of the fetus by adaptive immune responses is therefore a rare event. The reproductive success of eutherian mammals, in which the maternal immune system is in direct contact with the semi-allogeneic fetus, depends on the ability to control allogeneic immune responses. Multiple, overlapping mechanisms exist to prevent maternal allogeneic immune responses towards the fetus while maintaining the capacity to mount a defense against infectious organisms.

Since sperm is a foreign entity in the female reproductive tract, the immune system should attack and destroy them before fertilization. In reality, however, the sperm is protected and stored to allow fertilization. In the case of sperm cells, the antigen markers that play a crucial role in recognition of foreign cells are different. As they are sugar-based they are recognised by everyone's immune system, and no immune response is triggered during reproduction between any two people. Scientists suggest that the female reproductive tract is equipped with sensory systems that recognize sperm and alert the ancient, non-specific "innate" immune system to dampen its reaction towards them.

Proteins in semen may smooth the way for fertilization, damping down mother's immune response to the implanting embryo, a crucial step in the success of pregnancy. The sperm exempted from immunological reaction of mother fuse with egg resulting in fertilization. Following fertilization the fertilized egg rapidly divides to form the blastocyst, a hollow ball of cells with an inner cell mass and outer layer. The inner cell mass gives rise to the embryo, which develops into a fetus about eight weeks after conception. The outer layer of the blastocyst becomes the so-called trophoblast. The trophoblast cells aggressively invade the mother's uterus lining, anchoring the placenta and widening the maternal arteries to enhance its blood supply. Cells from the implanted blastocyst migrate in massive numbers into the decidualized maternal endometrium. Within a few weeks of making its home in the uterus, the trophoblast further transforms into the fetal part of the placenta, the conduit for the passage of nutrients and oxygen from mother to fetus. (Some of the mother's cells form a second part of the mature placenta).

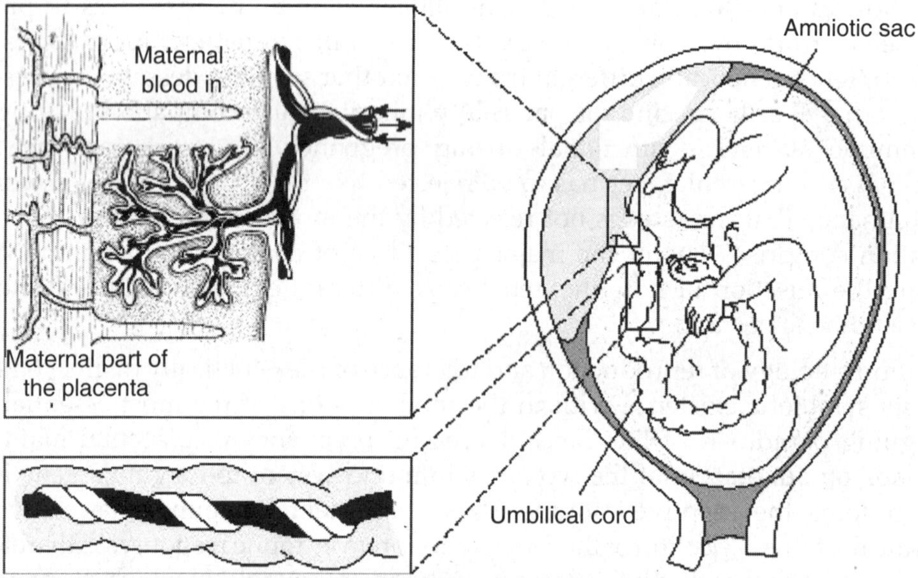

Fig: 23.1

This process of invasion of the extravillous trophoblast cells into the uterus is well balanced and finely controlled. There are delicate interactions at the implantation site with uterine natural killer (uNK) cells, macrophages and CD3-T cells. This results in production of the right balance of cytokines and chemokines, which control the extent of trophoblast infiltration and ultimately determines reproductive success. Trophoblast over-invasion endangers the mother. Trophoblast under-invasion and failure to modify the maternal spiral arteries leads to reproductive failure or complications.

On the fetal side of the interface, a specialized epithelial surface within the placenta, fetal syncytiotrophoblast cells directly contact maternal blood for nutrient exchange. On the maternal side of the interface, the uterine tissue (decidua) in contact with the placenta and fetal membranes is rich in specialized maternal immune cells including lymphocytes and macrophages. Despite the prolonged direct exposure of decidual leukocytes and maternal blood to fetal antigens, the immune system does not recognize the fetus as foreign.

The decidua is the maternal part of the placenta in which there is a close contact between maternal and fetal cells. Consequently, the decidual cells may play an important role in acceptance of the fetus and the control of trophoblast invasion. The deciduas contain a diverse population of cells, including decidualized stroma cells, lymphocytes, uterine NK cells (uNK cells), monocytes and epithelial cells

Many hypotheses have been proposed to explain the mechanisms of maternal-fetal immune tolerance. It is still however 'work in progress' since the early works of Medawar and his colleagues. Medawar in 1953 suggested that the immunological interaction between the mother and fetus is suppressed to allow survival of semi-allogeneic fetus till delivery. He articulated that this was due to anatomical separation of foetus from mother, antigenic immaturity of the foetus; and immunological indolence or inertness of the mother. Even though these theories have been refined and not correct to certain extent, somewhat they remain central to the present information in the area of reproductive immunology research.

Since various fetal cells (eg. trophoblasts) are in close contact with maternal (immune) cells there is no anatomical separation between the mother and the fetus as suggested by Medawar. However the fetal trophoblast cells do not express major histocompatibility complex (MHC)- the antigens required for antigen stimulation of maternal lymphocytes. Even though there is no general immune suppression, lymphocyte function indeed changes during pregnancy. This information strongly proposes that Medawar's suggestions cannot be discarded completely. The immunological paradox of pregnancy appears therefore to be extremely complex, and despite the vast body of knowledge about the subject there remain very many questions.

The mechanisms by which this state of tolerance is achieved are numerous and research continues to determine whether factors other than those described below are involved. These mechanisms work synergistically with an array of cytokines acting centrally to control the actions of cells, hormones and specialised immune system recognition and effector molecules.

Cytokines and TH1/TH2: Cytokines seem to play a key role in the maintenance of pregnancy via modulation of the immune system and associated cells. During the early stages of pregnancy, the conceptus and placental tissues produce a wide variety of cytokines, including interferons (IFN), interleukins (IL), tumour necrosis factor and granulocyte macrophage colony-stimulating factors (GM-CSF). These cytokines are believed to modulate the immune system in order that the foetus is not rejected.

Constitutive IL-4 expression has been reported in human amniotic and decidual tissues. IL-4 acts to suppress the TH1 response by inhibiting the production of IL-12 by macrophages and dendritic cells. Many studies have reported on the specific importance of IL-4 in the maintenance of pregnancy. Since TH1 cells are involved in delayed-type hypersensitivity reactions and associated with cytotoxic T cell functions they exert deleterious effects on pregnancy by inhibiting embryonic and fetal development. Decidual leukocytes and the preimplantaion embryo secrete IL-10, a cytokine that inhibits the proliferation and secretion of TH1 lymphocytes. As Th2 cytokines are associated with successful pregnancy shift towards Th2 cytokine production seems to be important for the continuation of pregnancy. Research data in reproductive immunology illustrate that various groups show significantly higher concentrations of the Th2 cytokines IL-6 and IL-10 at normal pregnancy. Conversely significantly increased concentrations of the Th1-type cytokine TNF- α were found in women with recurrent spontaneous abortions. In abortion-prone women who had a successful pregnancy, significantly higher concentrations of IL-6 and significantly lower concentrations of TNF- α were found as compared with abortion-prone women who had another abortion, supporting the notion that Th2- and Th1-bias are associated with successful and unsuccessful pregnancy respectively. The dramatic increase in pregnancy hormones (eg. progesterone and estrogen) may directly affect lymphocytes by shifting their cytokine production towards type 2. A progesterone induced blocking factor in lymphocytes might play an indirect role in shifting cytokine production towards type 2.

However, Th_1 responses may still be necessary to protect mother and foetus from pathogens, suggesting a systemic shift towards a Th_2 environment but not a complete suppression of Th_1 responses. They are able to function to protect the mother from a wide range of external pathogens for the term of her pregnancy, indicating that parts of her immune system must remain active to a greater or lesser degree.

Leukaemia inhibitory factor (LIF), synthesised and secreted by maternal endometrial and stromal cells, and its receptor are necessary for the implantation, differentiation and growth of trophoblast cells. LIF mRNA has also been demonstrated in decidual natural killer (NK) cells and T-cells (mainly of the Th^2 subset). Progesterone, IL-4 and IL-1 have been shown to up-regulate LIF production by endometrial cells while down-regulation is achieved via the actions of both IL-12 and IFN-γ (cytokines that induce Th_1 cells).

Leukaemia Inhibitory Factor: Leukaemia inhibitory factor (LIF), a cytokine of the interlukin- 6 family, is essential in blastocyst implantation. It is synthesised and secreted by maternal endometrial and stromal cells, and its receptor is necessary for the implantation, differentiation and growth of trophoblast cells. It also promotes the shift to TH_2. The embryo, prior to implantation sends signals to the endometrium. The expression of LIF and other cytokines in the uterine epithelium are gradually increased. LIF mRNA has also been demonstrated in decidual natural killer (NK) cells and T-cells (mainly of the TH_2 subset). Progesterone, IL-4 and IL-1 have been shown to up-regulate LIF production by endometrial cells while down-regulation is achieved via the actions of both IL-12 and IFN-γ (cytokines that induce TH_1 cells).

Major Histocompatibility Complex (MHC): During pregnancy mother's immune system has to remain tolerant of paternal major histocompatibility (MHC) antigens and yet maintain normal immune competence for defense against microorganisms. An unusual subset of major histocompatibility complex (MHC) Class I proteins of both maternal and paternal origin appears to play a key role in the mediation of tolerance at the maternal/fetal interface and in the control of preimplantation embryonic growth rate. Trophoblast cells fail to express MHC class I or class II molecules, essential for antigenic recognition by T-cells. The invasive extravillous cytotrophoblast and endovascular trophoblast cell subsets, however, express a unique subset of MHC Class I products HLA-C, HLA-G and HLA-E. HLA-G molecules appear to resemble classical HLA class I molecules in terms of intracellular assembly with β 2-microglobulin (β2m) and peptide fragments. Primary role of HLA-G may be the modulation of myelomonocytic cell behavior in pregnancy. It exhibits greatly decreased polymorphism when compared to other HLA and specifically binds natural killer cells via their killer-cell immunoglobulin-like receptors thus blocking their cytotoxity.

Coexpression of HLA-E and HLA-G in the invasive extravillous and endovascular trophoblast cells therefore suggests that either HLA-G itself interacts with an inhibitory receptor in NK cells, or both molecules act coordinately with HLA-C expressed in the same cell to regulate interactions with inhibitory and activatory NK receptors. Studies have shown that IL-10 produced by TH2 cells increases HLA-G production, thus protecting the foetus via the inhibition of NK cell medicated lysis. Some researchers suggest that HLA-E also have similar properties to HLA-G.

NK cells: In pregnant women, NK cells appear to be embryo toxic. The number of peripheral NK cells is decreased in pregnant women as compared with non-pregnant women. Besides a decrease in the number of NK cells, their production of IFN-g is also decreased. These changes in NK cell number and activity during pregnancy are also consistent with a shift from a cellular to a humoral immune response during pregnancy. In contrast to NK cells the number of uterine natural killer (uNK) cells which are normally present in the endometrium increases markedly during early pregnancy.

Uterine NK cells comprise the major lymphocyte population at implantation sites accounting for 30 – 90 % of the total number of cells during the first trimester. They are found only in the uterus and exhibit very limited killing mechanisms. These cells produce cytokines namely IFN-▯ necessary for the implantation of trophoblast cells early on in pregnancy. After implantation has taken place, these cells are thought to contribute to the modification of the uterine vasculature. Although the uNK cells are present in the decidua in large amounts, they do not attack the semi-allogeneic non-villous cytotrophoblast. This is due to the fact that uNK cells express inhibitory receptors. These receptors bind to the MHC Ia and b (HLA-C, HLA-E and HLA-G) on trophoblast, by binding to these MHC I antigens, the inhibitory receptors inhibit the lytic activity of the uNK cells. There are several types of inhibitory receptors on uNK cells, namely Ig-like killer cell inhibitory receptor (KIR) (eg. KIR2D, KIR2DL4) and lectin-like KIRs.

Because of the large number of uNK cells in the uterus during early pregnancy, it is suggested that they play an important role in protection against infections or in the regulation of immunity. uNK cell proliferation can be stimulated by either cytokines produced by other decidual cells, or by (steroid) hormones. The presence of uNK cells in the decidua may be explained by two mechanisms. The First mechanism is that peripheral blood uNK cells are selectively homing to the uterine mucosa, because they can interact with adhesion molecules on the decidual blood vessels. The second mechanism is insitu proliferation, as uNK are actively dividing.

It is well recognized that one function of the uNK cells is the production of cytokines. These uNK cell-derived cytokines influence placentation. Granulocyte colony-stimulating factor (G-CSF), granulocyte-macrophage colony-stimulating factor (GM-CSF), macrophage colony-stimulating factor (M-CSF) and leukaemia inhibitory factor (LIF) stimulate growth of the trophoblast. Colony-stimulating factors also promote trophoblast cell proliferation and differentiation, while LIF stimulates implantation.

The uNK cells undergo phenotypic transformation as gestation progresses. Midway through the gestation period, they characteristically display an absence of cytolytic activity and an increased production of effector molecules. Once pregnancy progresses into the second trimester, the numbers of these cells greatly decrease. Differentiation and proliferation of uNK cells is regulated by decidual stromal cell derived IL-15.

Uterine NK cells also act at the maternal-foetal interface to provide protection against attack from microorganisms that, if allowed to cross the placenta, would risk the viability of the foetus.

Macrophages: During implantation, apoptosis is critical for the appropriate tissue remodeling of the maternal decidua and invasion of the developing embryo. Yet the regulation of apoptosis is also imperative for a successful pregnancy. The quick and effective removal of apoptotic cells by tissue macrophages represents an essential process, which prevents the release of self-antigens and, in the case of pregnancy, paternal alloantigens. Hence macrophages have roles in the endometrial tissue remodeling and acquisition of epithelial cell adhesiveness which underpin the receptive state.

In humans, macrophages are spread through the pregnant uterus, including the decidua and are also associated with trophoblast cells of the placenta and extraplacental membranes. The macrophages that exhibit anti-inflammatory effects in placenta comprise 10 – 15 % of the total cell population. These cells, termed Hofbauer cells once activated, produce anti-inflammatory cytokines such as IL-10 and the level of cytotoxic free-oxygen species produced is greatly reduced (in some situations the levels are barely detectable) when compared to the amounts produced by "normal" macrophages.

The number of macrophages in the uterus may be affected by estrogens, as these hormones stimulate the influx of leukocytes (including macrophages) into the uterus. Moreover, cytotrophoblast can attract macrophages into the decidua by producing monocytes inflammatory protein-1 alpha. It seems clear that the number of uterine macrophages must be tightly controlled. Since significantly more macrophages were seen in pre-implantation endometrium of patients with recurrent miscarriage, than, in patients without these miscarriages. Because of the relative absence of other immune defence systems within the placental tissue, decidual macrophages are thought to have an important role in non-specific host defence in the placenta.

As they may be involved in the removal of cell and tissue debris associated with trophoblast invasion, macrophages play phagocytic role also. Macrophages are also suggested to have a role in placentation and in produced cytokines (TNF-a, TGF-b and colony stimulating factors). As indicated in the previous section, these cytokines are of major importance in successful pregnancy. Beside cytokines, macrophages can also produce immunosuppressive prostaglandins, which may block the function of Tc lymphocytes and uNK cells.

Regulatory T cells (Treg): Treg cells are potent suppressors of autoimmunity and allograft rejection. Treg cells are implicated in immune tolerance of the conceptus tissues, oocytes and spermatozoa.

They are reportedly present in the endometrium and decidua during normal pregnancies and absent in early pregnancy failure. Regulatory T cells (Treg) are believed to have a crucial role in maintaining pregnancy by creating a transient tolerant micro environment within the maternal uterus. Experimental study shows that Treg cells expand in lymph nodes of normal pregnant mice from day 2 of pregnancy. Abortion-prone mice present diminished numbers of Treg cells in immune organs throughout pregnancy. An enormous augmentation in the number of Treg cells in vaginal mucus of normal pregnant woman after conception is followed by an increase in Treg cell numbers in lymph nodes.

The raise of Treg cells suggests that they might be activated by male antigens for being protective. The antigen presentation would take place in the periphery of vaginal mucus - the first site of contact with paternal antigens, directly after insemination. Therefore Treg cells transfer might be effective in preventing abortion if done on days 0–2 of pregnancy. Treg cell-induced tolerance is transient, as Treg came back to the normal levels after the disappearance of the paternal/ fetal antigens (14 days post-partum). Treg cells might modulate the maturation and/or function of dendritic cells (DCs) required for effector T-cell activation.

Treg cells induce DCs to produce immunosuppressive molecules. Experimental study suggested that Treg cells may also downmodulate the capacity of DCs to activate effector T cells. Studies with human Treg cells have also indicated that Treg cells may also modulate the function of monocytes and macrophages. Treg cells could condition DCs, through a mechanism dependent on interactions with other cells to express indoleamine 2,3-dioxygenase (IDO), which is a potent regulatory molecule that induces the catabolism of tryptophan into pro-apoptotic metabolites that in turn cause suppression of effector T cells.

Lastly, Treg cells can also influence immune responses by modulating the recruitment and function of other cell types. For instance, Treg-cell-derived IL-9 has been shown to recruit and activate mast cells which were shown to be essential regulatory intermediaries in the establishment of peripheral allograph tolerance. As both pregnancy combinations (normal pregnancy and abortion-prone) present similar levels of progesterone, estriol and estrone, hormones do not seem to be involved in Treg expansion. However, they may be involved in their recruitment into the vaginal lumen. Unexplained infertility, miscarriage and pre-eclampsia are linked with numerical and functional Treg deficiency

Role of Indoleamine 2,-3-dioxygenase (IDO): The enzyme IDO, which degrades tryptophan, is expressed in syncytiotrophoblasts and macrophages during gestation. Indoleamine diogenase (IDO) is an enzyme that functions in the catabolism of tryptophan and indirectly suppresses maternal T-cell activity by tryptophan deprivation. In vitro, macrophages suppress T cell activity due to degradation of tryptophan by IDO, and the suppression is reversed by treatment with an IDO inhibitor. Likewise, the tryptophan concentration is significantly lower in pregnant women than in nonpregnant controls. IDO activity appears to protect the fetus by suppressing T-cell dependent inflammatory responses to fetal alloantigens, since syngeneic fetuses are not rejected after treatment with IDO inhibitor. Thus, trophoblasts and antigen-presenting cells in the placenta may protect the fetus via tryptophan catabolism, thus preventing a unique type of inflammation that involves T cell-dependent, antibody-independent complement activation. However, alternative mechanisms have been proposed to account for the results obtained with the IDO inhibitor, including indirect effects of IDO inhibition on vasoconstriction and macrophage activation, and death of T cells due to release of by-products of the IDO reaction, such as kynurerine, 3-hydroxykynurenine and 3-hydroxyanthranilic acid.

Apoptosis: Apoptosis is important for normal placental development. Trophoblast apoptosis increases in normal placentas as gestations proceeds. Apoptosis induction in immune cells has been proposed as a mechanism by which trophoblast cells are protected from anti-foetus immune cell destruction. Studies have suggested that, during the first trimester of pregnancy, Fas ligand (FasL) molecules are expressed on the inner cytotrophoblast and outer syncytiotrophoblast cells of the placenta as well as the maternal decidual cells of the placenta.

Fas/Fasligand systems play an important role in maintaining the balance at the implantation site as the mediators of programmed cell death. The trophoblast expresses Fas ligand, thereby conferring immune privilege: maternal immune cells expressing Fas will undergo apoptosis at the placenta/decidua interface. It is one of the pathways regulating T-cell proliferation and apoptosis and is sensitive to hormonal factors and cytokines. By way of expression of apoptosis-inducing ligands (FasL), trophoblast may escape attack by maternal immune cells. Induction of apoptosis by Fas Ligand (FasL) in invading lymphocytes acts as a mechanism of immune privilege.

The expression of FasL does not appear to be mandatory for pregnancy success, however. Other apoptosis-inducing pathways, such as binding of the TNF-related apoptosis-inducing ligand (TRAIL) to its receptor (TRAIL-R)

may play an immunoprotective role in the placenta, as TRAIL is expressed on trophoblast (especially syncytiotrophoblast). More recently, presence of other members of the death-inducing TNF superfamily ligands and their receptors have been shown to be expressed in the placenta. Thus, Fas-FasL and TRAIL- R apoptosis induction in maternal immune cells in the decidua might be important in maternal immunotolerance of the fetal allograft during pregnancy.

Macrophages present at the maternal-fetal interface may also contribute to trophoblast survival by removing apoptotic cells and producing cytokines and growth factors, which influence the progression of the apoptotic cascade.

Progesterone-dependent immunomodulation: The placenta continues to produce both progesterone and estrogen for the duration of the pregnancy and the levels get higher and higher right up to just before the birth. Progesterone converts the endometrium to its secretory stage to prepare the uterus for implantation. At the same time progesterone affects the vaginal epithelium and cervical mucus, making it thick and impermeable to sperm. If pregnancy does not occur, progesterone levels will decrease, leading to menstruation. During implantation and gestation, progesterone appears to decrease the maternal immune response to allow for the acceptance of the pregnancy.

Progesterone decreases contractility of the uterine smooth muscle. In addition progesterone inhibits lactation during pregnancy. The fall in progesterone levels following delivery is one of the triggers for milk production. A drop in progesterone levels is possibly one step that facilitates the onset of labour.

Progesterone is liberated by corpus luteum, due to the actions of IL-4 and IL-6 from TH2 cells, after ovulation and acts on the endometrium to prepare it for implantation. Throughout pregnancy, progesterone produced by the placental cells inhibits T-cell mediated graft rejection in the uterus. Lymphocytes of pregnant women have been shown to be particularly sensitive to the effects of progesterone compared to those of non-pregnant women. The state of pregnancy itself causes an increase in the number of progesterone receptors that are displayed on peripheral blood lymphocytes (PBL) making them more susceptible to progesterone's inhibitory mechanisms. It has been reported that in the presence of progesterone, lymphocytes secrete a 34 KDa protein blocking factor that has a direct inhibitory effect on the cytolytic effects of NK cells and PBL. Thus the presence of progesterone is necessary for the state of immunosuppression that must be achieved in order for the maintenance of pregnancy. This immunosuppression is only required in the uterus while peripheral immune mechanisms must be maintained at normal levels. This is achieved by high progesterone levels only being high enough to inhibit lymphocytes in the uterine environment only due to production by cells within the placenta. Additionally, other peripherally produced molecules regulate the actions of progesterone so as not to affect lymphocytes in an unwanted way. Progesterone also acts on syncytiotrophoblast cells driving them to produce cytokines that favour the TH2 environment necessary for successful pregnancy.

Complement System: Normal human pregnancy is associated with evidence of complement activation. It is determined by increased concentrations of the anaphylatoxins C3a, C4a and C5a in the maternal circulation. Complement components found in the placental tissue derive to a large extent from blood circulating in placental vessels. However, some complement components may also be produced locally by macrophages and other cell types. Presence of paternal antigens on the surface of placental cells would almost certainly initiate complement-mediated destruction of the placenta and foetus if there is no inhibitory mechanism. Successful pregnancy is maintained by the expression of complement regulatory proteins expressed on trophoblast, which prevent damage inflicted by complement activation. These complement regulators are localized in a strategic position on the surface of villous trophoblast protecting the fetus from the damage that may derive from uncontrolled complement activation. Decay-accelerating factor (CD55) and membrane cofactor protein (CD46) are complement regulatory proteins expressed on human trophoblast and are crucial for sustaining pregnancy. Hence physiologic activation of the complement system during pregnancy is a compensatory mechanism aimed to protect the host against infection.

Research suggests that complement activation (or failure of its suppression) in early gestation leads to a greater risk of preterm labor. By measuring serum levels of one of the complement activation fragments (called Bb), the researchers were able to show an association between abnormally high levels and spontaneous preterm delivery prior to 34 weeks of gestation. Complement activation or inhibition may be crucial in the treatment of unexplained recurrent pregnancy losses.

Blocking Antibodies: Serum blocking factors during pregnancy period may also help in successful continuation of the fetus as an allograft. In vitro cellular-immune reactivity to paternal alloantigens was demonstrated in multigravid women by production of lymphocyte migration inhibitory factor. Study of serum from normal multigravid women showed the presence of a factor that blocked production of migration inhibitory factor by maternal lymphocytes to paternal antigens in a specific manner. The blocking factor was an IgG antibody. Women who experience idiopathic spontaneous abortions produce lymphocyte migration inhibitory factor to paternal alloantigens, but their serums lack the blocking factor, whose activity was removed by absorption with paternal lymphocytes but not with pooled human platelets. Research data support the concept that PIBF may play an important role in early implantation, possibly by inhibiting the destructive function of natural killer lymphocytes. The percentage of PIBF expressing lymphocytes increases as a result of pregnancy and that the stimulus for PIBF induction occurs soon after implantation.

Miscarriage or spontaneous abortions

The term miscarriage is used to describe any pregnancy loss before 20 weeks of gestation. Miscarriages are often referred to as "spontaneous abortions", because they can happen without warning. Up to 25% of women will experience at least one miscarriage during their childbearing years. Some women will experience more than one miscarriage in their lifetime. Up to 50% of pregnancies are actually thought to end in miscarriage, however, many of these pregnancy losses occur before the woman even knows she is pregnant. The risk of miscarriage increases with age; women over the age of 40 have a 30% chance of experiencing a miscarriage.

Most miscarriages occur before the end of the first trimester that is before the twelfth week of pregnancy. These miscarriages are called early miscarriages. Though less common, some miscarriages do occur into the second trimester.

Any woman can experience a miscarriage; however, certain women are at increased risk. Risk factors include smoking during pregnancy, consumption of alcohols; narcotics etc., having certain sexually transmitted diseases, or infections, thyroid problems, diabetes, suffering from certain autoimmune diseases etc.

Symptoms of Miscarriage: Symptoms of a miscarriage include:

Vaginal bleeding that doesn't stop within a few days, abdominal cramping, lower backache, heavy bleeding accompanied by clots or tissue.

CAUSE OF RE OCCURING MISCARRIAGE: There are several factors which cause reoccurring miscarriages. Some of them are as follows:

(1) Hormaonal Imbalences: These include

(a) LutealPhase Defect (LPD): In this case the woman does not produce enough progesterone after ovulation to prepare the uterine lining for implantation. Low progesterone level is the most common problem.

(b) Thyroid hormone. Hypothyroidism and hyperthyroidism are two different problems associated with thyroid hormone. Only hypothyroidism is believed to be a threat to pregnancy. Hyper is suspected, but not yet proven. Inadequate levels of Thyroid hormone may interfere with Follicle Stimulating Hormone (FSH) and this will affect the ovaries.

(c) Insulin hormone/ Diabetes: when the pancreas isn't producing enough insulin to control glucose levels in blood, the irregular blood glucose levels can cause miscarriage.

Chromosome Defects: Chromosome defects that cause a newly fertilized egg to die can account for as much as 60 percent of early miscarriages. Even if both the egg and sperm come with perfect chromosomes, the first few cell divisions can see an abnormality crop up that would certainly be devastating. Miscarriage due to chromosome defects increase with an increase of age.

Physical Problem with the Uterus or Cervix: Some women have a uterus that does not have the usual shape. Others have a cervix that may be weakened by a number of causes, including multiple D&C(dilation and curettage) procedures or their mother taking DES when she was pregnant. Both of these problems can cause early labor, usually during a critical period from 12-24 weeks. This cause is responsible for 12 percent of miscarriages during this period. As the baby grows, especially during the very rapid growth spurt during this time frame, the irregularly shaped uterus may not be able to expand or the weak cervix may start to open up and let the baby out.

Immune Disorders: Antiphospholipid antibodies can cause blood clots in the placenta that block or slow down the baby's blood supply, causing growth to slow or the baby to die altogether. While a miscarriage due to this problem can happen at any time, often the baby will grow past the first trimester. 10 to 15% of recurring miscarriages are caused by these antibodies. Fetal-Blocking Antibodies work to protect the baby from the mother's immune system, which will recognize the father's genetic material as foreign to her body and attack it. Failure of Fetal-Blocking Antibodies by mothers immune system usually causes an early miscarriage, well before 12 weeks, and is often suspected when several miscarriages have occurred at exactly the same time in the pregnancy

Premature Rupture of Membranes and Early Labor (PROM): Most women who have leaking or gushing amniotic fluid face early Labor due to PROM. It is thought largely to be caused by infections or inflammation of the uterus or fetal membranes. How these infections come or why they cause the membrane rupture is not completely understood.

Others - Infections, Age, Chronic Disease

Many infections can cause miscarriage, but they are the big ones like syphilis, mycoplasma, toxoplasmosis, and malaria. Infections that directly affect the uterus are bigger risk. This does not include yeast infections, which are extremely common in pregnancy.

Sometimes a pregnancy ends unhappily, but it is not technically a miscarriage. This occurs on the following situations:

1. Blighted Ovum is a condition where the gestational sac grows, the woman gets all the pregnancy symptoms, but the baby itself never develops. A blighted ovum is believed to be caused by an egg or sperm with poor genetic material. When the egg is fertilized, instead of creating both a sac and a baby, the baby never grows.

2. Ectopic Pregnancy is a normal fertilized egg that gets stuck in the fallopian tube (although occasionally it will fall into the abdominal cavity) and implants there. This type of pregnancy cannot survive and puts the mother at great risk for severe hemorrhaging and possibly even death as the baby grows and eventually bursts the tube. When the ectopic is discovered based on pain and symptoms rather than an early ultrasound, the mother should immediately have surgery to remove the baby. Ectopics are usually caused by scar tissue in the fallopian tubes that could have been caused by: previous surgery in the pelvic region, uterus, or tubes; a pelvic infection such as pelvic inflammatory disease; or endometriosis that blocks the entrance to the tubes.

3. Molar Pregnancy is a very rare type of pregnancy where an abnormal mass forms inside the uterus after the egg is fertilized. The baby usually does not form, but the uterus is filled with big bubble clusters. A molar pregnancy is caused when a sperm fertilizes an empty egg (called a complete molar pregnancy) and no baby grows, or when two sperm fertilize an egg and both the baby as well as an abnormal placenta grow (called a partial molar.) Even if a baby does grow, it cannot survive. In about 15% of molar pregnancies (usually complete molars and not partial), the moles spread to other parts of the body like cancer. A mild form of chemotherapy will have to be used (with methotrexate), but rest assured that the cure rate for this type of disease is very high. The signs of a molar pregnancy include: bleeding in the 12th week of pregnancy, a uterus that is larger than normal, and HCG levels are too high.

4. Stillbirth is technically any pregnancy that ends after the 20th week and the baby does not survive. Some babies die in uterus and are discovered when the heartbeat is not found. The most common causes of this are: uterine abnormalities, a knot or other umbilical cord accident, infections of the lining of the gestational sac or cord, and placental abruptions that cause the placenta to pull away from the uterine wall. These babies are usually born through the induction of labor

Other babies are lost through early labor. The causes of early labor are premature rupture of membranes, uterine abnormalities that make the uterus too small to hold the baby, and an incompetent cervix, which opens up and lets the baby out. Sometimes a stillbirth occurs during the birth, by an umbilical cord that gets pinched between the baby's head and the cervix, or the cord wraps around the baby's neck.

GLOSSARY

Accessory cell: A cell required to initiate immune response often used to describe antigen-presenting cell (see also ***antigen-presenting cell***).

Accessory molecules: Molecules other than the antigen receptor and major histocompatability complex (MHC) that participate in cognitive, activation, and effector functions of t lymphocyte responsiveness.

Acquired immune response / Adaptive immune response: The response of antigen-specific lymphocytes to antigen including the development of immunologic memory; also known as acquired immune response. (See ***antibody-dependent, cell-mediated cytotoxity***).

Acute-phase proteins: A series of proteins, found in the blood shortly after the onset of an infection, that participates in the early phases of host defense against infection.

Acute-phase response (apr): An early response stimulated by cytokines which include interleukin-1, interleukin-6, interferons and tumor necrosis factor.

Adenosine deaminase (ada) deficiency: A form of severe combined immunodeficiency (scid) in which affected individuals lack an enzyme, adenosine deaminase (ada), which catalyzes the deamination of adenosine as well as deoxyadenosine to produce inosine and deoxyinosine, respectively.

Adhesion molecules: Molecules that mediate the binding of one cell to other cells or to extracellular matrix proteins, integrins, selectins, and members of the immunoglobulin gene superfamily. These molecules are important in the operation of the immune system.

Adjuvant: A substance, given with antigen that enhances the response to the injected antigen.

Adoptive transfer: The transfer of the capacity to make an immune response by transplantation of immunocompetent cells.

Affinity: A measure of the binding constant of a single antigen combining site with a monovalent antigenic determinant.

Affinity maturation: The sustained increase in affinity of antibodies for an antigen with time following immunization.

Agammaglobulinemia: See x-linked agammaglobulinemia.

Agglutination: The aggregation of particulate antigen by antibodies.

Alleles: Two or more alternate forms of a gene that occupies the same position or locus on a specific chromosome.

Allelic exclusion: The ability of heterozygous lymphoid cells to produce only one allelic form of antigen-specific receptor (Ig or TCR) when they have the genetic endowment to produce both.

Allergen: An antigen responsible for producing allergic reactions by inducing IgE formation.

Allergic asthma: It is constriction of the bronchial tree due to an allergic reaction to inhaled antigen.

Allergic rhinitis: It is an allergic reaction in the nasal mucosa, also known as hay fever, that causes runny nose, sneezing and tears.

Allergy: A term covering immune reactions to non pathogenic antigens, which lead to inflammation and deleterious effects in the host.

Allogeneic: Genetically dissimilar within the same species.

Allograft: A tissue transplant (graft) between two genetically nonidentical members of a species.

Allotypes: Antigenic determinants present in allelic (alternate) forms.

Alternate (alternative) pathway: The mechanism of complement activation that does not involve activation of the C1, C4, C2 pathway by antigen-antibody complexes, and begins with the activation of C3.

Alveolar macrophage: A macrophage found in the lung alveoli that may remove inhaled particulate matter.

Anaphylatoxin: Substance capable of releasing histamine from mast cells and basophils.

Anaphylaxis: Immediate hypersensitivity response to antigenic challenge, mediated by IgE and mast cells.

Anergy: A state of antigen-specific non responsiveness in which a T or B cell is present but functionally unable to respond to antigen.

Ankylosing spondylitis: A chronic inflammatory disease affecting the spine, sacroiliac joints, and large peripheral joints.

Antibody: Serum protein formed in response to antigen and involved in immune response.

Antibody-dependent, cell-mediated cytotoxicity (ADCC): A phenomenon in which target cells, coated with antibody, are destroyed by specialized killer cells (NK cells and macrophages), which bear receptors for the Fc portion of antibody.

Antigen: Any foreign material that is capable of inducing immune response.

Antigen presentation: The display of antigen as peptide fragments bound to MHC molecules on the surface of a cell.

Antigen processing: Large foreign molecules are broken down (processed) within macrophages into peptides and presented through MHC molecules.

Antigen receptor: The specific antigen-binding receptor on Tor B lymphocytes.

Antigen-binding site: The part of an immunoglobulin molecule or T-cell receptor that binds antigen specifically.

Antigenic determinant: A single antigenic site or epitope on a complex antigenic molecule or particle.

Antigen-presenting cell (APC): A specialized type of cell, bearing cell-surface class II MHC (see ***major histocompatibility complex***) molecules, involved in processing and presentation of antigen to T cells.

Anti-immunoglobulin antibodies: Antibodies against immunoglobulin constant domins that are useful for detecting bound antibody molecules in immunoassays and other applications.

Antiserum (plural: antisera): The fluid component of clotted blood contain heterogeneous collections of antibodies, which bind the antigen used for immunization.

Antitoxin: Antibody specific for exotoxins produced by certain microorganisms such as the causative agents of diphtheria and tetanus.

Apc see ***antigen-presenting cell***.

Apoptosis: A form of programmed cell death caused by activation of endogenous molecules leading to the fragmentation of DNA.

Appendix: A vestigial prgan with gut-associated lymphoid tissue located at the beginning of the colon.

Arthus reaction: A hypersensitivity reaction produced by local formation of antigen-antibody aggregates that activate the complement cascade and cause thrombosis, hemorrhage, and acute inflammation.

Asthma: A disease of the lungs characterized by reversible airway obstruction (in most cases), inflammation of the airway with prominent eosinophil participation, and increased responsiveness by the airway to various stimuli.

Atopy: A term used to describe IgE-mediated allergic responses in humans.

Autograft: A tissue transplant from one area to another on a single individual.

Autoimmunity (autoallergy): An immune response to "self" tissues or components and the immune response may have pathologic consequences leading to autoimmune diseases.

Avidity: the summation of multiple affinities, for example when a polyvalent antibody binds to a polyvalent antigen.

B cell / B lymphocyte: Lymphocyte which develops in the bone marrow or in bursa of Fabricus and binds antigen with membrane antibody (immunoglobulin).

B7: A costimulatory homodimeric immunoglobulin superfamily protein whose expression is restricted to the surface of accessory cells (e.g. B cells and macrophages) that interact with T lymphocytes

Bare lymphocyte syndrome: Immune deficiency resulting from a deficiency of some or all MHC molecules.

Basophil: A polymorphonuclear leukocyte, whose granules contain heparin, histamine and other vasoactive amines. Within tissues, these cells are known as mast cells.

BCR B cell (antigen) receptor, also called membrane immunoglobulin (mIg).

Bence-jones protein: Dimers of immunoglobulin light chains in the urine of patients with multiple myeloma.

Blocking antibody: A functional term for an antibody molecule capable of blocking the interaction of antigen with other antibodies or with cells.

Bone marrow: The site of hematopoiesis, in which stem cells give rise to the cellular elements of blood, including red blood cells, monocytes, polymorphonuclear leukocytes, platelets, and lymphocytes.

Bone marrow transplantation: A procedure used to treat both non neoplastic and neoplastic conditions not amenable to other forms of therapy.

Bronchus-associated lymphoid tissue (Balt): Secondary lymphoid organs connected to the bronchial tree.

Bursa of fabricius: An outpouching of the cloaca in birds and is the site of development of B cells in birds.

CAM: Cell adhesion molecule; membrane molecule that allows cells to adhere.

Carcinoembryonic antigen (CEA): A membrane glycoprotein epitope that is present in the fetal gastrointestinal tract in normal conditions.

Carrier: A large immunogenic molecule or particle to which a hapten or other non immunogenic, epitope-bearing molecule may attach, allowing it to become immunogenic.

Carrier protein: Protein covalently linked with a small molecule (hapten) to increase the hapten's ability to induce immunity.

CD antigen or cluster of differentiation: Membrane proteins on immune system cells that allow for their identification and isolation.

CD3: Part of the Tcell (antigen) receptor complex. CD3 transduces the antigen binding signal outside the plasma membrane into chemical signals (phosphorylation) in the cytoplasm.

CD4: Co-receptor on helper T cells that binds class II MHC and participates in T cell activation by antigen.

CD8: Co-receptor on cytotoxic T cells that binds class I MHC and participates in Tcell activation by antigen.

CDNA library: Collection of cDNA (complementary DNA) sequences from the mRNA of an organism in vectors; includes only exon DNA sequences from expressed genes.

CEA see *carcinoembryonic antigen*.

Cell adhesion molecule: Membrane molecule that allows cells to adhere (cam).

Cell line: Cells which can be cloned and propagated indefinitely in tissue culture.

Cell-mediated cytotoxicity (CMC): Killing (lysis) of a target cell by an effector lymphocyte.

Cell-mediated immunity (CMI): Immune reaction mediated by T cells, in contrast to humoral immunity, which is antibody-mediated.

Cellular immunity: Immunity which can be transferred between individuals with the transfer of T cells.

Central lymphoid organs : Sites of lymphocyte development.

Chediak-Higashi Syndrome: A childhood disorder with an autosomal recessive mode of inheritance that is identified by the presence of large lysosomal granules in leukocytes that are very stable and undergo slow degranulation.

Chemokine: Cytokines released by a variety of cells and involved in the migration and activation primarily of phagocytic cells and lymphocytes.

Chemotaxis: Movement of a cell in a chemical gradient, promoted by chemokines and anaphylatoxins.

Chimera: Refers to an individual containing cellular components derived from another genetically distinct individual.

Chimeric antibody: Antibody encoded by genes from more than one species, usually with antigen-binding regions from mouse genes and constant regions from human genes.

Chronic desensitization: Exposure to very low doses of allergen over time to decrease allergic reactions to that allergen.

Chronic granulomatous disease: Disease characterized by the presence of many granulomas, small nodules of inflammatory cells, usually associated with persistent infections or autoimmune inflammation.

Chronic lymphocytic leukemia (CLL): A B cell leukemia in which long-lived small lymphocytes continually collect in the spleen, lymph nodes, bone marrow, and blood.

Class I MHC: MHC proteins that present antigen synthesized in an infected cell's cytosol to cytotoxic T cells.

Class II MHC: MHC proteins that present antigen taken up in phagocytic or endocytic vesicles to helper T cells.

Class II-associated invariant chain peptide: A peptide of variable length cleaved from the invariant chain by proteases.

Classical complement pathway: The mechanism of complement activation initiated by antigen-antibody aggregates and proceeding by way of C1 to C9.

Clonal anergy: The interaction of a B or T lymphocyte with an antigen leading to its functional inactivation. Anergy can result when the lymphocyte interacts with antigen in the absence of a second signal, usually required for cell activation.

Clonal deletion: Elimination of all lymphocytes that bind a particular antigen; mechanism that normally prevents autoimmune reactions.

Clonal selection: Stimulation of antigen-specific lymphocytes to proliferate and become active effector cells that eliminate that antigen.

Clone: Many identical copies of a gene or a cell, produced from a single precursor.

Cold agglutinin: An antibody that agglutinates particulate antigen, such as bacteria or red cells, optimally at temperatures less than 37°.

Colony-stimulating factors (CSF): Glycoproteins that govern the formation, differentiation and function of hematopoietic progenitor cells (stem cells).

Combinatorial joining: The joining of segments of DNA to generate new combinations of Ig or TCR genes during the development of B and T cells. Combinatorial joining allows multiple opportunities for two sets of genes to combine in different ways.

Common variable immunodeficiency (CVID): A relatively common congenital or acquired immunodeficiency that may be either familial or sporadic.

Complement: A series of serum proteins involved in the mediation of immune reactions.

Complement receptors (CR): Cell-surface proteins on various cells that recognize and bind complement proteins that have bound pathogens or other antigens.

Complete freund's adjuvant (cfa): see ***freund's complete adjuvant***.

Conformational epitopes: Discontinuous epitopes on a protein antigen that are formed from several separate regions in the primary sequence of a protein when brought together by protein folding. Antibodies that bind conformational epitopes bind only native-folded proteins.

Congenic (also coisogenic): Describes two individuals who differ only in the genes at a particular locus and are identical at all other loci.

Constant region (c region): The invariant carboxyl-terminal portion of an immunoglobulin or TCR molecule, as distinct from the variable region at the amino terminus of the chain.

Contact dermatitis: A Type iv, T lymphocyte-mediated hypersensitivity reaction of the delayed type that develops in response to an allergen applied in the skin.

Contact hypersensitivity: A form of delayed-type hypersensitivity (type iv) in which T cells respond to antigens that are introduced by contact with the skin.

Convertase: An enzymatic activity that converts a complement protein into its reactive form by cleaving it.

Coombs test: A test named for its originator, R.R.A. Coombs, used to detect antibodies by addition of an anti-immunoglobulin antibody.

Corticosteroids: Steroid hormones (e.g. cortisone) that are lympholytic and are derived from the adrenal cortex.

Costimulatory molecules: Membrane-bound or secreted products of accessory cells that activate signal transduction events in addition to those induced by MHC TCR interactions. They are required for full activation of T cells.

CR: see ***complement receptors***.

C-reactive protein (CRP): Is a serum protein produced by liver cells as part of the acute phase response. It binds to phosphatidylcholine, a component of the surface of many bacteria, as a result of CRP binding to its surface, the bacterium is more easily taken up ***(opsonized)*** by phagocytic cells.

Cross-reactivity: The ability of an antibody, specific for one antigen, to react with a second antigen; a measure of relatedness between two different antigenic substances.

Cyclosporin: A drug that suppresses the immune system, specifically T cell activation.

Cytokine antagonist: Molecule that interferes with cytokine function.

Cytokine pleiotropism: A cytokine has more than one function.More than one cytokine has the same function.

Cytokine receptors: Cellular receptors for cytokines. Binding of the cytokine to the cytokine receptor stimulates signal transduction resulting in new activities in the cell, such as growth, differentiation, or death.

Cytokine: Small molecule secreted from one cell that signals another cell by binding to its specific receptor.

Cytokine synergism: Ability of cytokines to act together to promote more activity than either can generate alone.

Cytotoxic T cell: T cell which kills virus-infected cells and tumor cells.

Cytotoxins: Proteins made by cytotoxic T cells that participate in the destruction of target cells.

D gene: A small segment of immunoglobulin heavy-chain and T-cell receptor DNA, coding for the third hypervariable region of most receptors.

Delayed type hypersensitivity (DTH): A T cell-mediated reaction to antigen, which takes 24-48 hours to develop fully, and which involves release of lymphokines and recruitment of monocytes and macrophages.

Determinant: Part of the antigen molecule which binds to an antibody-combining site or to a receptor on T cells.

Differentiation antigen: A cell surface antigenic determinant found only on cells of a certain lineage and at a particular developmental stage; used as an immunologic marker.

Domain: A compact segment of an immunoglobulin molecule, made up of about 110 amino acids around an s-s bond, and encoded by a unique segment of DNA, surrounded by nontranslated sequences.

DR antigens: MHC class II molecules found on B cells and antigen-presenting cells of humans.

D gene: A small segment of immunoglobulin heavy-chain or t-cell receptor dna, coding for the third hypervariable region of the receptors.

Decay-accelerating factor (DAF): A membrane glycoprotein of normal human erythrocytes, leukocytes, and platelets, but absent from the red blood cells of paroxysmal nocturnal hemaglobulinuria patients. It facilitates dissociation of classical complement pathway C3 convertase (C4b2a) into C4b and C2a.

Degranulation: A mechanism whereby cytoplasmic granules in cells fuse with the cell membrane to discharge the contents from the cell. A classic example is degranulation of the mast cell or basophil in immediate (type i) hypersensitivity.

Delayed-type hypersensitivity (DTH): A form of cell-mediated immunity elicited by antigen present in the body. The reaction is mediated by TD cells and involves release of cytokines and recruitment of monocytes and macrophages. It is called "delayed-type" because the reaction appears hours to days (usually 24-48 hours) after antigen is injected.

Dendritic cell: Cell with long processes (dendrites) that presents antigen. They are nterdigitating reticular cells, derived from bone-marrow precursors that are found in T-cell areas of lymphoid tissues. They have a branched or dendritic morphology and are the most potent stimulators of T-cell responses.

Desensitization: A procedure in which allergic individuals are exposed to increasing doses of allergen with the goal of inhibiting their allergic reactions.

Diapedesis: It is the movement of blood cells, particularly leukocytes, from the blood across blood vessel walls into tissues.

Digeorge syndrome: Is a recessive genetic immunodeficiency disease in which there is a failure to develop thymic epithelium, and is associated with absent parathyroid glands and large vessel anomalies.

Diphtheria toxoid: An immunizing preparation generated by formalin inactivation of *corynebacterium diphtheriae* exotoxins, used in the active immunization of children against diphtheria.).

DNA vaccine: vaccine in which antigen DNA is injected and expressed in host cells; the expressed antigen stimulates an immune response.

Domine: A compact segment of an immunoglobulin or TCR chain, made up of amino acids around an s-s bond.

Double negative T cell: Immature T cell which expresses neither CD4 nor CD8 on its membrane. Double-negative thymocytes are immature T cells within the thymus that lack expression of the two co-receptors, CD4 and CD8.

Double positive T cell: Immature T cell which empresses both CD4 and CD8 on its membrane. Double-positive thymocytes are an intermediate stage in t-cell development in the thymus and are characterized by expression of both the CD4 and the CD8 co-receptor proteins.

DTH: Delayed type (Type IV) hypersensitivity. TH1 cells activate macrophages to eliminate antigen.

EBV: Epstein barr virus; infects B cells.

Ecam: Endothelial cell adhesion molecule. see ***adhesion molecules***.

Eczema: Skin rash, often occurs in response to antigen.

Effector cell: Activated cell which participates in antigen elimination.

Electroporation: A technique used to get cloned DNA into a cell; an electric current causes pores to form in the cell's membrane through which DNA enters.

ELISA: Enzyme-linked immunosorbent assay, which detects antigen-antibody binding using antibody complexed with an enzyme that forms a colored product from a colorless substrate.

ELIspot assay: It is an adaptation of ELISA in which cells are placed over antibodies or antigens attached to a plastic surface.

Encapsulated bacteria: Thet have thick carbohydrate coats that protect them from phagocytosis. encapsulated bacteria can cause extracellular infections and are effectively engulfed and destroyed by phagocytes only if they are first coated with antibody and/or complement produced in an adaptive immune response.

Endocytosis: A mechanism whereby substances are taken into a cell from the extracellular fluid by pinching off plasma membrane vesicles.

Endogenous antigen: Antigen synthesized in the cell cytoplasm, presented on class I MHC.

Endogenous pyrogens: Cytokines (e.g. IL-1, TNF-□) that can induce a rise in body temperature. They are distinct form exogenous substances such as endotoxin from gram-negative bacteria that induce fever by triggering endogenous pyrogen synthesis.

Endotoxins: Bacterial toxins that are released when bacterial cells are damaged or destroyed.

Eosinophil: Granulocytic white blood cell with cytosolic granules that stain with acidic dyes (eosin). Eosinophils have FC receptors for IgE and are efficient at killing worm parasites.

Epidemiology: Study of disease transmission.

Epitope: An alternative term for antigenic determinant. It is a part of antigen bound by antibody or TCR.

Erythroblastosis fetalis: A human fetal disease induced by IgG antibodies passed across the placenta from mother to fetus that are specific for fetal red blood cells, leading to their destruction.

Erythropoietin: A glycoprotein produced by the kidney, based on the presence of substances such as heme in the kidneys which are oxygen sensitive. it stimulates red blood cell production.

Exocytosis: The release of intracellular vesicle content to the exterior of the cell. The vesicles make their way to the plasma membrane, with which they fuse to permit the contents to be released to the external environment.

Exogenous antigen: Antigen synthesized outside the APC, phagocytosed or endocytosed into vesicles, and processed for presentation on class II MHC.

Fab: Fragment of antibody containing the antigen-binding site, generated by cleavage of the antibody with the enzyme papain, which cuts at the hinge region n-terminally to the inter-H-chain disulphide bond and generates two Fab fragments from one antibody molecule.

Fc: Fragment of antibody without antigen-binding sites, generated by cleavage with papain; the Fc fragment contains the c-terminal domains of the heavy immunoglobulin chains.

Fc receptor (FcR): A receptor on a cell surface with specific binding affinity for the Fc portion of an antibody molecule. Fc receptors are found on many types of cells.

Fluorescent antibody: An antibody coupled with a fluorescent dye, used with a fluorescence microscope to detect antigen on cells, tissues, or microorganisms.

Freund's complete adjuvant: A water-in-oil emulsion that contains an immunogen, an emulsifying agent, and killed mycobacteria which enhance the immune response to the immunogen; termed "incomplete" freund's adjuvant if mycobacteria are not included.

FACS: Fluorescence-activated cell sorter; equipment used to count and separate leukocytes labeled with fluorescent-tagged antibodies to cell surface molecules.

Factor B: An alternative complement pathway component which combines with C3b and is cleaved by factor d to produce alternative pathway C3 convertase.

Factor H: A regulator of complement in the blood that unites with C3b and facilitates dissociation of alternative complement pathway C3 convertase.

Farmer's lung: It is a hypersensitivity disease caused by the interaction of IgG antibodies with large amounts of an inhaled allergen in the alveolar wall of the lung, causing alveolar wall inflammation and compromising gas exchange.

Fas: A member of the TNF receptor family that is expressed on certain cells and makes them susceptible to killing by cells expressing Fas ligand. Binding of Fas ligand to Fas triggers apoptosis in the Fas-bearing cells.

Fas ligand (FasL): A cell-surface member of the tnf family of proteins. Binding of fas ligand to fas triggers apoptosis in the fas-expressing cell.

Fever: Increase in body temperature over the normal 98.6f (37c).

Flow cytometry: Process used to detect and quantify fluorescent antibody bound to leukocytes.

Fluorescence-activated cell sorter (FACS): An instrument that uses a laser to differentially deflect cells bound to fluorochrome-linked antibodies thus sorting the cells into fluorescent-positive and fluorescent-negative populations.

Fluorescent antibody: An antibody coupled with a fluorescent dye, used to detect antigen on cells, tissues, or microorganisms.

Fluorochrome: Small fluorescent tag which allows for detection of antibodies.

Follicle: Circular or oval areas of lymphocytes in lymphoid tissues rich in B cells. They are present in the cortex of lymph nodes and in the splenic white pulp. Follicle in immunology is an area in spleen or lymph node occupied by B cells and FDC.

Follicular dendritic cells (FDC): Cells within lymphoid follicles which are crucial in selecting antigen-binding B cells during antibody responses.

Freund's complete adjuvant: An oil containing killed mycobacteria and an emulsifier, which, when emulsified with an immunogen in aqueous solution, enhances the immune response to that immunogen after injection.

Gag protein antigen(s): They are present in the virus capsid. *gag*, gene for viral capsid protein(s).

GALT: Gut-associated lymphoid tissues

Gamma delta T cells: T cells with TCR composed of gamma and delta chains instead of the more usual alpha and beta chains.

Gamma globulin: Fraction of serum which contains most antibody molecules.

Gel electrophoresis: Technique used to separate proteins and fragments of DNA or RNA.

Gel-shift analysis: Technique for identifying regulatory regions of DNA by their altered electrophoretic mobility in the presence of protein regulators.

Gene expression: Production of mRNA and synthesis of a functional protein

Genetic immunization: It is a novel technique for inducing adaptive immune responses in which a plasmid DNA encoding a protein of interest is injected, usually into muscle; the protein is then expressed in vivo and elicits antibody and t-cell responses to the protein encoded by the DNA.

Genome: Nucleic acids representing entire genetic information of an organism; in humans, all 46 chromosomes.

Germ line: Refers to genes in germ cells as opposed to somatic cells. In immunology, it refers to genes in their unrearranged state rather than those rearranged for production of immunoglobulin or TCR molecules.

Germinal center: Concentration of rapidly dividing B cells in the spleen and lymph nodes.

Glomerulonephritis: A group of diseases characterized by glomerular injury. Immune mechanisms are responsible for most cases of primary glomerulonephritis and many of the secondary glomerulonephritis group.

Goodpasture's syndrome: Autoimmune disease in which vascular disease is caused by auto antibodies to Type IV collagen or basement membrane.

Graft rejection: Immune process that kills transplanted non-self tissue.

Graft versus host reaction (GVH): The pathologic consequences of a response initiated by transplanted immunocompetent T lymphocytes into an allogeneic, immunologically incompetent host.

Granulocyte: A leukocyte with a lobed nucleus and prominent cytoplasmic granules.

Granulocyte-macrophage colony-stimulating factor (GM-CSF): A cytokine involved in the growth and differentiation of myeloid and monocytic lineage cells, including dendritic cells, monocytes and tissue macrophages, and cells of the granulocyte lineage.

Granuloma: An organized structure in the form of a mass of mononuclear cells at the site of a persisting inflammation.

Granzyme: Enzymes present in the granules of cytotoxic T cells and NK cells which induce apoptosis in the target cells.

Graves' disease: An autoimmune disease in which antibodies against the thyroid-stimulating hormone receptor cause overproduction of thyroid hormone and thus hyperthyroidism.

Guillain-barre syndrome: A type of idiopathic polyneuritis in which autoimmunity to peripheral nerve myelin leads to a condition characterized by chronic demyelination of the spinal cord and peripheral nerves.

Gut-associated lymphoid tissue (GALT): Lymphoid tissue situated in the gastrointestinal mucosa and submucosa which constitutes the gastrointestinal immune system.

H chain: see ***heavy chain***.

H-2 complex: The major histocompatibility complex situated on chromosome 17 of the mouse; contains subregions k, i, d, and l.

Haplotype: A particular combination of closely linked genes on a chromosome in herited from one parent.

Hapten: A compound, usually of low molecular weight, that is not itself immuno genic but, after conjugation to a carrier protein or cells, becomes immunogenic and induces antibody, which can bind the hapten alone in the absence of carrier.

Hashimoto's thyroiditis: An autoimmune disease characterized by persistent high levels of antibody against thyroid-specific antigens. These antibodies recruit NK cells to the tissue, leading to damage and inflammation.

Heavy chain (H chain): The larger of the two types of chains that comprise a normal immunoglobulin or antibody molecule.

Helper T cell: Regulatory T cell which used cytokines to stimulate B cells to produce antibodies, macrophages to become activated, or cytotoxic T cells to become effector cells.

Hemagglutinin: Any substance that causes red blood cells to agglutinate. The hemagglutinins in human blood are antibodies that recognize the ABO blood group antigens. Influenza and some other viruses have hemagglutinin molecules that bind to glycoproteins on host cells to initiate the infectious process.

Hematopoiesis: The generation of the cellular elements of blood, including the red blood cells, leukocytes, and platelets.

Hematopoietic stem cell: A bone marrow cell that is undifferentiated and serves as a precursor for multiple cell lineages. These cells are also demonstrable in the yolk sac and later in the liver of the fetus.

Hemolysis: Lysis of erythrocytes.

Hemolytic disease of the newborn or erythroblastosis fetalis: It is caused by a maternal IgG antibody response to paternal antigens expressed on fetal red blood cells. The usual target of this response is the Rh blood group antigen. The maternal anti-Rh IgG antibodies cross the placenta, and bind to and lead to the lysis of fetal red blood cells.

Herd immunity: The protection of unimmunized members of a community by the resistance of the majority of the population to a particular pathogen; generally conferred by vaccinating most of the susceptible individuals.

Hereditary angioedema: A disorder in which recurrent attacks of edema occur in the skin and gastrointestinal and respiratory tracts.

Heterodimer: A molecule comprised of two components that are different, but closely joined structures, such as a protein comprised of two separate chains.

Heterophile antigen: A cross-reacting antigen that appears in widely ranging species such as humans and bacteria.

Heterozygous: Having non-identical copies (alleles) of a gene from each parent.

Hev: High endothelial venules. Specialized cells lining the capillaries in the lymphoid organs, where leukocytes enter from the circulation.

Hinge region: A flexible, open segment of an antibody molecule that allows bending of the molecule. The hinge region is located between Fab and Fc and is susceptible to enzymatic cleavage.

Hinge region: Flexible region of IgG and IgA antibody molecules. The hinge region connects the Fc and Fab regions and facilitates binding of both Fab regions to nearby antigen epitopes.

Histamine: A vasoactive amine stored in mast cell granules, which is released by antigen binding to IgE molecules on mast cells, causing dilation of local blood vessels and smooth muscle contraction.

Histocompatibility: Literally, the ability of tissues to be compatible; in immunology, it means identity in all transplantation antigens. These antigens, in turn, are collectively referred to as histocompatibility antigens.

HIV: Human immunodeficiency virus, the virus that causes aids.

HLA complex: see 'major histocompatibility complex'.

Hodgkins's disease: It is a malignant disease in which antigen-presenting cells that resemble dendritic cells seem to be the transformed cell type. Hodgkin's lymphoma is a form of hodgkin's disease in which lymphocytes predominate, and it has a much better prognosis than the nodular sclerosis form of this disease in which the predominant cell type is non-lymphoid.

Homodimer a protein comprised of dual peptide chains that are identical.

Homozygous having identical copies (alleles) of a gene from both parents.

Human immunodeficiency virus (HIV): Retrovirus that infects human $CD4^+$ cells and causes Aids.

Human leukocyte antigen (HLA): The human major histocompatibility complex; contains the genes coding for the polymorphic MHC class I and class II molecules and many other important genes.

Humanization: A term used to describe the genetic engineering of mouse hypervariable loops of a desired specificity into otherwise human antibodies. The DNA encoding hypervariable loops of mouse monoclonal antibodies or v regions selected in phage display libraries is inserted into the framework regions of human immunoglobulin genes. This allows the production of antibodies of a desired specificity that do not cause an immune response in humans treated with them.

Humanized antibody: Genetically engineered mouse antibody in which the Fc (and sometimes the framework) regions have been replaced with human sequences to prevent human response.

Humoral immunity: Immunity that can be transferred from one individual to another through serum; i.e., antibodies.

Hybridization: Specific binding of two complementary strands of DNA or of DNA and RNA.

Hybridoma: An immortalized hybrid cell resulting from the in vitro fusion of an antibody-secreting B cell with a myeloma; it secretes antibody without stimulation and proliferates continuously, both in vivo and in vitro. The term is also used for a hybrid T cell resulting from the fusion of a T lymphocyte with a thymoma (a malignant t cell); the T-cell hybridoma proliferates continuously and secretes cytokines upon activation by antigen and APC.

Hyper IgM syndrome: Immune deficiency in which serum IgM levels are high and serum IgG is absent or very low.

Hyperacute graft rejection: It is an immediate reaction caused by natural preformed antibodies that react against antigens on the graft. The antibodies bind to endothelium and trigger the blood clotting cascade, leading to an engorged, ischemic graft and rapid loss of the organ.

Hypergammaglobulinemia: Elevated serum immunoglobulin levels. A polyclonal increase in immunoglobulins in the serum occurs in any condition where there is continuous stimulation of the immune system, such as chronic infection, autoimmune disease, systemic lupus erythematosus, etc. Hypergammaglobulinemia may also result from a monoclonal increase in immunoglobulin production, as in multiple myeloma, waldenstrom's macroglobulinemia, or other conditions associated with the formation of monoclonal immunoglobulins.

Hyperimmune: A descriptor for an animal with a high level of immunity that is induced by repeated immunization to generate large amounts of functionally effective antibodies, in comparison to animals subjected to routine immunization protocols, perhaps with fewer boosters.

Hypersensitivity: Inappropriate immune response that damages one's body. Hypersensitivity responses are directed against non-dangerous antigens (allergens or grafts) or against persistent pathogens (lyme arthritis).

Hypervariable regions: Portions of the light and heavy immunoglobulin chains that are highly variable in amino acid sequence from one immunoglobulin molecule to another, and that, together, constitute the antigen-binding site of an antibody molecule.

Idiopathic Hemochromatosis: Excessive iron absorption and deposition in the skin and tissues; idiopathic means the cause is unknown.

Ifn-α Alpha interferon: Cytokine produced in response to virus infection that interferes with virus replication.

Ifn beta interferon: Cytokine produced in response to virus infection that interferes with virus replication.

Ig domain: Globular fold in antibody and Ig superfamily molecules held in place by a disulfide bond.

Ig isotype: A class of antibody molecules which share a heavy chain fc region. there are five Ig isotypes: IgA, IgG, IgD, IgE and IgM.

Ig superfamily: A group of proteins with structures very similar to Ig domains. Includes antibody, TCR, several receptors for cytokines, and some adhesion molecules.

Immature B cell: IgM IgD cell in the B cell lineage; easily tolerized by exposure to antigen.

Immediate-type hypersensitivity: Type I hypersensitivity reaction occurring within minutes after the interaction of antigen and IgE antibody.

Immune adherence: The adherence of particulate antigen coated with C3b to tissue having cells with C3b receptors.

Immune complex: Molecules formed by the interaction of a soluble (that is, non-particulate) antigen with antibody molecules.

Immune deficiency: Congenital or acquired inability of the immune system to function correctly, usually due to lack of a molecule or cell.

Immune modulators: Substances that control the level of the immune response.

Immune response gene: A gene controlling an immune response to a particular antigen; most genes of this type are in the MHC (major histocompatibility complex), and the term is rarely used to describe other types of IR genes outside the MHC.

Immune surveillance: The constant process by which the immune system kills arising cancer cells.

Immunity: The general term for resistance to a pathogen.

Immuno histochemistry: Detection of cell-associated molecules in the light microscope with antibodies labeled with enzymes which change a substrate into a colored precipitate.

Immunoblot Western blot or dot blot; detection of proteins on nitrocellulose paper by binding of labeled antibody molecules.

Immunodeficiency: Decrease in immune response that results from absence or defect of some component of the immune system.

Immunodiffusion: Identifies antigen or antibody by the formation of antigen-antibody complexes in a gel.

Immunoelectron microscopy: Detection of cell-associated molecules in the electron microscope with antibodies labeled with electron dense metals (often gold).

Immunoelectrophoresis: Detection of proteins which have been separated by electrophoresis by adding antibodies to form a visible precipitate in the gel.

Immunofluorescence: Detection of cell-associated molecules in the light microscope with antibodies labeled with fluorochromes.

Immunogen: A substance capable of inducing an immune response (as well as reacting with the products of an immune response). compare with ***antigen***.

Immunoglobulin (Ig): A general term for all antibody molecules.

Immunoglobulin superfamily: Proteins involved in cellular recognition and interaction that are structurally and genetically related to immunoglobulins.

Immunophilin: Cytoplasmic proteins in T cells which are the targets of the immunosuppressant drugs.

Immunotoxin: Genetically engineered monoclonal antibody specific for a tumor cell.

***In situ* hybridization:** DNA – DNA or RNA-RNA hybridization done on whole cells which have been fixed to a surface such as a filter or microscope slide.

Inactivated vaccine: Vaccine composed of killed pathogen.

Inbred mice: Mice which are the progeny of many generations of brother-sister matings, so that they are homozygous for most genes.

Inflammation: An acute or chronic response to tissue injury or infection involving accumulation of leukocytes, plasma proteins, and fluid.

Inflammatory T cell: TH1 cell, which activates macrophages to kill vesicular pathogens.

Innate immunity: Immunity present from birth and not dependent on prior antigen exposure.

Inositol triphosphate: Second messenger in lymphocyte activation; increases intracellular calcium and activates calcineurin.

Integrins: A family of two-chain cell-surface adhesion molecules found on leukocytes; important in the adhesion of APC and lymphocytes, and in leukocyte migration into tissues.

Interdigitating dendritic cells: Leukocytes with long processes (dendrites) that present antigen to T cells.

Interferon: A group of proteins having antiviral activity and capable of enhancing and modifying the immune response.

Interleukin: Glycoproteins secreted by a variety of leukocytes which have effects on other leukocytes.

Isograft: Tissue transplanted between two genetically identical individuals (same as syngraft).

Isohemagglutinins: Naturally occurring IgM antibodies specific for the red blood cell antigens of the ABO blood groups.

Isotype: Class of antibody molecules which share a heavy chain Fc region.

Isotype switch: The process by which a B cell switches from making antibody of one isotype to another without altering the specificity of the antibody.

Janus kinases (jak): Tyrosine kinases activated by cytokines binding to their cellular receptors.

J chain (joining chain): A polypeptide involved in the polymerization of immunoglobulin molecules IgM and IgA.

J gene: A gene segment coding for the J or joining segment in immunoglobulin or T-cell receptor chains;

K cell: An effector lymphocyte with Fc receptors, which allow it to bind to and kill antibody-coated target cells.

Killed vaccine: Vaccine composed of killed pathogen.

Killer inhibitory receptor: A receptor expressed on NK cells that binds to MHC class I molecules on target cells.

Killer T cell: A T cell that kills a target cell expressing foreign antigen bound to MHC molecules on the surface of the target T cell.

Knock-out mice: Mice in which one particular gene has been inactivated.

L chain: see *light chain*.

LAK: Lymphokine-activated killer cell. Natural killer cell which has been activated by IL-2 to become cytotoxic.

Langerhans cell: Cell of the monocyte/dendritic cell family that takes up and processes antigens in the epidermal layer of the skin.

Late phase response: Part of type I hypersensitivity which requires protein synthesis and occurs several hours after the immediate histamine release.

Leukemia: Uncontrolled proliferation of a malignant leukocyte.

Leukocyte adhesion deficiency (LAD): Immune deficiency in which one or more adhesion molecules are not expressed.

Leukocyte common antigen: An antigen shared in common by both T and B lymphocytes.

Leukocytes: White blood cells; comprise monocytes/macrophages, lymphocytes and polymorphonuclear cells.

Light chain (L chain): The light chain of the immunoglobulin molecule; occurs in two forms: lambda or kappa.

Lymph: Extracellular fluid that bathes tissues; contains tissue products, antigens, antibodies and cells (predominantly lymphocytes).

Lymph nodes: Secondary lymphoid organs, in which mature B and T lymphocytes respond to free antigen, or antigen associated with apc, brought in via lymphatic vessels.

Lymphatic system: System of vessels through which lymph travels, and which includes organized structures - lymph nodes - at the intersection of vessels

Lymphocyte: Leukocyte which has specific receptors for antigen and participates in adaptive immunity.

Lymphoid progenitor: Precursor to both T and B lymphocytes.

Lymphokine: Cytokine produced by a lymphocyte.

Lymphokine-activated killer (LAK) cells: The heterogeneous population of lym phocytes, including NK cells, derived from the in vitro cytokine-driven activation of peripheral blood lymphocytes from a tumor-bearing patient.

Lymphokines: Soluble substances secreted by lymphocytes, which have a variety of effects on lymphocytes and other cell types.

Lymphoma: Lymphocyte tumors in lymphoid or other tissues; not generally found in the blood.

M cell: Specialized antigen-collecting cell in the intestinal tract mucosal epithelium.

Mab: Monoclonal antibody; antibody produced from a clone of b cells.

MAC: Membrane attack complex; complement proteins which form a pore leading to cell lysis.

Macrophage: Phagocytic white blood cell found in the tissues; the circulating form of the cell is called a monocyte.

Macrophage-activating factor (MAF): Actually several lymphokines, including interferon, released by activated T cells, which together induce activation of macrophages, making them more efficient in phagocytosis and cytotoxicity.

Major Histocompatibility Complex (MHC): A cluster of genes encoding polymorphic cell-surface molecules (MHC class I and class II) that are involved in antigen presentation to T cells.

MALT: Mucosal-associated lymphoid tissue; collections of lymphoid cells found along the mucus membranes of the respiratory, digestive, and urogenital tracts.

Mast cell: Bone-marrow derived granule-containing cell found in connective tissues; releases mediators such as histamine and cytokines following cell activation.

Mature B cell: B cells with IgM and IgD on their surface.

MCP: Macrophage chemoattractant and activating protein; a chemokine.

Memory cell: Lymphocyte which can respond more quickly and efficiently to antigen than a naive lymphocyte.

Memory: In the immune system memory denotes a second interaction with antigen, leads to a more effective and more rapid response than the first interaction (primary response).

Memory response: Repeat response to an antigen which is faster and larger than a primary response.

MHC: Major histocompatibility complex; refers to the proteins used to present antigen to T cells or the genes which encode them.

MHC class I molecule: A molecule encoded by genes of the MHC that participates in antigen presentation to $CD8^+$ (cytotoxic) T cells.

MHC class II molecule: A molecule encoded by genes of the MHC that participates in antigen presentation to $CD4^+$ T cells.

MHC class II molecule: A molecule encoded by genes of the MHC which participates in antigen presentation to helper T (CD4+) cells.

MHC class III molecules: Proteins including complement components C2, C4, and factor B encoded by genes in the major histocompatibility complex (MHC).

MHC restriction: The property of T lymphocytes to respond only when they are presented with the appropriate antigen in association with either self MHC class I or class II molecules.

Migration inhibition factor (MIF): A lymphokine that inhibits the motility of macrophages in culture.

Minor Histocompatibility Antigen: Tissue antigens besides MHC, which are involved in graft rejection, usually to a lesser extent.

MIP: Macrophage inflammatory protein, a chemokine.

Mitogen: A substance that stimulates the proliferation of many different clones of lymphocytes.

Mixed lymphocyte reaction (MLR): Proliferative response occurring when leukocytes from two individuals are mixed in vitro.

Molecular mimicry: Identity or similarity of epitopes expressed by a pathogen and by a self molecule.

Monoclonal antibody: Means antibodies derived from a single clone.

Monoclonal: Literally, coming from a single clone. A clone is the progeny of a single cell.

Monocyte: White blood cell with a single (non-lobed) nucleus; lymphocytes and the circulating form of macrophages are monocytes.

Monokine: Cytokine made by a monocyte.

Motif: A pattern of amino acids in the sequence of a molecule critical for the binding of a ligand.

Mucosal-associated lymphoid tissue (Malt): System that connects lymphoid structures found in the gastrointestinal and respiratory tracts; includes tonsils, appendix, and peyer's patches of the small intestine.

Multiple myeloma: Plasma cell tumor, often characterized by high levels of monoclonal antibody in the circulation.

Multiple sclerosis: Disease of the central nervous system believed to be autoimmune in nature, in which an inflammatory response results in demyelination and loss of neurologic function.

Myasthenia gravis: Autoimmune disease in which antibody specific for the acetyl choline receptor expressed in muscle blocks function at the neuromuscular junction.

Myeloma: A tumor of plasma cells, generally secreting a single monoclonal immunoglobulin.

Myeloma protein: The monoclonal antibody produced by myeloma cells.

Natural killer (NK) cells: Large granular lymphocyte-like cells that kill various tumor cells in vitro and may play a role in resistance to tumors.

Negative selection: Step in development of B and T cells at which cells with potential reactivity to self molecules are functionally inactivated.

Neutralization: The ability of an antibody to block or inhibit the effects of a virus.

Neutrophil: White blood cell, a granulocyte that stains with neutral dyes.

Nrthern blotting: Process used to identify mRNA with a particular nucleotide sequence.

Nude mice: Mice with an epithelial cell defect which results in hairlessness and also lack of a thymus.

Null cells: An early population of lymphocytes bearing neither T-cell nor B-cell differentiation antigens.

Opsonin: Molecule which coats a pathogen and promotes its phagocytosis.

Opsonization: The coating of a particle such as a bacterium with antibody and/ or a complement component (an opsonin) that leads to enhanced phagocytosis by phagocytic cells.

Oxidative burst: Chemical process yielding toxic oxygen radicals and peroxides.

PAGE: Polyacrylamide gel electrophoresis, a technique for separating proteins by size using an electric current.

paracortical area (or paracortex): The T-cell area of the lymph node.

Paratope: an antibody combining site that is complementary to an epitope.

Passive cutaneous anaphylaxis (PCA): The passive transfer of anaphylactic sensitivity by intradermal injection of serum from a sensitive donor.

Passive hemagglutination: Technique for measuring antibody, in which antigen-coated red blood cells are agglutinated by adding antibody specific for the antigen.

Passive immunization: Immunization of an individual by the transfer of antibody synthesized in another individual.

Pathogen: An agent which causes disease.

Pathogenesis: The process of causing disease.

PBMC: Peripheral blood mononuclear cell (lymphocyte or monocyte)

PBMl: Peripheral blood mononuclear leukocyte

Peptidoglycan: Bacterial cell wall material

Perforin: A molecule synthesized by cytotoxic Tcells and NK cells that polymerizes on the surface of a target cell and creates a pore in the membrane, resulting in target cell death.

Peripheral lymphoid organ: Organs where lymphocytes are exposed to antigen: lymph nodes and spleen.

Peripheral tolerance: Tolerance induced in mature lymphocytes outside the thymus.

Peyers patch: Lymphoid tissue in the peritoneal cavity, associated with the digestive tract.

Phagocyte: Cell which engulfs particles: macrophages and neutrophils are the principal phagocytes of the immune system.

Phagocytosis: The engulfment of a particle or a microorganism by leukocytes such as macrophages and neutrophils.

Phagosome: Cytoplasmic vesicle containing the engulfed particle.

Phytohemagglutinin (pha): A mitogen that polyclonally activates T cells.

Pinocytosis: Ingestion of liquid or very small particles by vesicle formation in a cell.

Plasma: Fluid part of the blood, containing all proteins including clotting factors.

Plasma cell: The antibody-producing end-stage of B-cell differentiation.

Platelets: Bone-marrow derived cells crucial in blood clotting.

Pluripotent stem cell: Hematopoietic stem cell that can give rise to all blood cells.

PMN leukocytes: Polymorphonuclear leukocyte, a white blood cell with a lobed nucleus. usually refers to a neutrophil.

Pokeweed mitogen: A mitogen that polyclonally activates B cells.

Polyclonal activation: Activation of B cells or T cells with several different antigen specificities.

Polyclonal activator: A substance that induces activation of many clones of either T or B cells.

Polyclonal antibody: Antibody molecules with several different antigen-binding specificities.

Poly-Ig receptor: Binds to IgA at one surface of an epithelial cell, transports it through the cell, and releases it at the opposite lumenal surface,

Polymerase: DNA or RNA synthesizing enzyme

Polymerase chain reaction (PCR): Produces large amounts of DNA from a sequence by repeated cycles of synthesis.

Polymorphism: Literally, having many shapes; in genetics.

Polymorphonuclear leukocyte: white cell, granular cytoplasm. neutral staining (neutrophil) - most frequent, phagocytic. basophilic staining - basophil q.v. eosinophilic staining – eosinophil.

Positive selection: Selection process that allows a cell to survive or persist in a mixed population.

Pre B cell: A lymphocyte which has undergone H chain but not L chain somatic recombination.

Precipitin reaction: An assay for antibody-antigen complexes.The mixing of soluble antigen and antibody at different proportions can result in the precipitation of insoluble antigen-antibody complexes.

Pre-T cell: Cell in T-lymphocyte differentiation in the thymus that has rearranged TCR alpha genes and expresses TCR alpha polypeptide on the surface.

Primary cell culture: Cultured cells which recently came from an animal, plant, or person.

Primary follicle: Region of a secondary lymphoid organ containing predominantly unstimulated B lymphocytes; develops into a germinal center following antigen stimulation.

Primary lymphoid organ: Lymphoid organ in which lymphocytes mature (bone marrow and thymus).

Primary responses: The immune response to a first encounter with antigen. The primary response is generally small, has a long induction phase or lags period.

Priming: It is a process in which Pro B cell the developing lymphocyte which has undergone d-j joining in the Ig gene region and expressed CD45 (B22) but had not yet become a pre B cell.

Pro-B cell: Earliest stage of B cell differentiation in which a heavy chain d-gene segment rearranges to a j-gene segment.

Productive rearrangement: Somatic recombination of BCR or TCR gene segments those results in synthesis and membrane expression of a functional (antigen-binding) receptor.

Properdin (factor P): Plasma regulator of alternative pathway complement function; stabilizes the C3bBb3b complex.

Prophylaxis: protection.

Proteasome: Cytoplasmic organelle which processes (cuts into peptides) cytoplasmic proteins for transport and display on membrane class I MHC.

Protein kinase C: Enzyme activated by calcium and diacylglycerol during T- and B-lymphocyte activation.

Proto oncogenes: Cellular genes regulating growth control; mutation or aberrant expression can lead to malignant transformation of the cell.

Provirus: DNA form of a retrovirus integrated into the host DNA.

Pseudo gene: Sequence of DNA resembling a gene but containing codons that prevent transcription into full-length RNA species.

Pyogenic: Refers to the generation of pus at the sites of response to bacteria with large capsules.

Pyrogen: A substance that causes fever.

Radiation chimera: An individual whose immune system has been destroyed by irradiation and replaced by hematopoietic stem cells from another individual. The name comes from the mythological beast which is part lion, part goat, and part snake (see chimera).

Radioallergosorbent test (RAST): A solid-phase radioimmunoassay for detecting IgE antibody specific for a particular allergen.

Radioimmunoassay (RIA): A technique for measuring the level of a biologic substance in a sample, by measuring the binding of antigen to radioactively labeled antibody (or vice versa).

Reagin: Allergist's term for IgE antibodies.

Receptor: Generally a transmembrane molecule that binds to a ligand on the exterior surface of the cell, leading to biochemical changes inside the cell.

Receptor editing: Process by which the rearranged genes of a cell in the B-cell lineage may undergo a secondary rearrangement, generating a different antigenic specificity.

Recombinase: Enzyme which catalyzes somatic recombination of BCR and TCR gene segments.

Recombination signal sequence: DNA sequence that allows for correct recombinase joining of different gene segments.

Repertoire: The complete library of antigenic specificities generated by either B or T lymphocytes to respond to foreign antigen.

Reporter gene: Gene whose protein product can be easily measured, usually by its enzymatic activity, included with cloned DNA to demonstrate integration of DNA into a transformed cell.

Respiratory burst: oxygen dependent increase in metabolic activity within phagocytic cells stimulated by bacteria or parasites, to be microbicidal.

Restriction endonuclease: Bacterial enzyme which cuts DNA at particular DNA sequence; several hundred have been isolated.

Restriction mapping: Technique using two or more restriction endonucleases separately and together to cut DNA into segments of different sizes, then separating segments by gel electrophoresis to determine the location of the restriction sequences in the DNA.

Reticuloendothelial system (RES): A general term for the network of phagocytic cells.

Reverse transcriptase: Enzyme which transcribes the RNA genome of a retrovirus into DNA.

Rh antigen: Rhesus antigen, protein antigen on erythrocytes.

Rheumatoid arthritis: Autoimmune, inflammatory disease of the joints.

Rheumatoid factor: IgM anti-IgG, found in the serum of individuals with rheumatoid arthritis.

Rhogam: Human antibody to Rh antigen given to women to prevent hemolytic disease of the newborn.

RIA: Radio immuno assay; assay for antigen-antibody binding which is detected using radioactive ligand.

Scid mice: Mice with severe combined immune deficiency resulting from the failure to develop mature T and B lymphocytes.

Scid-human mice: SCID mice in which the immune system has been restored with human cells, so they have mature human B and T cells.

Secondary lymphoid organ: Lymphoid organ in which lymphocytes are activated by antigen and accessory cells and become effector cells and memory cells.

Secondary response: Repeat immune response to an antigen.

Secretary component: Cleaved component of the poly-Ig receptor that attaches to dimeric IgA and protects it from proteolytic cleavage as it is transported through an epithelial cell.

Secretory IgA: IgA which is secreted from mucosal epithelial cells in the digestive, respiratory, and genital tract.

Selectins: A family of cell-surface adhesion molecules found on leukocytes and endothelial cells; bind to sugars on glycoproteins.

Self antigen: Antigen normally present in one's own body, especially that with which the immune system has contact.

Sensitization: Initial contact with an allergen that results in IgE production and binding to mast cells, so that subsequent contact leads to rapid allergic symptoms.

Sepsis: Infection of the bloodstream.

Septic shock: Shock caused by immune response to infection.

Serology: Use of antibodies to detect antigens.

Serotype: Antigenic specificity of a pathogen.

Serum: Residual fluid derived from clotted blood; contains antibodies.

Serum sickness: A Type III hypersensitivity reaction resulting from deposition of circulating, soluble, antigen-antibody complexes leading to complement and neutrophil activation in tissues such as the kidney.

Severe combined immune deficiency (SCID): Disease resulting from early block in differentiation pathways of both B and T lymphocytes.

Signal transducers and activators of transcription (STATS): Intracellular proteins phosphorylated by janus kinases as a consequence of cytokine-cytokine receptor engagement.

Signal transduction: Enzymatic cascade which follows ligand binding to receptor and results in change in cell function.

Single positive T cell: T cell with either CD4 or CD8 on its membrane.

Slow-reacting substance of anaphylaxis: A group of leukotrienes released by mast cells during anaphylaxis that induces a prolonged contraction of smooth muscle.

Somatic gene conversion: Nonreciprocal exchange of sequences between genes: part of the donor gene or genes is "copied" into an acceptor gene, but only the acceptor gene is altered.

Somatic hypermutation: Change in the variable region sequence of an antibody produced by a B cell following antigenic stimulation, resulting in increased antibody affinity for antigen.

Somatic recombination: Process of cutting and splicing DNA segments to produce functiona BCR or TCR genes.

Southern blotting: Process used to identify specific pieces of DNA carrying a particular sequence

Spleen: Largest of the secondary lymphoid organs; traps and concentrates foreign substances carried in the blood.

Stem cell: Cell which can develop into different functional cells.

Strain: Set of animals (particularly mice and rats) in which every animal is bred to be genetically identical.

Subunit vaccine: Vaccine in which only parts of the antigen or pathogen are administered.

Suppression: A mechanism for producing a specific state of immunologic unresponsiveness by the induction of suppressor T cells.

Suppressor T cell: T cell which inhibits the function of b cells or other T cells.

Surrogate alpha chain: Alpha chain produced in pre T cells.

Surrogate light chain: Light chain produced in pre B cells.

Switch region: Region of B cell heavy chain DNA at which recombination occurs in an antigen-stimulated cell; allows isotype switch (e.g., IgM to IgE).

Switch region sequence: DTA sequence that allows a plasma cell to recombine v region DNAwith a different c region.

Syncytia: Multi-nucleate cells formed when cells fuse their plasma membranes.

Syngeneic: Literally, genetically identical; e.g., monozygotic twins or mice of the same strain.

Syngraft: Same as isograft.

Systemic lupus erythematosis: Systemic autoimmune disease characterized by facial rash (wolf-like markings, hence "lupus"), high levels of anti-DNA antibodies, and joint and kidney damage from immune complexes.

T cell activation: Biochemical process of stimulating a resting T cell to become an effector cell.

T cell development: Development of T cells in the thymus.

T cell education: Selection of T cells which can bind self MHC with appropriate affinity to be MHC-restricted.

T cell: Lymphocyte which has developed in the thymus and has membrane TCR that binds antigen plus self MHC. Tcells are either helper (CD4) or cytotoxic (CD8) phenotype.

T cell: A lymphocyte which undergoes a developmental stage in the thymus.

T cells: The set of lymphocytes whose differentiation requires the thymus.

Tap: Transporter of antigen peptide; protein complex that moves peptides from the cytoplasm into the endoplasmic reticulum where that can bind class I MHC.

Tap-1 and Tap-2: Molecules that selectively transport peptides from the cytoplasm to the endoplasmic reticulum of cells for binding to MHC class I molecules.

Target: A cell killed by one of the body's killer cells, such as a CTL or NK cell.

Target cell: Cell to be lysed by a cytotoxic cell; usually a virus-infected cell.

Tc: T cytotoxic cell.

T-cell receptor (TCR): A two-chain structure on T cells that binds antigen:

TCR: T cell (antigen) receptor, membrane molecule that binds antigen peptide plus MHC.

T-dependent antigen: An immunogen that requires T helper cells to interact with B cells in order to induce antibody synthesis.

T-dependent antigen: Antigen which generates T cell help for B cells.

T-dependent antigen: An immunogen that is able to induce antibody synthesis only in the presence of lymphokines released by helper t cells.

Template: Instructions for synthesis; mRNAis synthesized from a DNA template by an RNA polymerase which reads the DNA sequence and inserts complementary RNA bases.

Terminal deoxynucleotidyl transferase (TDT): Enzyme that inserts nontemplated nucleotides at the junctions of v, d, and j gene segments of ig and tcr locus dna; these N-nucleotides increase the diversity of antigen-specific receptors.

Th1: A subset of $CD4^+$ T cells that synthesizes the cytokines IL-2.

Th1 cell: Helper T cell that activates macrophages and cytotoxic T cells.

TH2: A subset of $CD4^+$ Tcells which synthesizes the cytokines IL-4, IL-5, IL-10, and IL-13.

Thymocyte: Cell which resides in the thymus

Thymus: Primary lymphoid organ in which T lymphocytes mature

T-independent antigen: An immunogen that induces antibody synthesis in the absence of T cells or their products.

Titer: Quantification of antibody, often expressed as the highest dilution to give a positive response.

Tolerance: Antigen-specific unresponsiveness of B or T cells.

Tonsils: Lymphoid tissue in the throat.

Toxic shock syndrome: The systemic reaction produced by the toxin derived from the bacterium *staphylococcus aureus.*

Toxoid: A nontoxic derivative of a toxin used as an immunogen for the induction of antibodies capable of cross-reacting with the toxin.

Transcription: Synthesis of mRNA from DNA template.

Transfection: Transfer of foreign DNA into a cell.

Transformation: Transfer of a recombinant plasmid vector into a bacterial cell, or conversion of a normal cell into a cancer cell.

Transgene: Cloned foreign gene inserted into a cell.

Transgenic mice: Mice which have a foreign gene in their cells.

Translation: Synthesis of protein from messenger RNA (mRNA)

Transplantation: Grafting solid tissue (such as a kidney or heart) or cells (particularly bone marrow) from one individual to another.

Trypan blue: Dye which can enter dead cells, used for determining viability.

TSST: Toxic shock syndrome toxin, a super antigen produced by *staphylococcus aureus* that causes toxic shock syndrome.

Tuberculin test: Antigens derived the organism causing tuberculosis are injected subcutaneously.

Tumor immunology: Subspecialty of immunology dealing with immune responses to tumors.

Tumor infiltrating lymphocyte (TIL): Mononuclear cells derived from the inflam matory infiltrate of solid tumors.

Tumor necrosis factor (TNF): A cytokine with various actions including the selective killing of tumor cells.

Tumor-specific transplantation antigen (TSTA): Antigens uniquely expressed by certain tumor cells.

Tyrosine kinases: A family of enzymes which phosphorylates proteins on tyrosine residues, a critical step in lymphocyte activation.

Unresponsiveness: Inability to respond to antigenic stimulus.

Urticaria: Also called hives: small areas of local inflammation in the skin.

cells.

Vaccination: Originally referred to immunization against smallpox with the less virulent cowpox (vaccinia) virus.

Vaccination: Originally referred to immunization against smallpox with the less virulent cowpox (vaccinia) virus;

Vaccine: Killed microorganisms, weakened living organisms, fully virulent living organisms, or subunit proteins of a microbe, administered to produce or artificially increase immunity to a particular disease.

Vcam: Vascular cell adhesion molecule cam found on the endothelial cells lining blood vessels

Variable (v) regions: The N-terminal portion of an Ig or TCR which contains the antigen-binding region of the molecule; V regions are formed by the recombination of V(d) and J gene segments.

Vascular endothelium: Endothelial cells lining the blood vessels.

V (d)J recombination: Mechanism for generating antigen-specific receptors of T and B

Vector autonomously replicating DNA molecule which can be used to clone and move inserted DNA from cell to cell.

Vector vaccines: *Vaccines* made by inserting protective *antigen* genes into harmless bacteria or viruses (vectors).

Viability stain: Stain that differentiates between live and dead cells.

Virion: A complete virus particle.

Virus: An organism comprising a protein coat and DNA or RNA genome.

Vitronectin: Plasma protein (also called s protein) that block binding of complement C567.

Western blot: Polyacrylamide gel electrophoresis of proteins followed by blotting and, binding of enzyme-tagged specific antibodies; used to detect specific antigens.

Wheal and flare: Itchy reaction at skin site where antigen is injected into an allergic individual.

Xenogeneic: Originating from a foreign species.

Xenograft: A tissue transplantation between individuals belonging to two different species.

Xenotransplantation: Transplantation of tissue from another species

Xla : linked agammglobulinemia, an immune deficiency caused by lack of bruton's thymidine kinase and resulting in recurring infections due to nearly complete absence of serum Ig.

X-linked agammaglobulinemia: Disease in boys manifesting as absence of mature B cells.

X-linked hyper-IgM syndrome: Disease in boys manifesting as inability to synthesize Ig isotypes other than IgM; result of defect in either CD40 or CD154.

X-scid: X -linked severe combined immune deficiency, due to defect in IL-2 receptor alpha chain.

Zap-70: A T-cell specific tyrosine kinase (second messenger) involved in T cell activation.

INDEX

A

B

C

D

E

F

G

H

I

P

R

S

T

U

V

W

X

NOTES

NOTES